BENDING THE AGING CURVE

The Complete Exercise Guide for Older Adults

JOSEPH F. SIGNORILE, PhD

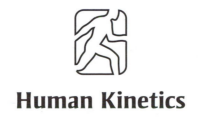

Human Kinetics

Library of Congress Cataloging-in-Publication Data

Signorile, Joseph F.
 Bending the aging curve : the complete exercise guide for older adults / Joseph F. Signorile.
   p. ; cm.
 Includes bibliographical references and index.
 ISBN-13: 978-0-7360-7445-2 (soft cover)
 ISBN-10: 0-7360-7445-7 (soft cover)
 1. Exercise for older people. I. Title.
 [DNLM: 1. Aging--physiology. 2. Exercise Therapy--methods. 3. Exercise--physiology. WT 104]
 RA781.S5643 2011
 613.7'10844--dc22

                         2010039248

ISBN-10: 0-7360-7445-7
ISBN-13: 978-0-7360-7445-2

Permission notices for material reprinted in this book from other sources can be found on page xiii.

The Web addresses cited in this text were current as of September, 2010, unless otherwise noted.

Acquisitions Editors: Judy Patterson Wright, PhD, and Myles Schrag; **Developmental Editor:** Christine M. Drews; **Assistant Editor:** Steven Calderwood; **Copyeditor:** Jocelyn Engman; **Indexer:** Andrea J. Hepner; **Permission Manager:** Dalene Reeder; **Graphic Designer:** Fred Starbird; **Graphic Artist:** Denise Lowry; **Cover Designer:** Keith Blomberg; **DVD Face Designer:** Susan Rothermel Allen; **Photographer (cover):** Neil Bernstein; **Photographer (interior):** Neil Bernstein, unless otherwise noted; **Photo Asset Manager:** Laura Fitch; **Visual Production Assistant:** Joyce Brumfield; **Photo Production Manager:** Jason Allen; **Art Manager:** Kelly Hendren; **Associate Art Manager:** Alan L. Wilborn; **Illustrations:** © Human Kinetics; **Printer:** Versa Press

We thank Truly Fit in Urbana, Illinois, for assistance in providing one of the locations for the photo shoot for this book.

The contents of this DVD are licensed for private home use and traditional, face-to-face classroom instruction only. For public performance licensing, please contact a sales representative at www.HumanKinetics.com/SalesRepresentatives.

Printed in the United States of America   10 9 8 7 6 5 4 3 2 1

The paper in this book is certified under a sustainable forestry program.

Human Kinetics
Web site: www.HumanKinetics.com

United States: Human Kinetics, P.O. Box 5076, Champaign, IL 61825-5076
800-747-4457
e-mail: humank@hkusa.com

Canada: Human Kinetics, 475 Devonshire Road Unit 100, Windsor, ON N8Y 2L5
800-465-7301 (in Canada only)
e-mail: info@hkcanada.com

Europe: Human Kinetics, 107 Bradford Road, Stanningley, Leeds LS28 6AT, United Kingdom
+44 (0) 113 255 5665
e-mail: hk@hkeurope.com

Australia: Human Kinetics, 57A Price Avenue, Lower Mitcham, South Australia 5062
08 8372 0999
e-mail: info@hkaustralia.com

New Zealand: Human Kinetics, P.O. Box 80, Torrens Park, South Australia 5062
0800 222 062
e-mail: info@hknewzealand.com

E4456

First and foremost, this book is dedicated to my friend and colleague Dr. Bernie Roos, whose belief, support, and mentoring have provided me with the opportunities and intellectual environment to develop the concepts presented in this book. I will always treasure the countless hours we have spent discussing aging and exercise. This book is also dedicated to my wife, who supported me and provided direction and encouragement; to my dear friend Sam Hollander, who taught me that dreams can become reality; to Julie, Colin, and Jennifer Milner at the International Conference of Active Aging, Sara Kooperman of Sara City Workout, and Tom Trebotich of the International Sports and Conditioning Association, who provided the opportunity for me to polish my presentation skills; to all students and colleagues with whom I shared my research; and to the thousands of fitness professionals who have attended my lectures throughout the years and asked, "Is there a book we can read that gives us this information?"

Contents

Preface   vii

About the DVD   ix

Acknowledgments   xi

Credits   xiii

Part I
Understanding the Aging Curves and Training Older Adults
1

Chapter 1   The Aging Curves   3

The Concept of Age   4
The Diamond Analogy   4
The Aging Curves   5
Using Exercise to Bend the Aging Curves   12
Frailty and Physical Vulnerability   12
Prehab or Rehab: Changing the Oil
   or Changing the Engine?   16
Exercise as a Targeted Intervention:
   Matching the Program to the Need   17
Summary   19
Topical Bibliography   19
References   20

Chapter 2   Testing   23

The Exercise Diagnosis and Prescription
   Model   23
The Exercise Diagnosis: Analysis of Needs   24
What Makes an Effective Test?   28
When to Test   29
Testing Activities of Daily Living   32
Summary   33
Topical Bibliography   33
References   35

Chapter 3   Training Principles   37

Overload and Adaptation   37
Exercise Specificity   38
Summary   43
Topical Bibliography   44
References   44

Part II
Training Exercises: From Theory to Practice
45

Chapter 4   Body Composition   47

The Prevalence of Obesity and Its
   Consequences   48
The Obesity Paradox   48
Sarcopenic Obesity
   and Activities of Daily Living   49
Sarcopenic Obesity and Fall Probability   50
Testing Body Composition   51
Training Interventions
   for Sarcopenic Obesity   57
Summary   63
Topical Bibliography   63
References   67

Chapter 5   Flexibility   69

Defining Flexibility and the Stress–Strain
   Curve   69
Possible Causes of Declining Flexibility
   With Aging   70
Why Train for Flexibility?   70
Types of Stretching   71
Do Stretching and Flexibility Training
   Increase Flexibility?   72
Stretching, Flexibility Training, and Injury
   Prevention   74
Stretching, Flexibility Training, and
   Performance   74
Practical Aspects of Flexibility
   Training   75
Testing Flexibility   76
Flexibility Program Design   80
Flexibility Training Exercises   81
Summary   100
Topical Bibliography   100
References   104

Chapter 6 Bone, Falls, and Fractures   105

Structure of Bone   105
Factors Affecting Bone Strength   106
Osteopenia and Osteoporosis   110
Exercise Training to Prevent Osteoporosis   112
Better Balance and Agility   115
Testing Balance   121
Balance Training   124
Summary   126
Topical Bibliography   127
References   132

Chapter 7 Muscular Strength, Power, and Endurance Training   133

Sarcopenia: What Makes It Happen?   133
Effects of Resistance Training on the Causes of Sarcopenia   135
Resistance Training to Reduce the Effects of Sarcopenia   137
Testing Neuromuscular Performance   148
Resistance Training Exercises   155
Summary   196
Topical Bibliography   196
References   207

Chapter 8 Cardiovascular Training   209

Increasing Cardiovascular Fitness: Benefits and Methods   209
Testing Cardiovascular Fitness   218
Cardiovascular Training and Program Design   219
Summary   231
Topical Bibliography   231
References   235

**Part III
Putting the Program Together   237**

Chapter 9 Periodized Training   239

Periodization: The Underlying Theories   239
Fatigue During Time-Based Training Cycles   242
Controlling the Fitness–Fatigue Balance During Training   243
Applied Periodization Using Specific Training Cycles   248
Summary   253
Topical Bibliography   254
References   254

Chapter 10 The Translational Cycle: Active Recovery Meets Functional Practice   255

Basic Concept of the Translational Cycle   256
Translational Cycles and Periodization   256
Timing of Translational Cycles   257
Motor Learning Drills: The Need for Progression   257
Matching Translational and Training Cycles   262
Translational Exercises   263
Summary   296
Topical Bibliography   297
References   298

Appendix: Normative Data   299
Index   307
About the Author   312

Preface

Bending the Aging Curve looks at exercise intervention for aging adults in a unique way. While this book is written for fitness and health professionals, its distinctive blend of research and readability makes it accessible to anyone, from the layman trying to bend his personal aging curves to the college student studying exercise intervention in order to serve this growing segment of the population. Unlike many of the texts addressing the older population, which tend to concentrate on a single aspect of physical decline, such as strength, cardiovascular fitness, or mobility, *Bending the Aging Curve* recognizes that maintaining independence means addressing a multitude of factors and developing a multifaceted solution. Therefore, this book presents exercise as a targeted prescription that is based on a diagnosis that takes into account the many factors, or aging curves, associated with age-related loss of function.

This text also recognizes the importance of using training cycles that target diagnosed needs, allowing the proper mix of work and recovery, and providing skill practice that simulates daily activities. This periodization model has been shown to be the most effective way to maximize improvement while reducing the potential for overtraining and overuse injuries.

Because I believe that the *why* is as important as the *how,* I have divided this book into three parts. Part I looks at the natural aging curves and how they can affect the overall aging curve that reflects our independence and safety throughout our lives. Part II presents exercise interventions that have been shown to be effective at bending the aging curves. Finally, part III shows how to structure a periodized program that includes a unique translational cycle designed to translate a client's physiological improvements into improvements in daily life.

To this end, the book is organized in a logical progression. Chapter 1 presents the diverse physiological curves associated with aging and their effects on independence and injury risk. We know from research as well as experience that most physiological functions decline sharply in our older years. The concept behind this book is to intervene with an appropriate exercise prescription that can bend, or straighten, those curves, making the declines less drastic and extending the years of independent living. Chapter 2 explains the concept of using physical testing as a diagnostic tool that reveals the individual needs that an effective exercise prescription must target. Chapter 3 presents an overview of training theory and explains how it applies to interventions for older clients.

Part II of this book establishes the link between diagnosis and prescription that is the basis of the text. Chapters 4 through 8 provide specific training strategies for targeting each of the physical factors associated with successful aging, including body composition, flexibility, bone density, muscular strength and power, and cardiovascular fitness, respectively. Each chapter provides an overview of why the physical factor is important to your older client; describes effective, efficient, and cost-effective testing methods; and provides proven exercise interventions.

Chapters 9 and 10 make up part III of *Bending the Aging Curve.* Chapter 9 presents periodization theory and explains how that theory can be applied to programs designed to bend specific aging curves. Chapter 10 shows how active recovery periods can be used to improve performance and exercise adherence and at the same time be used to translate increases in physical performance into improved daily living and reduced fall probability.

I hope that this book provides you with a logical and somewhat whimsical picture of how targeted exercise interventions can be used to improve the lives of your clients as they face off with Father Time. If you finish reading this book with "Of course!" on your mind, "What if?" in your imagination, and "I can!" in your heart, I will have been successful in its writing.

About the DVD

*T*he DVD that accompanies this book contains ideas for applying the concepts from the book to individual clients, videos of the translational exercises, and the actual diagnostic testing battery in an Excel spreadsheet. I first introduce the need to bend the aging curve and discuss the exercise diagnosis and prescription model. I also explain how to use the diagnostic testing battery, which you can access from the DVD. Be sure to save it to your hard drive before using it. Instructions for saving the diagnostic testing battery are on the last page of this book.

The diagnostic testing battery is divided into 14 age ranges. Select the appropriate age range for your client's gender. The red cells are the data you need to replace with your client's information and test results. The black cells should not be changed. After entering your client's information and test results, the diagnostic testing battery will show your client's percentile for each test. You can use the test results to make an exercise prescription for your client.

As a unique feature, I introduce four clients as case studies. After identifying a client's weaknesses via the testing battery, I explain how the training cycle for that client might be designed. Then you can see the client performing the translational exercises that a fitness professional might choose for that client during the active recovery phase of the training cycle. You can also see how the translational exercises can be modified to meet the needs of your individual clients.

The DVD includes an index of the 73 translational exercises and variations. To view video of a translational exercise, select that exercise from the submenu of the translational exercises index.

My hope is that this DVD will bring the exercises to life and illustrate how you might individualize exercise prescription to bend each client's unique aging curve.

DVD Menu

Introduction

The Exercise Diagnosis and Prescription Model

Using the Diagnostic Testing Battery

Case Studies

Translational Exercises Index

Balance Drills

  Heel Stand

  Heel Walk

  Functional Reach Drill

  Pillow Stands

  Triple-Line Drill

Line Drills

  Lateral Line Drill

  Truckin' Drill

Agility Drills

  Lateral Shuffle Drill

  Forward and Backward Cone Drill

Zigzag Drill

Up-and-Go Drill

In-and-Out Agility Drill

Skating Drill

Ladder Drills

  Between-Every-Rung Drill

  Two-Between-Every-Rung Drill

  Between-Every-Other-Rung Drill

  Two-In, Two-Out Drill

  In-and-Out-the-Window Drill

  Lateral Advances

ADL Drills: Chair Stands

  Chair Stand Drill

  Straight-Line Chair Drill

  Musical Chairs Drill

  In-and-Out Chair Drill

ADL Drills: Step Drills

  Step-Up Drill

  Lateral Step-Up Drill

Speed and Stride Drill

IADL Drills

  Scarf Drill

  Book Drills

  Ball-and-Pylon Drills

  Coin Pickup Drill

  Gallon Jug Drill

  Dot or Grid Drills

  Hexagon Drill

  Star Excursion Drill

Ball Drills

  Back-to-Back Handoff

  Chest Pass

  Overhead Throw

  Lateral Throw

Accessing the Diagnostic Testing Battery

Credits

Acknowledgments

I would like to acknowledge all the researchers and clinicians whose hard work and dedication produced the information that allowed me to formulate this training system. I would also like to acknowledge Chris Drews, Myles Schrag, Neil Bernstein, Doug Fink, Roger Francisco, Steven Calderwood, and Judy Wright of Human Kinetics, whose expertise helped transform this book into its final form. To paraphrase a famous saying, it truly does take a village to raise a writer.

Credits

Figure 1.2: Reprinted from *Journal of Neurophysiological Science*, Vol. 84, J. Lexell, C.C. Taylor, and M. Sjostrom, "What is the cause of the ageing atrophy? Total number, size and proportion of different fiber types studied in whole vastus lateralis muscle from 15-to 83-year-old men," pgs. 284 and 286, Copyright 1988, with permission from Elsevier.

Figure 1.3: Data from Lexell, Taylor, and Sjostrom 1988.

Figure 1.4: Reprinted, by permission, from F.R. Noyes and E.S. Grood, 1976, "The strength of anterior cruciate ligament in humans and rhesus monkeys: Age-related and species-related changes," *Journal of Bone and Joint Surgery* 58A: 1074-1082.

Figure 1.5a and 1.5b: Based on Pimentel et al. 2003; Tanaka et al. 1997; Fleg et al. 2005; and Hull et al. 2010.

Figure 1.5c: Data from S.S. Guo et al., 1999, "Aging, body composition, and lifestyle: The Fels Longitudinal," *American Journal of Clinical Nutrition* 70: 405-411.

Figure 1.6: Data from Department of Medicine, University of Washington.

Figure 1.7: Reprinted, by permission, from B. Sharkey, 2010, *Fitness illustrated* (Champaign, IL: Human Kinetics), 248.

Figure 1.9a and 1.9b: Based on Pimentel et al. 2003; Tanaka et al. 1997; Fleg et al. 2005; and Fitzgerald et al. 1997.

Figure 4.1: Based on data from Centers for Disease Control.

Figure 4.2: Based on data from Administration on Aging.

Figure 4.3: Data from Curtis et al. 2005

Figure 4.4: Reprinted by permission from Macmillan Publishers Ltd: OBESITY RESEARCH, R.N. Baumgartner et al., "Sarcopenic obesity predicts instrumental activities of daily living disability in the elderly," 12: 1995-2004. Copyright 2004.

Figure 4.5: Reprinted by permission, from National Strength and Conditioning Association, 2008, Administration, scoring, and interpretation of selected tests, by E. Harman and J. Garhammer. In *Essentials of strength training and conditioning*, 3rd ed., edited by T.R. Baechle and R.W. Earle (Champaign, IL: Human Kinetics), 268.

Figure 4.6: Reprinted by permission, from National Strength and Conditioning Association, 2008, Administration, scoring, and interpretation of selected tests, by E. Harman and J. Garhammer. In *Essentials of strength training and conditioning*, 3rd ed., edited by T.R. Baechle and R.W. Earle (Champaign, IL: Human Kinetics), 269.

Figure 4.7: Reprinted by permission, from National Strength and Conditioning Association, 2008, Administration, scoring, and interpretation of selected tests, by E. Harman and J. Garhammer. In *Essentials of strength training and conditioning*, 3rd ed., edited by T.R. Baechle and R.W. Earle (Champaign, IL: Human Kinetics), 269.

Figure 4.8: Reprinted by permission, from National Strength and Conditioning Association, 2008, Administration, scoring, and interpretation of selected tests, by E. Harman and J. Garhammer. In *Essentials of strength training and conditioning*, 3rd ed., edited by T.R. Baechle and R.W. Earle (Champaign, IL: Human Kinetics), 268.

Figure 4.9: Reprinted by permission, from National Strength and Conditioning Association, 2008, Administration, scoring, and interpretation of selected tests, by E. Harman and J. Garhammer. In *Essentials of strength training and conditioning*, 3rd ed., edited by T.R. Baechle and R.W. Earle (Champaign, IL: Human Kinetics), 268.

Figure 4.10: Reprinted by permission, from National Strength and Conditioning Association, 2008, Administration, scoring, and interpretation of selected tests, by E. Harman and J. Garhammer. In *Essentials of strength training and conditioning*, 3rd ed., edited by T.R. Baechle and R.W. Earle (Champaign, IL: Human Kinetics), 268.

Figure 4.11: Reprinted by permission, from National Strength and Conditioning Association, 2008, Administration, scoring, and interpretation of selected tests, by E. Harman and J. Garhammer. In *Essentials of strength training and conditioning*, 3rd ed., edited by T.R. Baechle and R.W. Earle (Champaign, IL: Human Kinetics), 269.

Figure 4.14: Data from Haltom et al. 1999.

Understanding the Aging Curves and Training Older Adults

Part I of this book presents the premise that the curve that illustrates our loss of physical capacity with aging is the total of several distinct curves representing the physical attributes of strength, power, flexibility, and aerobic capacity. Chapter 1 explains the curves and how exercise can be used to bend the overall aging curve. The diagnosis and prescription model described in this part provides a process by which you can target your clients' specific needs. To that end, chapter 2 talks about testing theory and its relationship to effective exercise prescription. Finally, training theory is discussed in chapter 3 as the conceptual framework for the focused exercise techniques presented in chapters 4 through 8.

The Aging Curves

As we age our physical capacity declines. For example, strength, cardiovascular endurance, and flexibility all show distinct patterns of change during the aging process and affect our lives to varying degrees. This chapter examines the unique patterns of change, which I call aging curves, that occur in each of these physical parameters. The combination of each of these curves is your client's overall aging curve. The chapter also discusses how aging curves influence successful aging and explains how you can structure the most effective training program to address your client's specific pattern of decline.

After reading these first few pages, you may find the changes described depressing and you may want to change professions or throw the book out the window. Please fight this urge and think back to the scene in the classic movie *A Christmas Carol* (the black-and-white version with Alastair Sim, please) where the Ghost of Christmas Future whisks Scrooge forward in time (remember the spinning hourglass?) to a graveyard. His bony finger emerges from under his cloak as he points to a gravestone—Scrooge's gravestone. Scrooge falls to the ground, weak and horrified at the sight of his own grave, and asks if this future is inevitable or if there is something he can do to change it. We all remember how the story ends. Scrooge did change that vision of the future by keeping Christmas as well as any man in England might keep it.

This chapter shows the way things might be if a person decides to age gracefully, quietly accepting the future as it comes. But the rest of this book shows you how you can change this future for your clients and yourself. Remember that this book is called *Bending the Aging Curve* and not *Bending Under the Aging Curve*. Just as it would have been useless for the Ghost of Christmas Future

to show Scrooge an inevitable future, it would be foolish to present to you a description of inevitable decline with no hope of change. This first chapter shows what can be so that you can understand the changes that must be made to reduce the effects of aging on your clients' health and performance. This book is not about preventing death. It's about using exercise to twist your clients' aging curves so far out of shape that the scientists who drew them won't recognize them. This is not a book about not aging; it's a book about helping clients to function and feel as young as their sons, daughters, nieces, nephews, and even grandchildren.

I can still remember a wonderful woman, Maria, who participated in one of my first studies more than 20 years ago. The study began, as most university studies do, in early September. During the Thanksgiving holidays most of the participants got together with their children for a traditional celebration, and Maria was no exception. When she returned to the lab, she was very excited and told me this story. She, her son, her daughter-in-law, and her grandson were in the kitchen preparing dinner, and her daughter-in-law couldn't remove the top from one of those vacuum-packed jars—you know, the jars with the lids screwed down like the lug nuts on a tractor trailer. Her daughter-in-law asked Maria's son to help her with the jar. But before he could, Maria's grandson interceded, saying, "Don't give it to daddy. Give it to grandma. She looks stronger than he does!" Maria beamed as she told me the story and I still tear up when I tell it to others (in fact I'm leaning back from the keyboard right now). This feeling is what you can expect when you use the information in this book to bend your clients' aging curves. So let's look at the curves before we turn them into nothing more than a flawed vision of an unnecessary future.

THE CONCEPT OF AGE

The definition of *age* might seem obvious. It is, quite simply, the length of time you have lived. But if we look at the term within the context of this book, that definition should be modified to express more than the simple chronological concept of existence. In addition to a *chronological age,* we have other ages that are important when we consider exercise intervention for older clients. Possibly the best known of these other ages is *functional age.* Your older clients cannot simply be classified by their chronological ages; they need to be defined by how they function in their daily lives, their jobs, and their community interactions. We often use expressions such as "She doesn't look 60!" or "He runs like a kid!" to describe our own observations of functional age. In this text we will take this concept one step further and examine how functional age can be used to assess a client's specific needs and gauge a client's progress during targeted exercise interventions. In fact, functional age has often been called *physiological age* because it is affected by how well we function physiologically. In this book we use assessments of physiological function to provide targeted prescriptions throughout clients' training seasons—also known as their *lives.*

The final age we should discuss is *training age.* Training age is how long a client has been exercising on a regular basis. For example, if your client is 65 and either has never trained before or hasn't trained since high school or college, your client is in training infancy. Clients who are training infants can tolerate a much lower workload than they would be able to tolerate if they had exercised regularly throughout their life. Training age is one of the strongest modifiers of any training program. All too often we jump into an exercise program with no preparation, trying to regain in a few weeks what took years to lose. The least insidious result of these reckless charges into fitness is usually discomfort, pain, and a feeling

that exercise is just too hard—but all too often this mistake leads to acute or even chronic injury. Before I leave the concept of training age I'd like to insert one more training anecdote. When my graduate students and I were screening subjects for a study back in 1995, we ran into Betty. Betty was about 5 foot (1.5 m) nothing and weighed in at a whopping 99 pounds (45 kg). Her questionnaire indicated that she did no formal training and therefore qualified for our study. On the first day of that study we began testing our participants, and Betty blew the doors off women 10 years her junior and 20 to 30 pounds (9-14 kg) heavier than her. We again asked her if she trained, and again she told us that she did not. After a somewhat protracted conversation we were informed by Betty that she had no time to train because she was too busy working on her farm. This story has two morals. First, physical activity can be incorporated into every aspect of life, from taking the stairs rather than the elevator to walking or biking instead of jumping into the car. Second, you can never tell how fit your "Betty" is until you test her and find out how you can best help her bend her own unique aging curves.

> **APPLICATION POINT**   People have different patterns of aging and different life experiences. Don't make the mistake of thinking you know what your clients need based solely on how long they have lived on this earth.

THE DIAMOND ANALOGY

Three famous songwriters, Wright, Waters, and Gilmour, wrote a well-known song about aging. Those of you who are reading this book so you can bend your own aging curves, and you younger trainers who have acquired good taste in rock and roll, know these songwriters by the name of their group, Pink Floyd. Their song was entitled "Shine

Definitions of Age	
chronological age	The number of years a person has lived.
functional, or physiological, age	How well a person functions in daily life, on the job, and in community interactions.
training age	How long a person has been exercising on a regular basis.

on You Crazy Diamond." The first few lines of the song go as follows:

> Remember when you were young,
>
> you shone like the sun.
>
> Shine on you crazy diamond.

Although Pink Floyd may not have intended it, they provided the perfect template for successful aging. If you think about what makes a diamond shine, you can come up with a number of factors: the color, the clarity, or the absence of flaws. Optimizing any or all of these features will cost you big bucks when you buy that engagement ring or those diamond earrings (or earring). But these qualities mean very little if the diamond is not cut correctly. For a diamond to truly reach its potential, for it to reflect the light and look alive, all of its facets must bring the light together and then disperse the light properly so the diamond can reveal its highest level of brilliance. As Pink Floyd said, we are like that diamond. If you want your client to shine with the greatest brilliance possible while aging, you must address all the factors that affect performance in daily life (see figure 1.1). For this reason, the diagnostic model that is used in this text is based on the analyses of numerous physiological factors, each of which contributes to a client's overall performance and well-being. This book shows you how to check each facet of the diamond by identifying specific physiological limitations. Then it teaches you to set up a training program that can cut and polish each facet so you can get the highest level of brilliance out of each client's genetic gemstone.

> **APPLICATION POINT** A good exercise prescription polishes all facets of the fitness diamond for a brighter future.

THE AGING CURVES

By looking at the changes that occur in our bodies over time, we can begin to understand the transformations that result from the aging process. An aging curve is a picture of a specific transformation across time, and the interactions of each of these "physiological" aging curves dictate each client's unique overall aging curve. Recognizing the validity of the old saying "A picture is worth a thousand words," I have provided individual curves for each of the physiological factors addressed in this book.

Neuromuscular Curves

John Lexell gave us the now-famous picture of the aging curve for human skeletal muscle (1988). The curve shows that after the age of 50 the size

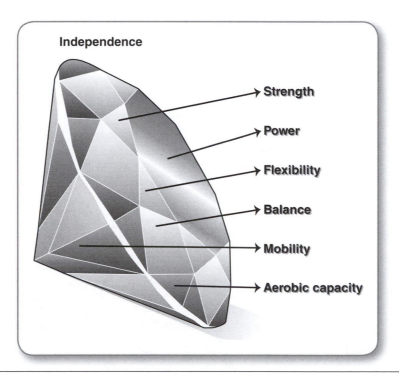

Figure 1.1 The diamond analogy: Factors associated with successful aging.

of our muscle doesn't just go down; it drops like a stone off the edge of a cliff (see figure 1.2a). The loss in muscle size that accompanies aging is called *sarcopenia,* from the Greek roots *sarco,* meaning "flesh," and *penia,* meaning "abnormal reduction" or "deficiency." As one of the baby boomers staring into the muscle mass abyss, I'm not any happier about the prospect of sarcopenia than your older clients are, but we must face this reality in order to change it.

Let's look at why sarcopenia occurs. Our muscles lose size, or atrophy, for two reasons. First, each muscle cell, called a *muscle fiber,* shrinks. Since these muscle fibers are all wrapped together in connective tissue, when individual fibers lose their size, the entire muscle shrinks. But that's not the end of the story. Every muscle fiber has a nerve, called a *motor nerve,* that innervates it. This nerve allows our brain to communicate with the muscle, telling it what we want it to do and also what it must do in order to stay alive. To make our bodies more efficient, a motor nerve innervates more than one muscle fiber by sending off branches, much like the way the main power line that carries electricity into your neighborhood branches into the smaller lines that go to each home. These lines then branch again to supply electricity to each electrical socket. A motor nerve

and all the muscle fibers it innervates are called a *motor unit.* As we age, our motor nerves and their associated muscle fibers die off at an ever-increasing rate. A small percentage of these fibers are rescued by neighboring motor units, but the number of living fibers still drops exponentially. In fact, the shape of the curve that shows the loss in muscle fibers that occurs with aging is very close to the shape of the aging curve for the whole muscle (see figure 1.2b). The bottom line is that as we age we not only have smaller but also fewer muscle fibers.

Just in case things don't sound bleak enough, let's look a little more closely at aging muscle. You've probably heard that we have two major types of skeletal muscle fibers: slow twitch (called *type I*) and fast twitch (called *type II*). Obviously, fast-twitch fibers contract faster than slow-twitch fibers do; otherwise the names would be pretty silly. As we age, the motor units that we lose are mainly the fast-twitch variety. You can see in figure 1.3 that while the number of fast-twitch fibers decreases steadily with age, the number of slow-twitch fibers shows practically no change. This phenomenon is due to the rescue process that I mentioned earlier. During the rescue process, slow-twitch motor units rescue fast-contracting fibers and change them into slow-contracting

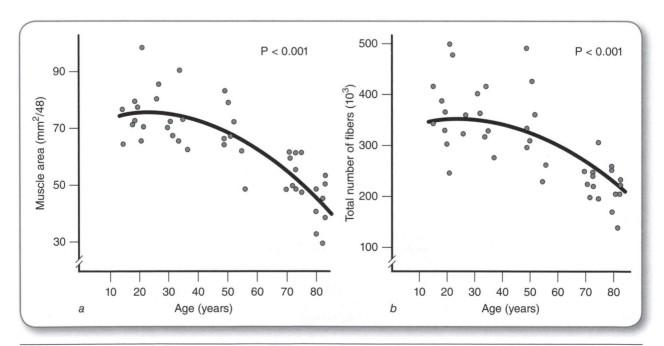

Figure 1.2   The relationships between age and *(a)* cross-sectional area of muscle and *(b)* muscle fiber number. Data are from the vastus lateralis muscles of men 15 through 83 years of age.

Reprinted by permission from Lexell, Taylor, and Sjostrom 1988.

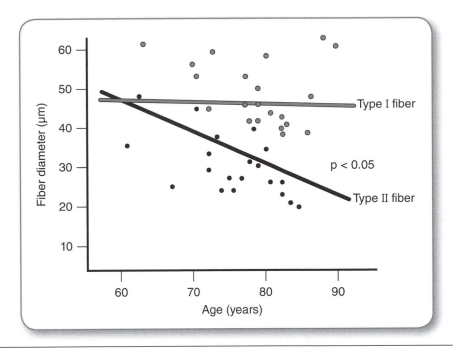

Figure 1.3   The age-associated patterns of change in mean cross-sectional areas of type II (fast-twitch) and type I (slow-twitch) muscle fibers. Data are from the vastus lateralis muscles of men 15 through 83 years of age.

Data from Lexell, Taylor, and Sjostrom 1988.

fibers. So the cost of rescuing a few fibers is that aging muscle shows a predominance of slow-twitch fibers.

What's the bottom line? The smaller the muscle, the less force it can produce, and so the more muscle mass we lose with age, the weaker we become. Also, the more fast-twitch fibers we lose with age, the slower we become. But more important than the loss of strength and speed is the loss of the product of the two, which is *power.* We examine the importance of power in the preservation of independence and the prevention of falls later in chapters 7 and 10.

> **APPLICATION POINT**   The combined loss of muscle size and fast-twitch fibers means that we become weaker, slower, and less powerful as we age.

Connective Tissue Curves

What doctors and scientists call *connective tissue* is simply the stuff that holds you together, supports and protects your body's structure, and provides lubrication to your joints. There are four major types of connective tissue: loose connective tissue, dense connective tissue, adipose (or fat) tissue, and reticular connective tissue. *Loose connective tissues* support internal organs and connect epithelial (surface) tissues to underlying tissues. *Dense connective tissues* are composed mainly of collagen fibers and make up our ligaments and tendons. Ligaments attach bone to bone, and tendons attach muscle to bone. *Adipose tissue* is used mechanically for insulation and padding and metabolically for energy storage. *Reticular connective tissue* is found mainly in the lymph nodes, thymus, spleen, and bone marrow. The most important connective tissues for our discussion on aging are tendons, ligaments, and adipose tissue.

Our tendons and ligaments become stiffer and lose their elasticity and strength as we age. This is because the structures of our connective tissue change with age. For example, collagen, the structural protein that gives strength to connective tissue, comes in two types, a more elastic type III collagen and a less elastic type I collagen. As we age, the levels of our type I, or stiffer, collagen increase and the levels of our type III, or elastic, collagen decrease. In addition, as we age our most elastic connective protein, elastin (good name!), degenerates. It's not difficult to guess the consequences of these changes. Your older clients will

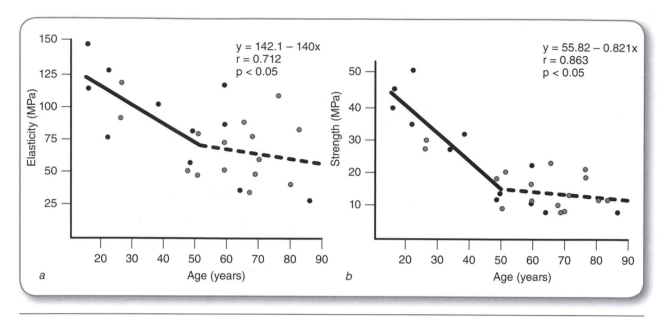

Figure 1.4   Changes in anterior cruciate ligament *(a)* elasticity and *(b)* strength with age.

Reprinted, by permission, from F.R. Noyes and E.S. Grood, 1976, "The strength of anterior cruciate ligament in humans and rhesus monkeys: Age-related and species-related changes," *Journal of Bone and Joint Surgery* 58A: 1074-1082.

tell you about them! They feel stiff, find it harder to move (especially in the morning!), and enjoy less range of motion (ROM). Figure 1.4 shows the aging curves for the elasticity and strength of the anterior cruciate ligament. You should also know that older women's ligaments and tendons typically have lower strength and less elasticity than older men's have.

APPLICATION POINT   Loss of flexibility is one of the most important and least addressed physical factors that change with aging. Be sure to include flexibility training as part of your client's training program.

So what are the implications of these changes? They include, but are not restricted to, reduced ROM, increased metabolic cost of movement, reduced mobility, decreased stored elastic energy, and increased risk of injury. Additionally, the joints themselves, as well as their lining and lubricating surfaces, degenerate with age.

Now let's look at the most unusual connective tissue, adipose tissue. Our body weight typically increases from early adulthood to approximately 60 years of age. At that point it begins to decline (see figure 1.5*a)*, but a sneaky thing happens that we can't see on the scale. From our 20s until our late 50s our lean body mass remains fairly stable,

but thereafter it shows an exponential decline (see figure 1.5*b)*. In contrast, our percentage of body fat gradually increases throughout our lives (figure 1.5*c)*. The combination of reduced muscle mass and increased body fat illustrated by these aging curves has been termed *sarcopenic obesity*. Sarcopenic obesity has extensive health and functional consequences, as you will see later in chapter 4.

There are three other tissues that you might not think of as connective tissues: bone, cartilage, and blood. Bones are vital for shape and support. They also serve as the levers that muscles use to move your body parts. Without them you'd have to slither or ooze along the ground like a worm or a slug. Our bones are also affected by the aging process. Nearly everyone has heard of osteoporosis, which is the loss of bone with aging. However, most of us think of osteoporosis as a condition that's either there or not there, when in reality the aging curve for bone density shows an exponential drop similar to that seen for skeletal muscle (see figure 1.6).

Any bone at any age can break if the stress placed on it exceeds its tensile strength. Many of us have broken our bones as kids when falling off a bike or out of a tree. As the strength and density of our bones decrease with age, the probability of breaking them increases. So we adjust our walking patterns, our posture, and

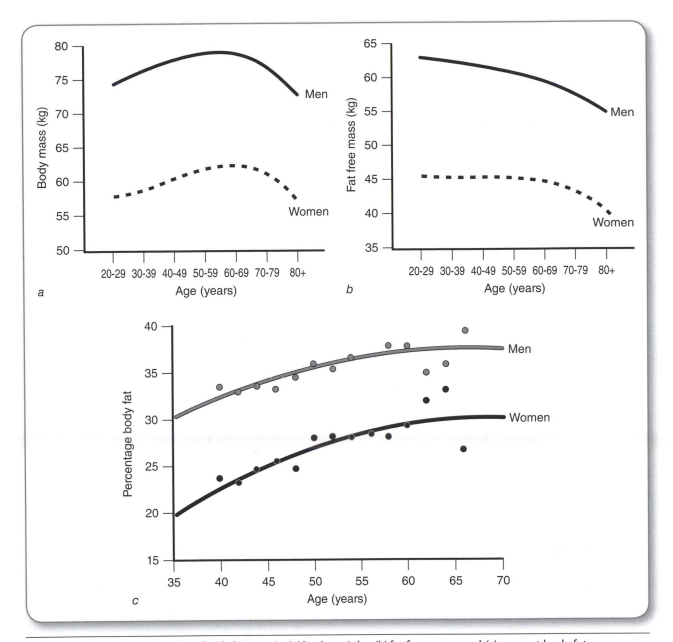

Figure 1.5 Age-related longitudinal changes in *(a)* body weight, *(b)* fat free mass, and *(c)* percent body fat.

Figure 1.5*a-b* Based on Pimentel et al. 2003; Tanaka et al. 1997; Fleg et al. 2005; and Hull et al. 2010.

Figure 1.5*c* Data from Guo et al. 1999.

our very lifestyle to protect ourselves from falls. Unfortunately, in doing this we often increase our likelihood of falling by drastically cutting back on one of our most effective preventative therapies: physical activity.

Different types of cartilage can be found in specific locations throughout the body. Hyaline cartilage covers the surfaces of joints, where it serves as a cushion and reduces bone-to-bone friction. It also holds the ribs to the sternum. Elastic cartilage can be found in the external ear, epiglot-

tis, and larynx. Finally, fibrocartilage is found in intervertebral discs, in the symphysis pubis (the fusion point of the pubic bones), and in many bone–ligament junctions. Age-associated loss in the integrity and compliancy of these tissues leads to specific conditions that negatively affect health, performance, and quality of life (see figure 1.7). These conditions include arthritis, bursitis, avulsed or protruding discs, and other degenerative conditions that can negatively affect mobility, balance, and activities of daily living (ADL).

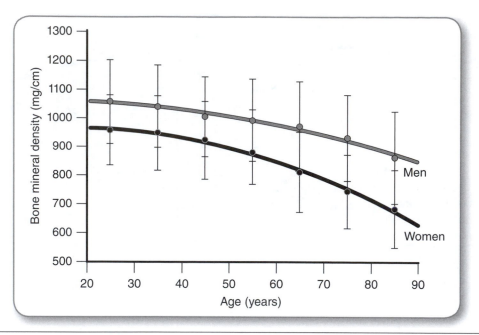

Figure 1.6 Declines in bone mineral density across age for men and women.

Data from Department of Medicine, University of Washington.

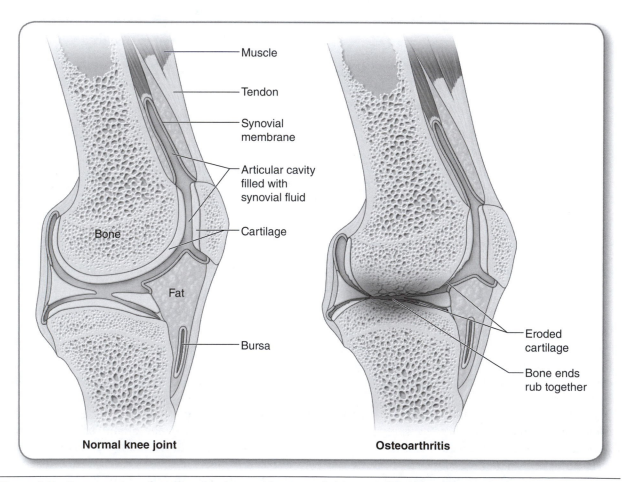

Figure 1.7 Degeneration of cartilage in a knee with osteoarthritis, a condition that commonly occurs with aging.

Reprinted by permission from Sharkey 2010.

Due to the loss of connective tissue strength and elasticity that accompanies aging, your older clients must begin their training gradually to allow for tissue adaptation. This reduces the potential for injury when your clients first begin training.

Blood is the other specialized connective tissue. It is composed of plasma, red blood cells (erythrocytes), white blood cells (leucocytes), and platelets (thrombocytes). Plasma carries dissolved gases and nutrients as well as the hormones that direct specific functions within the body. Erythrocytes contain hemoglobin and carry oxygen to support aerobic metabolism in the body's tissues. Leukocytes help fight disease and infection. Finally, thrombocytes are small cell fragments that are integral to blood clotting. Since blood is the delivery tissue for the cardiovascular system, it is discussed in detail in chapter 8.

Cardiovascular Curves

The cardiovascular system is the basis for our final set of aging curves. Cardiovascular capacity is the ability of the heart and blood vessels to deliver oxygen to our body tissues. The most common measure of this capacity is maximal oxygen uptake ($\dot{V}O_2$max). It is a measure of the maximal rate at which your body can use oxygen, or simply your aerobic power. Since obtaining this measurement requires a person to work at progressively higher workloads until oxygen utilization reaches a plateau, many people, especially older individuals, cannot reach $\dot{V}O_2$max. Therefore, $\dot{V}O_2$peak, the rate of oxygen use at volitional stoppage of an oxygen consumption test, is often used.

Jerome Fleg and colleagues (2005) presented aging curves for $\dot{V}O_2$peak and other cardiovascular factors across a median time of 7.9 years. Figure 1.8 shows the aging curves for $\dot{V}O_2$peak adjusted for body weight in men and women aged 20 through 80. These curves illustrate that declines in oxygen consumption accelerate with age. So what controls $\dot{V}O_2$peak?

$\dot{V}O_2$peak is controlled by two factors: heart rate (HR), which is the number of times the heart beats per minute, and oxygen pulse (O_2pulse), which is the amount of oxygen extracted by the body from a single heartbeat. If we examine the aging curves for HR and O_2pulse (figures 1.9*a* and 1.9*b*, respectively), we can see that there is a nearly linear decline in HR and an exponential decline in O_2pulse with age. This means that the ability of your client's working tissues to extract oxygen from the blood is the factor dictating the *exponential* drop in $\dot{V}O_2$peak. In chapter 8 we'll look at how training can improve this ability. But before we look at interventions, let's look at the consequences all of these aging curves will have in store for us if we don't intervene.

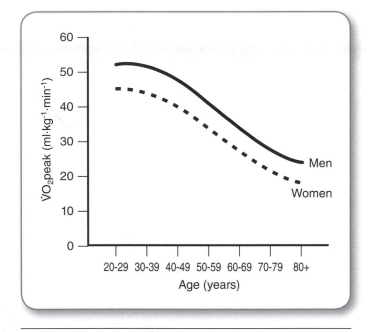

Figure 1.8 Declines in $\dot{V}O_2$peak relative to body weight in men and women across age groups.

Oxygen Consumption	
$\dot{V}O_2$max	Maximal oxygen uptake as indicated by a plateau of oxygen consumption even as work increases during a graduated exercise test.
$\dot{V}O_2$peak	Highest oxygen consumption level reached at the voluntary stoppage of a graduated exercise test prior to reaching $\dot{V}O_2$max.

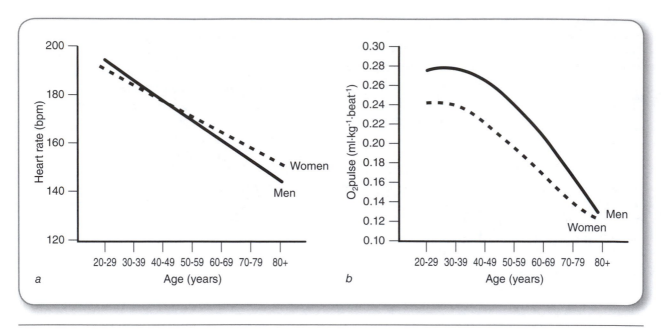

Figure 1.9   Declines in *(a)* maximum HR and *(b)* O$_2$pulse in men and women across age groups.
Based on Pimentel et al. 2003; Tanaka et al. 1997; Fleg et al. 2005; and Fitzgerald et al. 1997.

USING EXERCISE TO BEND THE AGING CURVES

Since we have examined some of the aging curves that affect your clients' independence, metabolic health, and fall probability, I think this is a great time to revisit the title of this book, *Bending the Aging Curve.* As you have seen, the majority of the curves show an exponential drop as we age as does the overall aging curve. The idea behind the title of this book, and its underlying philosophy, is that you can use targeted exercise prescriptions to improve your client's wellness and "bend" his or her aging curves. The solid line in figure 1.10 is redrawn from the neuromuscular aging curve presented in figure 1.2*a*. What would this line look like if you were able to improve your client's neuromuscular condition? Let's say you could produce a 30% improvement in your client at 60 years of age, a 50% improvement in your client at 75 years of age, and an 80% percent improvement in your client at 90 years of age. As you can see from the dashed line in figure 1.10, the new curve would be "bent" upward illustrating this improvement. But what about the client who has been training his or her entire life? Will that client still show an exponential drop in performance with age? The answer is yes. But as you can see from the

dotted line in figure 1.10, your client that regularly exercised will have a curve that begins at a much higher level than an untrained person, and the decline often will still place the client at a level equivalent to an untrained person years younger.

FRAILTY AND PHYSICAL VULNERABILITY

For years we have used the word *frailty* to describe the weakness and disability associated with aging. In recent years scientists and clinicians have applied operational definitions to the term. These operational definitions not only help us to understand frailty, they also allow us to select the correct curve-bending treatments to address the problem. So let's look at the complex nature of frailty and the consequences if you don't provide an intervention that can effectively "bend" your clients' aging curves.

Definitions of Frailty

The word *frail* brings to mind a weak and brittle body that can barely support its own weight without breaking. The Merriam-Webster online dictionary in part supports this image through the following entry:

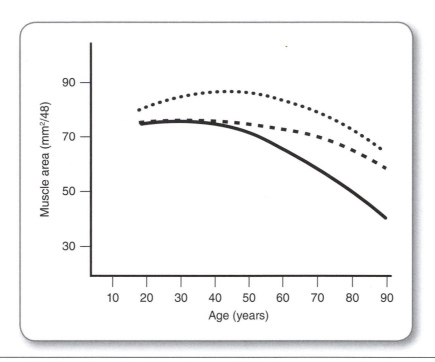

Figure 1.10 The capacity of exercise to "bend the aging curve" using the neuromuscular aging curve as an example. The long solid line shows the neuromuscular aging curve as originally presented in figure 1.2a. The dashed line shows how that curve may be "bent" through exercise training. The dotted line shows what an aging curve might look like for a person who has been a lifelong exerciser.

Frail

Etymology: Middle English, from Anglo-French *fraile*, from Latin *fragilis* fragile, from *frangere*

1: easily led into evil < frail humanity >

2: easily broken or destroyed: fragile

3 a: physically weak b: slight, unsubstantial

Synonyms: see *weak*

Although these descriptions may define the word *frail*, they cannot begin to address the clinical concept of frailty, especially as it relates to aging. In fact, the term itself has been used in so many ways that it has no single clinical definition. So let's look at this moving target called *frailty* and see what makes a simple definition so problematic.

Frailty as a Syndrome

Although there is no clear consensus among clinicians or researchers concerning the definition of *frailty*, most agree that it is by nature a *syndrome*. A syndrome is a group of signs and symptoms that occur in concert to characterize a particular abnormality or condition. *Frailty syndrome* is made up of a number of interactive factors. In fact, in his editorial "Frailty and Its Definition: A Worthy Challenge," Kenneth Rockwood (2005) uses the term *complexity of frailty* to express the elaborate interplays among the factors associated with the syndrome. We can break these factors down into theoretical and empirical. The most common theoretical factors include physical inactivity, disease, nutritional status, cognitive and psychological condition, socioeconomic status, spirituality, residential and legal issues, and aging. Of these factors, the physical ones such as reduced physical activity are those most commonly cited.

The empirical factors mirror the theoretical ones, with the physical factors at the top of the list as indicators of frailty. The most common measures used to assess physical declines are deficits in sensory perception, ADL decrements, and reductions in mobility and agility. The importance of physical performance as a marker of frailty is further emphasized in a consensus report (Ferrucci et al., 2004) that recommends that the definition of *frailty* be based on physical factors such as muscle strength, balance, mobility, motor processing, cognition, cardio-vascular endurance, physical activity, and nutritional status (especially as it relates to weight loss).

In the past, a loss in body weight was considered a marker of tissue wasting and, therefore, a marker of frailty. In our modern societies, however, with our reduced levels of physical activity and increased availability of food, we often maintain or even increase our body weight by adding adipose tissue as we lose muscle mass. Chapter 4 discusses this sarcopenic obesity and its treatment.

Is Frailty an Absolute?

Frailty is often thought of as a condition that either exists or does not exist, like an on–off switch. This concept is inaccurate for a number of reasons. First, frailty is really the later stage of a continuum; therefore, it should be defined by *level* and not *state*. Second, the pattern of decline associated with frailty is different for each person, so we cannot assume that one person has the same degree of frailty as another has simply because they are both diagnosed as frail. And third, frailty is multifactorial, so different factors may decline at different rates and contribute at different degrees to the overall level of frailty. This *individualized, multidimensional continuum* is one of the bases of the diagnostic model I present in this book. It demonstrates that exercise interventions must be tailored to the specific needs of the individual if they are to be effective and efficient.

> **APPLICATION POINT** Each client has personal patterns of decline and personalized definitions of physical vulnerability; therefore, one-size-fits-all programs can be ineffective and potentially harmful.

Vulnerability and the Evolution of Frailty

Your client's level of frailty may be seen as the balance between a stable capacity to perform daily activities and a state of physical vulnerability in which your client is losing independence (see figure 1.11). Additionally, frailty is clearly

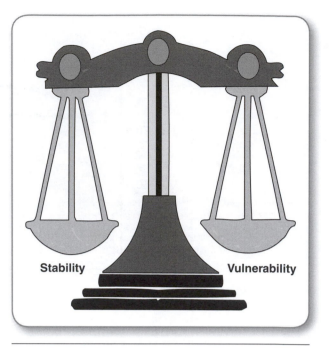

Figure 1.11 Frailty is the balance between stability in performing daily activities and a state of physical vulnerability.

not an instantaneous process. With the possible exception of experiencing a catastrophic event, your client won't wake up one morning instantaneously frail. Frailty evolves over time as physical reserves decline and your client becomes less able to deal with changes in the internal or external environments. To appreciate this concept, let's examine some of the terminology associated with it. First of all, *physical reserve* or *functional reserve capacity* can be defined as the difference between a person's maximal capacity and the minimal capacity required to perform a specific task or maintain a specific level of activity. For example, if the leg extension power required to climb stairs is 2.0 W/kg bw (Watts per kilogram of body weight) and an individual can produce 4.0 W/kg bw, he has a physical reserve of 2.0 W/kg bw. However, if a second person has a maximal leg extension power of 2.2 W/kg bw, his physical reserve is only 0.2 W/kg bw. Thus the second person is at greater risk for dependency (see figure 1.12).

The terms *internal environment* and *external environment* should be considered both independently and interactively. Everything in life, from the basics such as breathing and maintaining blood flow to the extremes such as running a

Activities of Daily Living

| ADL | Activities of daily living, such as walking, dressing, and transferring from bed to chair. |
| IADL | Instrumental activities of daily living, meaning activities that involve complex movements like doing housework, taking medications, shopping, using the telephone, and paying bills. |

marathon or an all-out sprint, requires energy. Therefore, even the most basic activities cause a disruption in our body's internal environment that our systems must correct. This maintenance of a fairly constant internal environment is called *homeostasis,* which comes from the Greek roots *homoios* meaning "the same" and *stasis* meaning "stance" or "posture." Changes in our body's internal environment are corrected by an interactive network of feedback mechanisms that hold each system within specific physiological limits. When the physical reserve of any of these systems declines to the extent that the system can no longer compensate for changes, the system becomes vulnerable to the adverse effects of

disruption, increasing the level of frailty of the individual. Challenges in the external environment may be the factors disturbing homeostasis. For example, think about climbing three flights of stairs. In order to meet this challenge, you must increase your HR, breathing, and muscle activity. If your cardiovascular or neuromuscular reserves are too small to meet the challenge, climbing the stairs becomes impossible. It is these failures in a person's ability to perform common daily activities that are used as common markers of frailty.

Perhaps our most intimate acquaintance with the term *physical vulnerability* comes from its antithesis, *invulnerability.* Many of our mythical

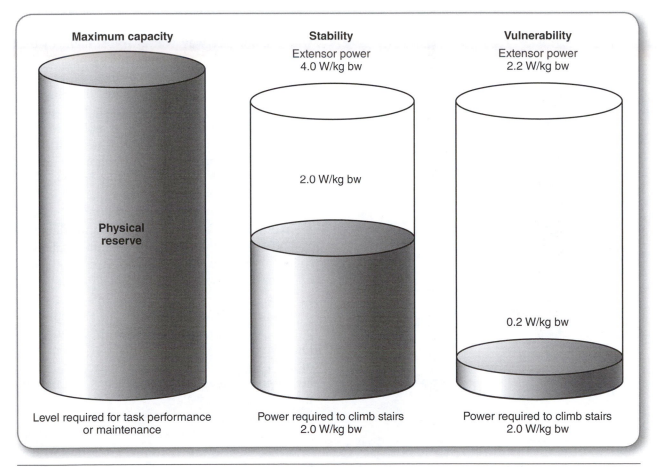

Figure 1.12 Physical reserve (shown as shaded cylinder) as it relates to lower-body power output and the ability to climb stairs.

heroes, from Achilles to Superman, are invulnerable to physical harm. Perhaps we have attached this attribute to our mythical heroes because it flies in the face of our own vulnerability. For this text I am using a modified definition of *physical vulnerability* presented by Debra Saliba and coworkers (2001). Physical vulnerability is a level of functional decline that puts a person in imminent danger of losing her ability to perform the necessary ADL and instrumental activities of daily living (IADL) required for independent living.

We have now examined the terms *independence, physical vulnerability,* and *frailty* as points along a continuum that increases in severity as physical reserve declines (see figure 1.13). Additionally, we've seen that a person's position along this continuum is determined by how well all of the physical factors associated with functionality work in concert.

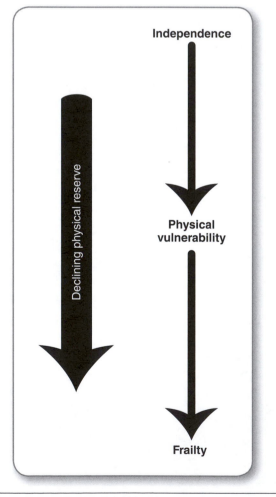

Figure 1.13   The relationship between declining physical reserve and the onset of frailty.

PREHAB OR REHAB: CHANGING THE OIL OR CHANGING THE ENGINE?

Because physical vulnerability results from declines in physical performance and activity, an intervention designed to improve these factors, such as exercise, can reduce frailty in older persons. Since the adaptations resulting from training are specific to the exercises provided by the training, we can tailor an exercise prescription to match an individual's needs, thereby maximizing the rate of improvement (see figure 1.14). Later chapters in this book provide the specifics of tailoring an exercise program and modifying it to meet the *evolving* needs of clients.

One of the most effective advertising campaigns has been that of the Castrol oil company. The basis of the campaign was that you could spend a few dollars to change your oil now or you could spend a few thousand dollars to change your engine later . . . sort of a corporate version of "an ounce of prevention is worth a pound of cure." Somewhere along the way we have lost sight of this simple concept in our health care system. Rather than using simple tools such as exercise and diet to help reduce the negative effects of aging, we allow physical declines to occur and then address them with prescription drugs, assistive devices, and rehabilitation. In other words, the industrialized nations of the world spend billions of dollars trying to change the engine when instead they could spend much less to change the oil.

This book is not about rehabilitation. It's about *pre*habilitation. It's about recognizing declines and addressing them early in the independence–frailty continuum, when you can have the greatest effect both physically and financially. This is not to say that exercise cannot help frail elders. The literature clearly demonstrates that the opposite is true. However, the earlier we intervene, the longer our clients have to enjoy a higher quality of life, a lower probability of catastrophic injury, and a greater level of independence throughout their stay on planet Earth.

The next few chapters describe how to accomplish this with the highest level of success and the lowest level of time commitment. In other words, this book shows you how to get the most *fitness* bang for your *exercise* buck.

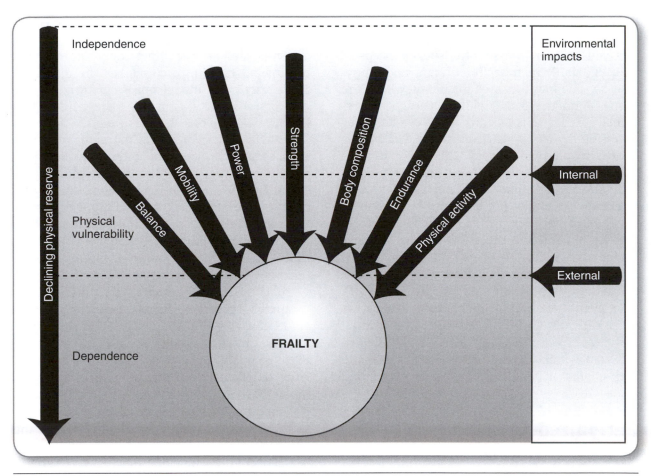

Figure 1.14 Declines in fitness variables due to internal and external environmental factors and their effects on frailty in older persons. Since not all variables show similar declines, targeted exercise prescriptions are needed to maximize results.

APPLICATION POINT When working with your older clients, you have the unique opportunity to prevent and even reverse their declines and improve their lives rather than waiting for those declines to happen and then trying to deal with them through extended care and nursing home care.

EXERCISE AS A TARGETED INTERVENTION: MATCHING THE PROGRAM TO THE NEED

This book presents an exercise intervention based on three concepts:

1. An exercise diagnosis and prescription model

2. A periodized system of application

3. A translational recovery period

Diagnosis and Prescription Model

As illustrated by the diamond analogy and reiterated by the aging curves, there are a multitude of factors associated with the declines in health, functional performance, and mobility that accompany aging. Therefore, in order to maximize efficacy, exercise prescriptions must target the specific needs of the individual. The concept of exercise specificity has appeared in the literature for decades; however, its application to specific populations is often weak and concentrates only on a single physiological system. As the medical community has shown us, a true prescription is based on a diagnosis. Therefore, chapter 2 lays the groundwork for diagnosis by presenting the concept of physical testing as a diagnostic tool that you can use to assess the specific needs of your clients. Remember that diagnosing injury, disease, or illness in a client is not within the scope of practice of a health and fitness professional. By *diagnosis* I clearly mean evaluating or assessing the client's strengths and weaknesses related to physical activity. Chapter 3 reviews the general training principles that are used to develop exercise programs. Chapters 4 through 8 provide the diagnostic tests and training tools needed to tailor programs to your clients' needs, thereby maximizing the effectiveness and efficiency of each training prescription. And finally, the appendix provides normative scores so you can assess each of the factors associated with your client's multifaceted functional diamond. For those of you who, like me, prefer a more automated approach, the DVD offers a spreadsheet file from which you can automatically evaluate your clients' needs using their gender, age, and test scores.

Periodized System of Application

Periodization is one of the most important training tools to come down the pike in the past five decades. It is based on three major concepts: targeted training cycles, training evolution, and recovery as a training tool. The concept of targeted training cycles takes the diagnosis and prescription model one step further, since it recognizes that exercise as a prescriptive tool is not instantaneous. It takes time for the body to reengineer itself to meet the demands of an exercise prescription. And often this biological retooling requires a number of different targeted training cycles. During these training cycles your client evolves into a new and improved system that more effectively deals with the aging process (see figure 1.15). And finally, the most important aspect of periodization is the recognition that the body requires time to reengineer itself. Take the example of the U.S. automotive industry. Major companies such as General Motors, Chrysler, and Ford know that the American public wants battery-, solar-, or hydrogen-powered vehicles, but these companies can't yet meet those demands since they must retool their plants to produce those cars. Humans, too, need time to retool. By manipulating exercise intensity, volume, and method, we can cycle our clients through the exercise process so that periods of recovery are available for the molecular retooling process. You will learn how to use the powerful training tool of periodization in chapter 9.

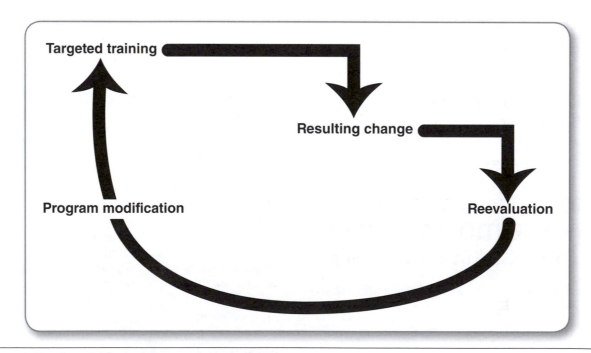

Figure 1.15 A model for evolving exercise prescription.

Translational Recovery Period

When I lecture on the topic of using recovery as a training tool, my audience often becomes a bit agitated, asking, "So what do I do with my clients . . . just send them away?" The answer to this question has both physiological and financial consequences, so I'll reply as succinctly as I can: No! One thing we know from empirical information and scientific studies is that the best way to get good at something is to do it. A few years back my colleagues and I looked at the factors that make a good tennis player and came to one conclusion that most tennis coaches already know: What makes a good tennis player is playing a lot of tennis. In other words, if you want to get good at something, you have to either do it or at the very least do something that imitates it—that uses motor patterns that reflect the skill you want to improve. That's one of the reasons why athletes spend more time on the field or on the court than they do in the weight room.

So the answer to the question of what to do with clients is quite simple. Once you have improved their physical conditioning, you must teach them to *translate* that new physical prowess into patterns that increase their independence and reduce their likelihood of falling. This *translational* process not only facilitates the recovery time so vital to a successful training program but also develops between you and your clients the coach–athlete relationship necessary for them to succeed in the most important game they will ever

play: the game of life. Chapter 10 will explain the concept behind translational training and how to properly structure these cycles using activities that address your clients' specific needs and that are related to the preceding training cycle. It will also provide descriptions of the drills and some case studies. The accompanying DVD offers a series of case studies showing how to proceed from exercise diagnosis to targeted training to the development of translational cycles. These cycles will effectively teach your clients to use their newly developed physical capacity in movements that are related to their daily needs and aspirations.

SUMMARY

Aging is an inevitable consequence of life, just like death and taxes. But since it sneaks up on us we sometimes don't notice until we're there (and sometimes not even then). But aging doesn't need to be associated with the specters of frailty, loss of independence, and morbidity. Using the diagnosis and prescription model presented in this text you can evaluate the declines in clients' aging curves and bend them back to levels associated with individuals that are decades younger. Now that we have looked at the aging curves and briefly examined their negative effects on health and well-being, it's time to examine the programs that are most effective at bending these aging curves and polishing every facet of the client's functional diamond.

Topical Bibliography

The Concept of Age

Sharkey, B.J. (1987). Functional vs chronologic age. *Medicine and Science in Sports and Exercise* 19:174-178.

Neuromuscular Curves

Brooks, S.V., & Faulkner, J.A. (1994). Skeletal muscle weakness in old age: Underlying mechanisms. *Medicine and Science in Sports and Exercise* 26:432-439.

Harman, E. (2006). Strength and power: A definition of terms. *National Strength and Conditioning Association Journal* 15:18-21.

Larsson, L., Li, X., & Frontera, W.R. (1997). Effects of aging on shortening velocity and myosin isoform composition in single human skeletal muscle cells. *American Journal of Physiology* 41: C638-C649.

Lexell, J. (1993). Aging and human muscle: Observations from Sweden. *Canadian Journal of Applied Physiology* 18:2-18.

Lexell, J., Taylor, C.C., & Sjostrom, M. (1988). What is the cause of the ageing atrophy? Total number, size and proportion of different fiber types studied in whole vastus lateralis muscle from 15-to 83-year-old men. *J Neurol Sci* 84:275-294.

Levy, D.I., Young, A., Skelton, D.A., & Yeo, A.I. (1994). Strength, power and functional ability. In M. Passeri (Ed.), *Geriatrics '94* (pp. 85-93). International Association of Gerontology, European Region Clinical Section Congress. Rome: CIC Edizioni Internationali.

Macalusa, A., & De Vito, G. (2004). Muscle strength, power and adaptations to resistance training in older people. *Eur J Appl Physiol* 91:450-472.

Skelton, D.A., Greig, C.A., Davies, J.M., & Young, A. (1994). Strength, power and related functional ability of health people aged 65-89 years. *Age and Ageing* 23:371-377.

Skelton, D.A., Kennedy, J., & Rutherford, O.M. (2002). Explosive power and asymmetry in leg muscle function in frequent fallers and non-fallers aged over 65. *Age and Ageing* 31:119-125.

Tomonaga, M. (1977). Histochemical and ultrastructural changes in senile human skeletal muscle. *Journal of the American Geriatrics Society* 25:125-131.

Connective Tissue Curves

Gregg, E.W., Pereira, M.A., & Caspersen, C.J. (2000). Physical activity, falls, and fractures among older adults: A review of the epidemiologic evidence. *Journal of American Geriatric Society* 48:883-893.

Howland, J., Lachman, M.E., Peterson, E.W., Cote, J., Kasten, L., & Jette, A. (1998). Covariates of fear of falling and associated activity curtailment. *The Gerontologist* 38:549-555.

Noyes, F.R., & Grood, E.S. (1976). The strength of anterior cruciate ligament in humans and rhesus monkeys: Age-related and species-related changes. *J Bone Joint Surg* 58A:1074-1082.

Stevens, J.A., Powell, K.E., Smith, S.M., Wingo, P.A., & Sattin, R.W. (1997). Physical activity, functional limitations, and the risk of fall-related fractures in community-dwelling elderly. *Ann Epidemiol* 7:61.

Seals, D.R., Monahan, K.D., Bell, C., Tanaka, H., & Jones, P.P. (2001). The aging cardiovascular system: Changes in autonomic function at rest and in response to exercise. *International Journal of Sport Nutrition and Exercise Metabolism* 11: S189-S195.

Wilmore, J.H., Green, J.S., Stanforth, P.R., Gagnon, J., Rankinen, T., Leon, A.S., Rao, D.C., Skinner, J.S., & Bouchard, C. (2001). Relationship of changes in maximal and submaximal aerobic fitness to changes in cardiovascular disease and non-insulin-dependent diabetes mellitus risk factors with endurance training: The HERITAGE Family Study. *Metabolism* 50:1255-1263.

Cardiovascular Curves

Fleg, J.L., Morrell, C.H., Bos, A.G., Brant, L.J., Talbot, L.A., Wright, J.G., & Lakatta, E.G. (2005). Accelerated longitudinal decline of aerobic capacity in healthy older adults. *Circulation* 112:674-682.

Frailty

Ferrucci, L., Guralnik, J.M., Studenski, S., Fried, L.P., Cutler, G.B., Walston, J.D., & The Interventions on Frailty Working Group. (2004). Designing randomized controlled trials aimed at preventing or delaying functional decline and disability in frail older persons: A consensus report. *Journal of the American Geriatrics Society* 52(4):625-634.

Rockwood, K. (2005). Frailty and its definition: A worthy challenge. *Journal of the American Geriatrics Society* 53(6):1069-1070.

Saliba, D., Elliott, M., Rubenstein, L.Z., Solomon, D.H., Young, R.T., Kamberg, C.J., Roth, C., MacLean, C.H., Shekelle, P.G., Sloss, E.M., & Wenger, N.S. (2001). The Vulnerable Elders Survey: A tool for identifying vulnerable older people in the community. *Journal of the American Geriatrics Society* 49(12):1691-1699.

References

Ferrucci, L., Guralnik, J.M., Studenski, S., Fried, L.P., Cutler, G.B., Walston, J.D., and The Interventions on Frailty Working Group. (2004). Designing randomized controlled trials aimed at preventing or delaying functional decline and disability in frail older persons: A consensus report. *Journal of the American Geriatrics Society* 52(4):625-634.

Fleg, J.L., Morrell, C.H., Bos, A.G., Brant, L.J., Talbot, L.A., Wright, J.G., & Lakatta, E.G. (2005). Accelerated longitudinal decline of aerobic capacity in healthy older adults. *Circulation* 112:674-682.

Lexell, J., Taylor, C.C., & Sjostrom, M. (1988). What is the cause of the ageing atrophy? Total number, size and proportion of different fiber types studied in whole vastus lateralis muscle from 15-to 83-year-old men. *J Neurol Sci* 84:275-294.

Noyes, F.R., & Grood, E.S. (1976). The strength of anterior cruciate ligament in humans and rhesus monkeys: Age-related and species-related changes. *J Bone Joint Surg* 58A:1074-1082.

Rockwood, K. (2005). Frailty and its definition: A worthy challenge. *Journal of the American Geriatrics Society* 53(6):1069-1070.

Saliba, D., Elliott, M., Rubenstein, L.Z., Solomon, D.H., Young, R.T., Kamberg, C.J., Roth, C., MacLean, C.H., Shekelle, P.G., Sloss, E.M., & Wenger, N.S. (2001). The Vulnerable Elders Survey: A tool for identifying vulnerable older people in the community. *Journal of the American Geriatrics Society* 49(12):1691-1699.

Testing

One of the many things this book describes is how to use the classic diagnosis and prescription model to bend the aging curves that affect your clients' independence and safety. This model allows you to evaluate each client's specific needs (the exercise diagnosis) and to tailor an activity program that addresses those needs (the exercise prescription). By *diagnosis* I mean evaluating or assessing the client's strengths and weaknesses related to physical activity. Diagnosing injury, disease, or illness in a client is not within the scope of practice of a health and fitness professional. This chapter examines the nature of the exercise diagnosis and prescription model and how it allows you to prepare the most effective exercise prescription for clients. In addition, it explains how you can use the model to monitor a client's progress in order to provide feedback and restructure the training program as your client progresses.

THE EXERCISE DIAGNOSIS AND PRESCRIPTION MODEL

In his article, "A Perspective on Exercise Prescription," Herb Weber (2001) noted that the concept of exercise prescription was introduced by the American College of Sports Medicine (ACSM) about 25 years ago. Weber's perspective on the term *exercise prescription* serves as an excellent starting point for our discussion:

> We do value the very beneficial side effects of exercise. Thus, the imagery of a prescription in its traditional or clinical sense is diametrically opposed to its

perception as a directive for exercise. To continue prescribing exercise for the apparently healthy and low risk adult population is to perpetuate a conflict of "having to" rather than "wanting to" engage in physical activity and can only lead to less effective compliance. (Weber, 2001, p. 2)

Weber is suggesting that the term *prescription* commonly is used to describe a pharmaceutical intervention that deals with an illness and that it may negatively influence the client's desire to exercise. However, the precedent for its use has been established in both physical therapy and cardiac rehabilitation.

If we examine the recent U.S. Congressional debates concerning how to improve the American health care system, we find that one term surfaces over and over again: *prevention*. In the context of our aging society, a prescription for prevention is more important than a prescription for rehabilitation. Perhaps the new American mantra should be, "An ounce of prevention is worth 300 billion dollars of cure."

In the context of a prescription for prevention, Weber's paper reinforces a number of major concerns I have had for years. First of all, the term *prescription,* especially as used by the medical profession, implies a response to a diagnosis. Unfortunately, this is not the case with most exercise prescriptions. Rather than providing exercise prescriptions in response to a diagnosis, we usually provide them by using general population guidelines, dictates of specific facilities, or personal beliefs. While general population guidelines can certainly be used to guide us in how we use a test or how we view a client, they cannot and should not be the basis of a prescription. Second, many exercise prescriptions concentrate on only one aspect of fitness (strength, cardiovascular endurance, and so on), often to the detriment of the others. For exercise diagnosis and prescription to be effective, they must reflect all the needs of the client. Third, we have engendered in the American population an environment of failure. Rather than helping the public to see exercise as a two-for-one special, providing both health benefits and recreation, we have made it a second job that a person must complete every day or be considered a failure. Fourth, if we are to use the exercise diagnosis and prescription model, we must be sure that our diagnostic tests are performed correctly. To that end you should carefully learn and practice the tests you will be using to assess clients' needs. And finally, we must understand the links between our diagnostic testing and the associated prescriptions. Only then can we use these powerful tools to maximize the benefits for our clients.

APPLICATION POINT   A prescription without a diagnosis is no prescription at all.

THE EXERCISE DIAGNOSIS: ANALYSIS OF NEEDS

An effective exercise prescription must be preceded by an exercise diagnosis. In actuality there are two diagnoses: a general diagnosis and a specific diagnosis. The general diagnosis is a face-value, first-impression analysis based on the specific characteristics of the client, such as age, gender, and appearance. The general diagnosis is represented by the aging curves presented in chapter 1. The curves show the declines in strength and power, speed, muscular and cardiovascular endurance, flexibility, balance, and agility that are associated with aging. They also show the age-related reductions in lean body mass and increases in body fat.

While the general exercise diagnosis may give you a broad framework for an exercise prescription, it does not reveal the specific needs that must be addressed to improve an aging client's quality of life. Figure 2.1 presents scatter plots showing the results for two functional tests, the 8-foot (2.4 m) up-and-go test and the gallon jug shelf test, performed by trained and untrained older persons at our laboratory. Each number

on the plots represents a different client. If you look across the horizontal axis, or x-axis, you'll notice that the further to the right a number is, the older that person is, and if you look up the vertical axis, or y-axis, you'll see that the higher up the number is, the longer it took to complete the task and so the lower the performance level. Notice that the regression lines, the lines that show the patterns of change in performance across age, show an exponential increase across age groups. But before you get excited about how wonderful aging is, remember that a higher number indicates a poorer performance. Therefore, these plots show the exponential drops in performance expected with age given the curves presented in chapter 1.

But let's take a more analytical look at these graphs. If you look at the subject numbers, you'll notice that very few of them fall on, or even near, a line. This is also demonstrated by the r^2 values presented on the graphs, which are .267 for the 8-foot (2.4 m) up-and-go test and .402 for the gallon jug shelf test. For those of you who are unfamiliar with r^2 values, an r^2 value of 1.0 means that all the numbers (i.e., data points) fall right on the line and that the line perfectly describes the exact amount of time it takes each subject to complete each test. But if a data point does not fit a line very well, and we use the lines, which present generalized views of aging, to diagnose the client, we'll be wrong more times than we are right in predicting performance. In fact, if you look at subject 102 on the 8-foot (2.4 m) up-and-go test, you'll notice that he's about 82 years old and can perform better than more than half of the people on the graph, many of whom are decades younger. A similar situation exists with subjects 46 and 140 for the gallon jug shelf test. These two 75-year-olds outperformed nearly half of the younger participants.

In looking at these results, something else should jump out at you: The subjects who performed best on the gallon jug shelf test were not necessarily the ones who did best on the 8-foot (2.4 m) up-and-go test. These data demonstrate that a client may show little or no decline in one physical factor while showing substantial deterioration in another. In other words, not everyone follows the same patterns of decline when aging. We can't evaluate a person's needs simply by knowing that person's age, and we can't assume that a low score on one test, such as flexibility, will mean a low score on another, such as cardiovascular endurance.

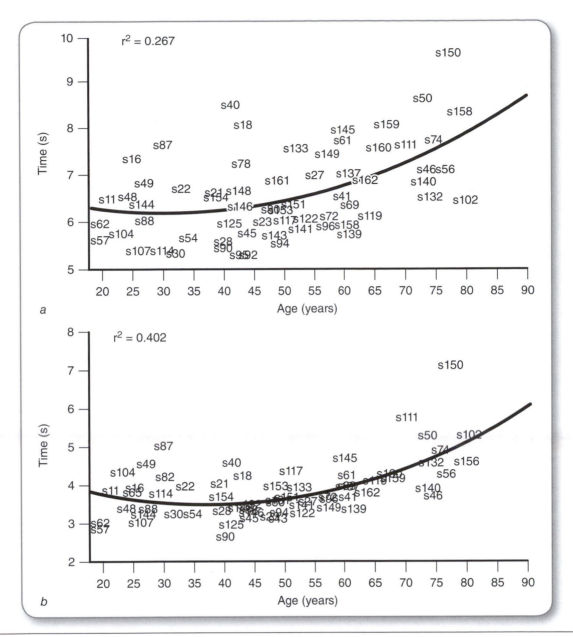

Figure 2.1   Performance times for subjects aged 18 to 85 years performing *(a)* the gallon jug shelf test and *(b)* the 8-foot (2.4 m) up-and-go test.

Each client needs a battery of diagnostic tests to assess the specific needs along the independence–frailty continuum for each physical factor. Over the years, I have assembled a testing battery that diagnoses the specific needs of clients and can be used to tailor training prescriptions to clients' unique requirements (see table 2.1). The latest version of this diagnostic testing battery is provided on the DVD that accompanies this text. When using the spreadsheet, be sure to use the proper sheet for your client's age group, as noted at the top of each sheet.

APPLICATION POINT   Clients change as they age and train. It's your job to follow those changes so you can provide the most effective prescriptions.

For your convenience, table 2.2 lists the tests that are included on the diagnostic spreadsheet, the physical parameter they measure, and how each parameter is related to bending the aging curve. The descriptions of how the individual tests should be performed are included in chapters 4

Table 2.1 Sample Diagnostic Sheet

For Females, 65 to 69 Years Old

Name or ID Number	4		Date	7/7/2010
Age (years)	67		Gender	F
Height (in.)	66		Weight (lb)	145
Height (m)	1.68		Weight (kg)	65.91

Note: The *Test* column shows the name of the test and the units you should use when entering each trial's result.

Test	Trial 1	Trial 2	Average	Percentile
Chair Sit-and-Reach, Left (in.)	2.5	2.5	2.50	50-75
Chair Sit-and-Reach, Right (in.)	2	2.5	2.25	50-75
Back Scratch, Left (in.)	0	0	0.00	50-75
Back Scratch, Right (in.)	0	-1	-0.50	50-75
Modified Trunk Rotation (in.)	27	26	26.50	50-75
Single-Leg Stance Balance (s)	26	25	25.50	50-75
Functional Reach (in.)	15	15.2	15.10	50-75
8-Foot (2.4 m) Up-And-Go (s)	5.6	5.5	5.55	50-75
30-Second Chair Stand (reps)	14	14	14.00	50-75
Modified Ramp Power (s)	1	0.9	0.95	50-75
30-Second Arm Curl (reps)	16	17	16.50	50-75
Gallon Jug Shelf (s)	9	8.9	8.95	50-75
6-Minute Walk (yards)	600	■■■■■■	600.00	50-75
15-Foot (4.6 m) Walk, Usual (s)	3.1	3.93	3.52	50-75
15-Foot (4.6 m) Walk, Maximal (s)	2.5	2.4	2.45	50-75
% Body Fat	28.3	28.3	28.3	50-75
BMI	■■■■■■	■■■■■■	23.40	50-75
Modified Ramp Power Test				
Ramp Height (m)	0.33			
Ramp Power (absolute)	224.73			
Ramp Power (per kg bw)	3.41			
Skinfolds	**Trial 1**	**Trial 2**		
Chest	20	19		
Midaxillary	22	21		
Suprailiac	18	19		
Abdominal	24	23		
Thigh	18	18		
Triceps	16	17		
Subscapular	18	19		
Sum	136.0	136.0		
Body Density	1.0	1.0		
% Body Fat	28.3	28.3		

Table 2.2 How the Testing Battery Relates to Bending the Aging Curves

Test	Performance factor	Relationship to ADLs
Chair sit-and-reach (right and left)	Hamstring and back flexibility	Ability to perform many daily activities, walking ability, movement speed, and adjustment of balance used to prevent a fall
Back scratch (right and left)	Shoulder flexibility	Ability to perform many instrumental activities of daily living such as dressing and bathing
Modified trunk rotation	Trunk flexibility	Related to nearly every activity of daily living and recreational sports
Single-leg stance balance	Balance	Ability to recover from a stumble, which reduces the probability of falling
Functional reach	Balance	Ability to recover from a stumble, which reduces the probability of falling
8-foot (2.4 m) up-and-go	Balance, gait, leg strength, and agility	Ability to rise from a chair, walk at moderate to high speeds, and navigate around objects while maintaining balance
30-second chair stand	Lower-body strength and power	Ability to rise from a chair, bed or toilet, ability to catch oneself and thus prevent a fall
Modified ramp power	Walking power	Ability to climb stairs, to accelerate to high speeds when walking (e.g., when crossing a street), and to recover from a stumble and reduce the potential for a fall
30-second arm curl	Upper-body strength and power	Ability to perform many activities of daily living like lifting an object from a table, shelf, or counter
Gallon jug shelf	Object transfer power	Capacity to move an object from one location to another, especially when the surfaces are uneven (e.g., moving a gallon of milk or a roast from a refrigerator shelf to a counter)
6-minute walk	Cardiovascular endurance	Walking distances, such as when shopping in a mall, walking through your neighborhood, or hiking
15-foot (4.6 m) walk (usual speed)	Speed at which your client usually walks	Mobility and overall independence
15-foot (4.6 m) walk (maximal speed)	Maximal speed at which your client can walk	Ability to deal with more challenging activities, ability to recover from a stumble and reduce the probability of falling
Body composition	Percentage body fat	Ability of your client to effectively move his or her body during locomotion or when transferring (e.g., moving from the bed to a chair); also indicative of metabolic health
Body mass index	Your client's weight divided by the square of the client's height	Ability of your client to effectively move his or her body during locomotion or when transferring (e.g., moving from the bed to a chair); also indicative of metabolic health

through 8 along with the specific *facet* of aging that the individual tests measure.

WHAT MAKES AN EFFECTIVE TEST?

For a test to be of clinical value as a diagnostic tool, it must meet three criteria. It must be valid, reliable, and sensitive to change. While we use these terms very freely in everyday conversation, they have very specific meanings in the context of testing theory.

Let's begin with validity. As one of my students put it, "Validity means the test measures what it's supposed to measure." Now let's get a bit more precise. The first distinction we should make is between external validity and internal validity. External validity is the extent to which the norms developed for a test can be applied to a specific population. The tests presented in table 2.1 were developed using older people as subjects and are therefore valid for older clients. And what should make you feel even more confident about using these tests is that the norms are presented in five-year increments and by gender, which means you can expect valid results that can target your individual clients.

Internal validity has a number of subtypes, including face validity, content validity, predictive validity, concurrent validity, convergent validity, and discriminant validity (see table 2.3 for definitions). If you examine each term, you'll see that each fits my student's definition. They all ask the question, "Does the test actually measure what it's supposed to measure?"

Reliability is an equally important property for a test. A test is reliable if the results are repeatable or consistent. Think about it: If a test doesn't give you consistent results, how can you use it to compare your clients' performances to the norms or to check clients' progress? To ensure the reliability of your testing, you must adhere strictly to the testing techniques described in each chapter. And if you have helpers, they must perform the test exactly as you do. In the lab we call this *intertester reliability*.

The final quality that a test must have is sensitivity. The test must be able to detect the changes in the factor being measured. These changes may be due to something as potent as training or injury or as subtle as the aging process.

In addition to these academic markers of testing efficacy, I like to add my own more practical model of effectiveness, which is what I call my *testing triangle* (see figure 2.2). For a test to be valid, changes in ADL or IADL performance should cause related changes in the test result. If a person shows a reduction in an ADL or IADL performance factor, the test must be sensitive and specific to that change. Changes in test performance will indicate changes in performance in daily life. Finally, we must understand what physiological changes affect the ADL or IADL and test performances or we will not know what to target with our training prescription. This final element of the controlling physiological factor is

Table 2.3   Types of Validity

Type of validity	Definition
Face	The test is valid at face value. It obviously measures what it is intended to measure. For example, the 15-foot (4.6 m) walk test obviously measures how fast the client can walk 15 feet (4.6 m).
Content	The test does an effective and thorough job of measuring all the important information associated with the performance variable being measured.
Predictive	The test has the capacity to predict or forecast future performance.
Concurrent	The test shows the same results as other gold standard tests administered at the same time. Its ability to measure a specific trait is agreed upon by a group of experts.
Convergent	The test provides similar results to other tests that should provide similar results.
Discriminant	The test has the capacity to examine the differences between the factor it is measuring and other factors.

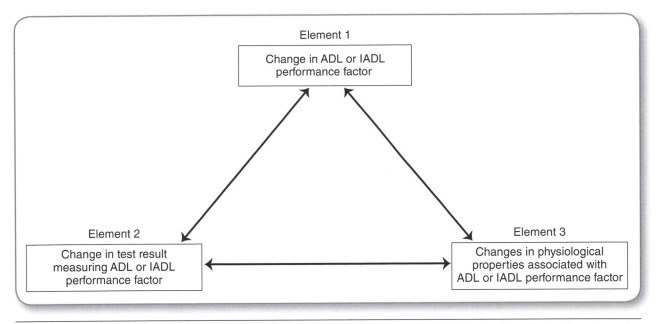

Figure 2.2 The testing triangle shows the connections among ADL or IADL performance, physiological factors, and testing necessary for an effective diagnostic test.

perhaps the most difficult element to isolate, and yet it is the most important component for ensuring an effective link between exercise diagnosis and exercise prescription. The difficulty arises from the fact that more than one factor is almost always associated with performing an ADL. Just like a diamond, an ADL takes more than one facet to make it shine. For example, getting up out of a chair clearly depends on lower-body strength and power, but balance, core strength, upper-body flexibility, and the correct neural firing patterns also contribute to rising successfully from a chair. Once you establish the link between the test and the controlling physiological factors, you can be fairly confident that the intervention you design will improve your client's functional performance.

APPLICATION POINT Performing a test incorrectly leads to false results and bad conclusions, something researchers like to call *garbage in, garbage out.* If you are going to take the time to do testing (and you should), take the time to do it right.

WHEN TO TEST

Now that I have discussed why you should test your clients and what makes a good test, there are still several questions that need to be answered.

These include the following:

- How do I design a testing calendar?
- How do I decide when to test?
- Do I repeat the test at the same time interval regardless of the training protocol and the fitness or wellness level of my client?

The answer to the first question hangs on two words: *when* and *why*. To write a prescription, you need a preliminary test. This test reveals the physiological factors that the exercise prescription should target. To explain the necessity of the preliminary test (or any subsequent test, for that matter), I would like to present my famous mall analogy:

I begin with the question, "When you go to a new mall, how do you find the store you're looking for?"

The answer that I always receive is, "I look at the directory."

The follow-up I ask is, "And what's on the directory?"

"A map."

"And what's on the map?"

"Oh, the positions of all the stores, with numbers so you know which store is which."

"And what else?"

"Sometimes different colors that tell you the type of each store or the wing of the mall each store is in."

"And what else?"

Usually at this point there is a protracted pause while the brain's search engine links to the visual memories of the mall directory. Then the answer comes hurling through the stagnating air to rescue the discussion: "There's the dot! You are here!"

And that is the point of the entire analogy: No matter how beautiful, colorful, or detailed the map, it's useless if it doesn't tell you where you are relative to all those stores! It's the same thing with providing your client with an exercise prescription. You don't know where to send her unless you know where she is. Testing is the "You are here!" that precedes training. Without knowing your starting location, you roam through the mall using pure chance as your GPS, hoping you'll run into the correct store.

Preliminary testing, however, is merely the beginning of the process. Throughout the training process your client is evolving, controlled by the conflicting influences of aging and training (see figure 2.3). At the same time the client is training, the client's body is also aging, and the two environments interact. Performance improvements, injuries, and illnesses all interact. Therefore, you must test the client periodically (more frequently at the beginning, when progress is fastest, and then at longer intervals as adaptations plateau) to evaluate progress and modify training according to changing functional status and fitness level.

You may ask why periodic retesting is necessary if you already understand the changes that should occur with your training prescription. There are sev-

eral reasons. The most obvious is to provide feedback to your client. I remember a number of years ago sitting in a lecture on exercise adherence and older persons. During the study being presented, the researcher had asked the question, "What do you find to be the most important quality in the caregiver providing exercise for you?" The answer was both simple and enlightening: "Don't just tell me what to do—tell me why I should do it!" A couple of years later my colleagues and I experienced this sentiment firsthand when we attempted to run a large-scale study incorporating diagnostic testing and exercise prescription. None of our subjects wanted to be tested. After a bit of convincing we managed to get the entire sample, with a few holdouts, through the initial testing. Then we sent the subjects, in a sort of menu-driven program, to the specific training modalities dictated by the primary and secondary needs that the testing battery had identified. After the first 8 weeks of training, we once again, a bit more easily this time, convinced our participants to be retested. It was at this point that we saw tangible proof of the effectiveness of providing feedback to a client. During the second wave of tests the participants noticed two things. First, they were showing improvements in nearly every test we gave them. But that wasn't the most important thing. The important thing was that the majority of them saw the greatest improvements in the performance variables we had targeted with our training—those very variables that our testing had indicated were the most important to train. This made a considerable impression on our participants, since they began to realize we could actually identify their weaknesses and then target those weaknesses with our exercise interventions. The other thing that made an impression was when we compared their values with the norms for indi-

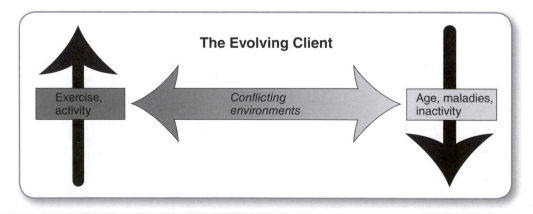

Figure 2.3 A client's performance depends on the conflicting effects of aging and training.

viduals within their gender and age groups. Many of them had reached the highest level possible (90th percentile) for their age group and were asking what the next step was. We explained that if they were 82, for example, and were being compared with norms for 80- to 84-year-olds, we were now going after the norms for 75- to 79-year-olds. It didn't take long for the word to spread that they were getting younger, especially in the specific factors we were targeting with our training. Of course we were not changing their chronological ages; rather, we were changing (lowering) what they perceived as their functional ages. This was a very pleasant realization and one that had a positive effect on the participants' desire to continue with the program.

The second reason for repeated testing is best explained by my analogy of tasting the sauce. As you can no doubt tell by my name, I am of Italian descent, and I've been told I make a pretty good tomato sauce. It typically takes me about 8 hours to complete this feat, since I start from scratch and simmer the sauce slowly for hours. During this simmering process, I constantly taste the sauce and add a bit of this and a bit of that so that the final product tastes as expected. You might ask, "Why is this necessary—don't you have a recipe?" Well, yes, there is a recipe float-ing around somewhere in the deep recesses of my mind, but there is a problem with always follow-ing the recipe: When I first add my ingredients, I never know how they may react with each other. Depending on the batch, the tomatoes may be riper or more acidic, the oregano may be stronger or weaker, the meat may be fatter or leaner, and the garlic may be milder or may have a bit more kick. So I cook and I taste and I modify until I get the desired result. What's the point of this cooking lesson? It's simple. I can guarantee that your clients have a much more complex genetic structure than a tomato or a garlic clove has. If, even after all these years, I can't predict how my sauce will come out without tasting it, how can any of us have the audacity to believe that we know the exact adaptation a client will make to an exercise prescription? We can't predict that outcome. I encourage you to taste the sauce.

Now let's switch from the why to the when. If testing is to provide a true picture of the improve-ments made by the client, it must be done after a taper period that provides the client with sufficient time to recover from the stresses of training. For this reason, I suggest you follow the pattern pre-sented in figure 2.4, which shows a high-intensity training period followed by a lower-intensity

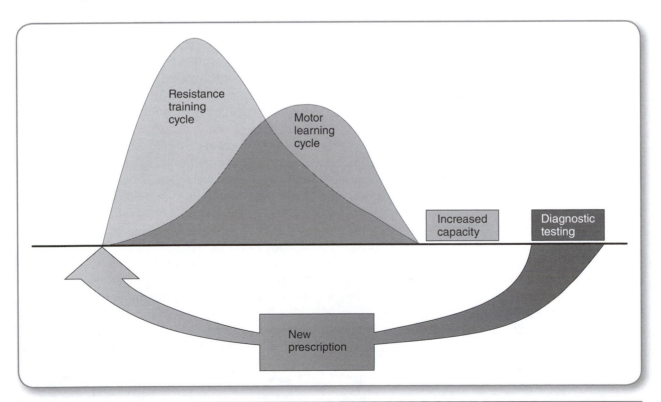

Figure 2.4 The training–testing sequence: Testing should follow the motor learning training period, when reduced intensity and frequency allow recovery and your client can be tested at his or her maximum level of training adaptation.

motor learning (translational) period and then diagnostic testing to determine the nature of the next training period. Without a recovery period, the testing results will be indicative of fatigue rather than training. Because a single targeted training cycle can have a duration of as few as 4 weeks and as many as 12 weeks, the time between diagnostic tests can vary accordingly. So don't worry about having regularly scheduled testing intervals. Additionally, as I mentioned earlier, the durations of your clients' training cycles and the degrees of change you see may vary considerably after a year or two of training. In this case you can spread the testing sessions further apart or even decide to run a number of training cycles without testing. If you do this, then be careful of two things. First, **never** skip over the motor learn-ing (what I call *translational cycle*) just because you are not going to test. Remember, recovery is a major tool for maximizing training. Second, don't get into the habit of ignoring diagnostic testing. Depending on your client's age, level of activity, intervening illnesses, and a plethora of other factors, you have to have a grasp on the client's evolving needs.

> **APPLICATION POINT**   Testing a client without first providing a recovery period produces artificially low results, especially in the performance factors targeted during the training cycle.

TESTING ACTIVITIES OF DAILY LIVING

In addition to measuring physical capacity, you may also wish to evaluate your client's ability to perform ADLs. The tests you can use for ADL evaluation include the seven-item and nine-item Physical Performance Tests (the PPT-7 and PPT-9, respectively) and the 10-item and 16-item Contin-uous-Scale Physical Functional Performance Tests (the CS-PFP-10 and CS-PFP-16, respectively). The PPT-7 includes writing a sentence, pretending to eat, turning 360°, putting on and removing a jacket, lifting a book and putting it on a shelf, picking up a penny from the floor, and walking 50 feet (15.2 m). To this the PPT-9 adds climbing stairs, which is scored as two items. The PPT takes an average of 10 minutes to complete and requires a pen and paper, a number of jackets of

varying sizes, a penny, a book, shelves, a table, chairs, stairs, and a place setting.

The CS-PFP-16 includes carrying a pot of water 3.3 feet (1 m), pouring water from a jug into a cup, putting on and taking off a jacket, placing a sponge on a high shelf and then retrieving it, sweeping the floor with a broom and dustpan, transferring clothes from a washer to a dryer and then to a basket, opening and closing a fire door, making a bed, vacuuming, placing a strap over a shoe, picking up scarves from the floor, carrying a bag up and down the stairs to a simulated bus stop, sitting on the floor and standing up again, climbing stairs, carrying groceries, and walking 6 minutes. Of these tasks, the CS-PFP-10 eliminates pouring water, opening and closing the fire door, making a bed, vacuuming, strapping on a shoe, and carrying groceries.

In addition to these testing batteries, there are a number of questionnaires that have been shown to predict ADL performance accurately. The Functional Status Questionnaire uses 48 ques-tions to evaluate your clients' functional status and incorporates eight general questions concern-ing ADL performance. Since it is a seven-page questionnaire and is not specifically designed to assess ADL performance, it may not be your most effective or efficient choice. The Rosow-Breslau Functional Health Scale measures three aspects of mobility: walking up and down a flight of stairs, walking half a mile (0.8 km), and doing heavy housework. The Lawton IADL Scale contains nine items that are scored from 0 (low function) to 8 (high function). This test takes 10 to 15 minutes to administer and evaluates a mix of physical and cognitive functions. The Modified Katz ADL Scale measures your client's ability to perform, without assistance, six basic ADLs. The Nagi Scale evalu-ates a client's difficulty in performing five activi-ties, including stooping, handling small objects, sitting or standing for prolonged durations, and carrying or lifting weights greater than 10 pounds (4.5 kg). All of these tests can be found on the Internet or in their original sources, which are listed in the topical bibliography.

While these questionnaires can evaluate a client's ADL capacity, they provide no assess-ment of the physiological variables that control specific ADL performances. Therefore, they are not substitutes for the diagnostic testing battery described in this chapter. The bottom line is that the individual tests presented in each chapter of this book are still the keystones for prescribing the highest quality of training to your clients.

SUMMARY

An effective and efficient exercise prescription hinges on an accurate exercise diagnosis of a client's needs. The tests presented in the following chapters of this book are included in my testing battery so that you can use them to quantify the decline observed in each of the facets of your client's successful aging diamond. When you use these tests at the onset of training, they provide an exercise diagnosis on which you can base your client's training prescription. When you administer these tests at the end of a training cycle, you can assess the changes that have occurred during that cycle and then modify your client's prescription so that you can polish all the facets of their diamond.

Topical Bibliography

The Exercise Diagnosis and Prescription Model

Weber, H. (2001). A perspective on exercise prescription. *J Exerc Physiol Online* 4:1-5.

The Exercise Diagnosis: Analysis of Needs

Alexander, N.B., & Goldberg, A. (2006). Clinical gait and stepping performance measures in older adults. *Eur Rev Aging Phys Act* 3:20-28.

Bassey, E.J., Fiatarone, M.A., O'Neill, E.F., Kelly, M., Evans, W.J., & Lipsitz, L.A. (1992). Leg extension power and functional performance in very old men and women. *Clinical Science* 82:321-327.

Booth, F.W., Weeden, S.H., & Tsend, B.S. (1994). Effect of aging on human skeletal muscle and motor function. *Medicine and Science in Sports and Exercise* 26:556-560.

Clarke, D.H., & Quint, M.Q. (1992). Muscular strength and endurance as a function of age and activity level. *Research Quarterly for Exercise and Sport* 63:302-310.

Evans, W.J. (1997). Functional and metabolic consequences of sarcopenia. *J Nutr* 127:998S-1003S.

Fleg, J.L., Morrell, C.H., Bos, A.G., Brant, L.J., Talbot, L.A., Wright, J.G., & Lakatta, E.G. (2005). Accelerated longitudinal decline of aerobic capacity in healthy older adults. *Circulation* 112:674-682.

Foldvari, M., Clark, M., Laviolette, L.C., Bernstein, M.A., Kaliton, D., Castaneda, C., Pu, C.T., Hausdorff, J.M., Fielding, R.A., & Singh, M.A. (2000). Association of muscle power with functional status in community-dwelling elderly women. *J Gerontol A Biol Sci Med Sci* 55(4): M192-M199.

Going, S.B., Williams, D.S., Lohman, T.G., & Hewitt, M.J. (1994). Aging, body composition, and physical activity: A review. *Journal of Aging and Physical Activity* 2:38-66.

Helbostad, J.L., & Moe-Nilssen, R. (2003). The effect of gait speed on lateral balance control during walking in healthy elderly. *Gait and Posture* 18:27-36.

Holland, G.J., Tanaka, K., Shigematsu, R., & Nakagaichi, M. (2002). Flexibility and physical functions of older adults: A review. *J Aging Phys Act* 10:169-206.

Hortobagyi, T., Zheng, D., Weidner, M., Lambert, N.J., Westbrook, S., & Houmard, J.A. (1995). The influence of aging on muscle strength and muscle fiber characteristics with special reference to eccentric strength. *Journal of Gerontology* 50A: B399-B406.

Izquierdo, M., Ibañez, J., Gorostiaga, E., Garrues, M,, Zúñiga, A., Antón, A., Larrión, J.L., Häkkinen, K. (1999) *Acta Physiol Scand.* 167:57-68.

King, M.B., Judge, J.O., & Wolfson, L. (1994). Functional base of support decreases with age. *J Gerontol A Biol Sci Med Sci* 49:M258-M263.

Kozak, K., Ashton-Miller, J.A., & Alexander, N.B. (2003). The effect of age and movement speed on maximum forward reach from an elevated surface: A study in healthy women. *Clinical Biomechanics* 18:190-196.

Liu-Ambrose, T., Khan, K.M., Eng, J.J., Janssen, P.A., Lord, S.R., & McKay, H.A. (2004). Resistance and agility training reduce fall risk in women aged 75 to 85 with low bone mass: A 6- month randomized, controlled trial. *JAGS* 52:657-665.

Mathias, S., Nayak, U.S.L., & Isaacs, B. (1986). Balance in elderly patients: The "get-up and go" test. *Arch Phys Med Rehabil* 67:387-389.

Mazariegos, M., Heymsfield, S.B., Wang, Z.M., Wang, J., Yasumura, S., Dilmanian, F.A., & Pierson, R.N. (1993). Aging affects body composition: young versus elderly women pair-matched by body mass index. In Ellis, K.J., & Eastman, J.D. (Eds.), *Human Body Composition* (pp. 245-249). New York: Plenum Press.

Pendergast, D.R., Fisher, N.M., & Calkins, E. (1993). Cardiovascular, neuromuscular, and metabolic alterations with age leading to frailty. *Journal of Gerontology* 48:61-67.

Schwendner, K.I., Mikeshy, A.E., Holt, W.S., Peacock, M., & Burr, D.B. (1997). Differences in muscle endurance and recovery between fallers and non-fallers, and between young and older women. *Journal of Gerontology: Medical Sciences* 52:M155-M160.

Skelton, D.A., Greig, C.A., Davies, J.M., & Young, A. (1994). Strength, power and related functional ability of healthy people aged 65-89 years. *Age and Ageing* 23:371-377.

Teasdale, N., Stelmach, G.E., & Breung, A. (1991). Postural sway characteristics of the elderly under normal and altered visual and support surfaces. *J Gerontol* 46:B238-B244.

What Makes an Effective Test?

American College of Sports Medicine. (1998). *ACSM's resource manual for guidelines for exercise testing and prescription* (3rd ed.). Baltimore: Williams & Wilkins.

Graham, J. (1994). Guidelines for providing valid testing of athletes' fitness levels. *Strength and Conditioning* December: 7-14.

Green, J., Forster, A., & Young, J. (2002). Reliability of gait speed measured by a timed walking test in patients one year after stroke. *Clin Rehabil* 16:306-314.

Jacob, G.M., & Palmer, R.M. (1998). Tools for assessing focuses on improving quality of life. *Postgrad Med* 104:135-153.

Jones, C.J., Rikli, R.E., Max, J., & Noffal, G. (1998). The reliability and validity of a chair sit-and-reach test as a measure of hamstring

flexibility in older adults. *Res Quar Exerc Sport* 69:338-344.

MacDougall, D., Wenger, H.A., & Green, H.J (1993). *Physiological testing of the high performance athlete.* Champaign, IL: Human Kinetics.

Resnick, B., & Nigg, C. (2003). Testing a theoretical model of exercise behavior for older adults. *Nursing Research* 52:80-88.

Rodgers, M.M., & Cavanagh, P.R. (1984). Glossary of biomechanical terms, concepts, and units. *Physical Therapy* 64:1886-1902.

Rossier, P., & Wade, D.T. (2001). Validity and reliability comparison of 4 mobility measures in patients presenting with neurologic impairment. *Arch Phys Med Rehabil* 82:9-13.

Rubin, S. (1987). *The principles of biomedical instrumentation.* Chicago: Yearbook Medical.

Van Genderen, F.R., De Bie, R.A., Helders, P.J.M., & Van Meeteren, N.L.U. (2003). Reliability research: Towards a more clinically relevant approach. *Phys Ther Rev* 8:169-176.

When to Test

Gibala, M., MacDougall, J.D., & Sale, D.G. (1994). The effects of tapering on strength performance in trained athletes. *Int J Sports Med* 15:492-497.

Testing Activities of Daily Living

Cress, M.E., Petrella, J.K., Moore, T.L., & Schenkman, M.L. (2005). Continuous-scale physical functional performance test: Validity, reliability, and sensitivity of data for the short version. *Phys Ther* 85:323-335.

Cress, M.E., Buchner, D.M., Questad, K.A., Esselman, P.C., deLateur, B.J., & Schwartz, R.S. (1996). Continuous-scale physical functional performance in healthy older adults: A validation study. *Archives of Physical Medicine and Rehabilitation* 77:1243-1250.

Jette, A.M., Davies, A.R., Cleary, P.D., Calkins, D.R., Rubenstein, L.V., Fink, A., Kosecoff, J., Young, R.T., Brook, R.H., & Delbanco T.L. (1986). The functional status questionnaire: reliability and validity when used in primary care. *J Gen Intern Med* 1(3):143-149.

Katz, S. (1983). Assessing self-maintenance: Activities of daily living, mobility, and instrumental activities of daily living. *Journal of the American Geriatrics Society* 231:721-727.

Lawton, M.P., & Brody, E.M. (1969). Assessment of older people: Self-maintaining and instrumental activities of daily living. *Gerontologist* 9:179-186.

Reuben, D.B., & Siu, A.L. (1990). An objective measure of physical function of elderly outpatients. The Physical Performance Test. *J Am Geriatr Soc* 38:1105-1112.

Rosow, I., Breslau, N., & Guttman, A. (1966). A health scale for the aged. *J Gerontol* 21:556-559.

References

Weber, H. (2001). A perspective on exercise prescription. *J Exerc Physiol Online* 4:1-5.

Training Principles

For centuries people have been studying how the human body adapts to different types, volumes, and intensities of exercise. The combined efforts of trainers, clinicians, and scientists have allowed us to formulate accepted training principles on which we can base our exercise prescriptions. Knowing these principles will allow you to provide exacting interventions to address the health and performance deficits of your older client.

OVERLOAD AND ADAPTATION

Let's begin with one of the pillars on which exercise training programs are built. For training to change the structure and function of the human body, it must provide a stress level over and above the client's normal daily activity level. This concept is called the *overload principle.* When the systems of the client's body face this *overload stress,* they receive the signal to change. The change that occurs is called an *adaptation,* since the body is reacting to the overload stimulus (see figure 3.1). This is a sort of minievolution in

which the change in the body's internal environment causes it to restructure itself.

I would like to make a distinction between exercise and training. Exercise is an event or a tool. Every time your clients exercise, they disrupt the internal environment of the body. This environment was first described by the French physiologist Claude Bernard in the mid-1800s. He called it the *milieu intérieur* (Noble, 2008). Toward the end of the 19th century biologists and other scientists began to apply Bernard's principle to the feedback mechanisms of the human body. They recognized that these mechanisms maintain the body's internal environment (remember homeostasis) through the upregulation and downregulation of different systems. They also recognized that the body is capable of self-engineering. That is, the body can sense the upregulation and downregulation of its systems and restructure them so they are better able to deal with the specific overloads applied. When you exercise, you disrupt your internal environment, and all the systems of the body spring into action to deal with the insult. We call this an *acute* or *immediate response* to exercise. Those of us who exercise are familiar with this response. Let's say you're going for a run. As you

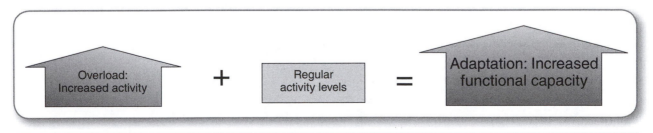

Figure 3.1   A model for increasing functional capacity by increasing activity (overload).

run, there are several changes that you experience. Your heart rate and breathing increase as your body deals with the need to take in and distribute more oxygen to support the increased workload. You sweat to deal with the excess heat you produce during exercise. Your skin becomes flushed as blood flow increases for greater cooling. These are all changes that you feel and recognize as the body acutely responds to the stress of exercise and attempts to stabilize its internal environment (see table 3.1). Regardless of your fitness level, these responses always occur.

Exercise that is applied in a repetitive, organized plan with a specific target in mind is called *training.* You can think of your client's body as a very intelligent machine. If it is forced to deal with the same disruption on a regular basis, it restructures itself. In fact, training can be defined as exercise that tells your DNA how to reengineer your body so it can deal more easily with the stresses being applied. This reengineering is called a *chronic* or *training response* to exercise. Let's return to our running example. The chronic changes induced by regular running are a reduction in heart rate at any level of exercise, a reduced energy requirement for breathing, an enhanced oxygen-carrying capacity, and an increased blood volume for improved cooling capacity (Plowman & Smith, 1996; see table 3.1). In addition, remember that when the body becomes more effective at dealing with exercise, it also becomes more effective at performing the activities necessary for daily life.

APPLICATION POINT   Although you need to provide sufficient overload to cause a training effect in your clients, you also need to cycle that training (as you will soon learn) so that your clients have sufficient time to recover and their bodies have time to restructure.

EXERCISE SPECIFICITY

Since training is the body reengineering itself in response to an exercise stimulus, you can dictate the changes you want by varying the exercise program you provide. Exercise scientists and practitioners have a very descriptive term for this stimulus–response scenario: *exercise specificity.* Exercise specificity provides the foundation for exercise prescription. Since different modes of exercise promote different changes in the body's structure and function, the exercise that is prescribed must match the diagnosed need if the prescription is to be effective. This need for proper diagnosis is the basis of the exercise diagnosis and prescription model presented in chapter 2.

Exercise specificity takes a number of forms. Table 3.2 lists the factors associated with the two major types of specificity: bioenergetic and biomechanical. These two types of specificity work in concert so that the exercise prescription you provide can effectively address the functional

Table 3.1 Acute (Immediate) and Long-Term (Training) Responses to Running

Single run (exercise)	Multiple organized runs (training)
Increased heart rate	Lower heart rate at similar exercise levels • Increased cardiac muscle contractile force • Increased capacity of the heart chambers to hold blood volume • Increased parasympathetic neural messages (signals to slow down) sent to the heart's pacemaker (sinoatrial node)
Increased breathing rate	Lower breathing rate at similar exercise levels • More efficient respiratory muscles • Better oxygen transfer from lungs to blood • Better capacity of the blood to carry oxygen
Increased sweat production	Increased sweat production • Higher blood volume • Reset of body's thermostat

Table 3.2 Bioenergetic and Biomechanical Variables Responding to Training

Bioenergetic specificity	Biomechanical specificity
Enzyme structure, concentration, and distribution	Specific muscles and muscle groups
Organelle structure, concentration, and distribution	Specific joints
Fiber type	Specific joint angles and related muscle lengths
Electrochemical systems	Specific movement speeds
Hypertrophy and hyperplasia	Specific loads
Hormones	Specific contractile states
	Specific motor patterns

needs that dictate the level of independence and the likelihood of falls in your client.

APPLICATION POINT Training specificity is the cornerstone of any prescription program. Once you have diagnosed your client's needs, you must apply the training that targets those needs or the diagnostic process will be meaningless.

Bioenergetic Specificity

In order to maintain itself, the human body must have energy. The immediate source of this energy is a molecule called *adenosine triphosphate*—or, for those of us who have limited time and like acronyms—*ATP*. ATP releases energy when the body breaks it down to ADP (adenosine diphosphate, which has two phosphates instead of three phosphates). Then the body uses the energy it receives from all the other fuels it breaks down to stick the third phosphate back onto the ADP and resynthesize the ATP (see figure 3.2). This process would be simple if it were not for the facts that

- we can increase our level of energy expenditure by nearly 700% during maximal exercise, and
- we continuously change our energy needs to meet the changing energy demands of daily living.

For this reason the human body has developed a number of different systems that can produce

energy and resynthesize ATP at different rates to meet the body's demands. These energy systems work in a continuum, with the rate of energy demand or metabolic power dictating their proportional use. The systems, in the order of their metabolic power (rate of energy production), are the creatine phosphate system (most powerful), anaerobic glycolysis, aerobic glycolysis, and the oxidative breakdown of fat, often called *beta-oxidation* (see figure 3.3).

These systems are all controlled by their own set of helper molecules called *enzymes*. Enzymes allow the energy systems to function at the speeds and levels of activity necessary to meet the body's energy demands, whatever they might be. When you train your client in a specific way, you can increase the activity, as well as the concentration, of certain enzymes. This in turn makes your client's body better at performing one type of exercise. An obvious example of how specific training improves specific types of exercise is comparing sprinters with long-distance runners. Sprinters do the majority of their training at high speeds. This means that they are stressing the faster, more anaerobic systems during training. Therefore, the activities and concentrations of the enzymes controlling these systems are increased in sprinters. In contrast, the marathoners, who predominantly train at slower velocities for longer durations, slide to the more aerobic end of the energy continuum during training. This means that the enzymes controlling aerobic glycolysis and beta-oxidation show the greatest degree of change in long-distance runners. If you apply this concept when training

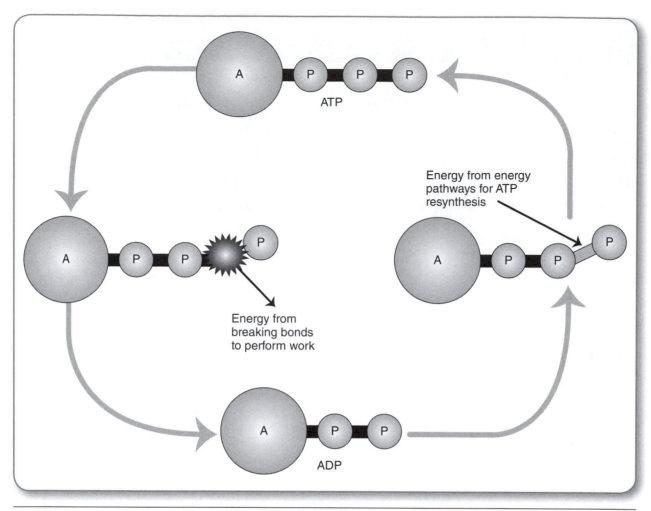

Figure 3.2 The breakdown and resynthesis of ATP.

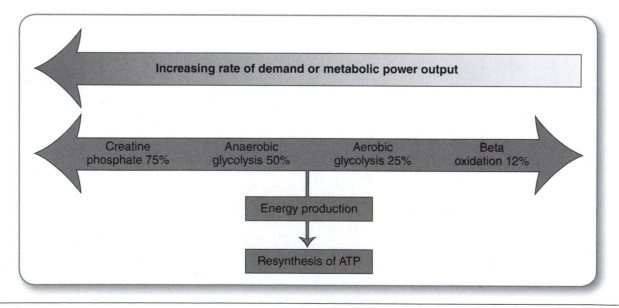

Figure 3.3 Energy systems and metabolic power. Percentages show approximate levels at which the systems can replenish ATP at maximal rate of utilization.

your client, you can target the specific metabolic needs that address the client's declines due to reduced activity levels or the aging process itself (Poehlman, 1992).

For example, we know that muscle size decreases with aging. We also know that this reduction is to a large degree the result of the loss of fast-twitch muscle fibers. Therefore, you might expect your older clients to show decrements in strength, speed, and power. If this diagnosis is confirmed by low normative scores on the 30-second chair stand, modified ramp power test, and gait speed test, your training prescription should contain exercise protocols that concentrate on the anaerobic systems. In contrast, if these tests show moderate normative scores while the 6-minute walk test shows low performance values, your prescription should lean toward improving the aerobic systems. As you read part II of this book, you will notice that the specific training interventions lean toward greater utilization of one energy system over another.

> **APPLICATION POINT** All exercise prescriptions are a mix of aerobic and anaerobic work. Your training program may favor one system over another, but there is no such thing as purely aerobic or anaerobic exercise.

Biomechanical Specificity

Although the principle of biomechanical specificity may be more tangible, and therefore easier to grasp, than bioenergetic specificity is, its complex nature requires far greater explanation. *Muscle, muscle group,* and *joint specificity* may seem like terms for bodybuilders, since they are commonly used in popular fitness and bodybuilding magazines. However, the concept of targeting specific muscles should go well beyond developing bulging biceps. For those of us interested in improving or maintaining the quality of life of our older clients, biomechanical specificity should be directed toward the muscles and muscle utilization patterns associated with increasing ADL performance and reducing fall probability. For years, physical therapists, physiatrists, and exercise scientists have been evaluating muscle-specific and joint-specific weaknesses and prescribing exercises to counteract them. This book expands

the practice of prescribing exercise from its limited clinical and rehabilitation application to one that encompasses preventing and counteracting the declines in the general aging population (which, by the way, is all of us).

Muscle specificity and joint angle specificity are important to our discussion of bending the aging curves for a number of reasons. The most obvious reason comes to light during flexibility training. Due to age-related changes in connective tissue (noted in chapter 1), joint ROMs decrease with age. This reduction can limit the range over which your clients can apply force and speed and therefore can limit their ability to produce power. It can also reduce their strength within certain ROMs, making specific daily tasks either difficult or impossible to perform. In addition, changes in ROM due to the age-associated exponential declines in the elasticity and compliance of connective tissue have an even more practical implication. Think about performing different ADLs such as making dinner, washing clothes, or mowing the lawn and consider the different muscle patterns utilized during each activity. If you wish to maximize your client's ability to perform these activities, you must target not only the specific muscles involved in each activity but also the specific sequences in which the muscles are used (Voight & Cook, 1996). For example, a skill as common as sweeping the floor uses your muscles in a set pattern. If you vary that pattern your sweeping won't go very well (see figure 3.4). To allow you to train your clients to "translate" their physical improvements into movement patterns that will help in their daily lives, I have included exercises that target functional muscle groups in chapter 7 and exercises that target patterns of use in chapter 10.

> **APPLICATION POINT** To give your client the most bang for the exercise buck, you must not only target the correct muscle groups but also translate increases in strength, power, and muscular endurance into movement patterns that are used in the client's daily activities and strategies for fall recovery.

Two additional biomechanical factors to consider when prescribing exercises are speed specificity and load specificity. The theory of speed specificity

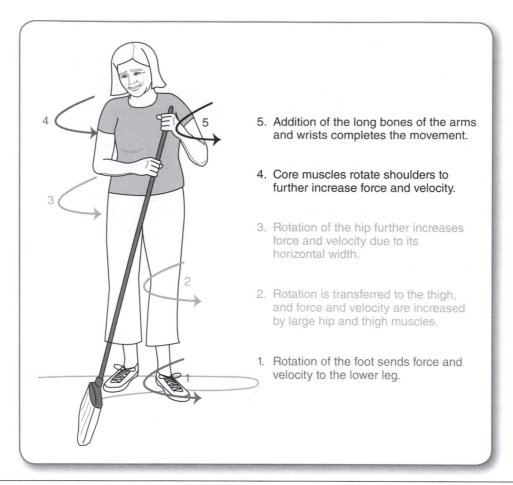

5. Addition of the long bones of the arms and wrists completes the movement.

4. Core muscles rotate shoulders to further increase force and velocity.

3. Rotation of the hip further increases force and velocity due to its horizontal width.

2. Rotation is transferred to the thigh, and force and velocity are increased by large hip and thigh muscles.

1. Rotation of the foot sends force and velocity to the lower leg.

Figure 3.4 The application of movement pattern training to sweeping the floor. Instead of performing this skill in the pattern shown, try 2, 3, 1, 4, 5 or 4, 3, 2, 1, 5 and see how well your sweeping goes.

states that performance improvements are greatest at the speed at which the training is applied (Behm & Sale, 1993). This theory is supported by scientific studies as well as practical application, although the results are at times confounded by differences in training speeds, loads, equipment, and testing methods. For your purposes as a trainer working with older individuals, speed specificity is a vital topic for a number of reasons. As I mentioned earlier, bioenergetic specificity and biomechanical specificity often overlap. Nowhere is this more clearly demonstrated than in speed specificity. Working at higher speeds not only increases your client's speed and power but also increases your client's capacity to generate anaerobic power. In chapters 6, 7, and 8 we'll see the importance of movement speed and anaerobic power in preventing falls and making daily activities easier to perform.

Load specificity is an important principle in resistance training since different loads can be used for selective improvement in muscle size, power, strength, and endurance (Campos et al., 2002). However, load specificity has implications that go well beyond targeting these characteristics. As we will see in chapter 7, the rate at which a muscle contracts during power training is dictated by the load it must move. Obviously the lighter the load, the faster it can be moved. Since power is the product of the load that is moved and the velocity at which the load is moved, maximizing power during training requires the use of a specific load called an *optimal load* (de Vos et al., 2005). However, certain exercises, due to the anatomical structures of the joints and muscles they target, require very different loads in order to maximize their power increases (Mow et al., 2008). Additionally, recent research has shown that different ADLs have different loads and movement speeds associated with their performance. Therefore it is best to modify training loads to match the specific ADLs you wish to improve.

Load can also be used to affect the proportional use of the different energy systems. Consider resistance training, in which using light loads with high repetitions targets aerobic metabolism, while lifting heavy loads at moderate to high speeds targets anaerobic systems.

APPLICATION POINT Changing the loading patterns during training can be quite complex since changes are affected by the client's specific needs, the physical performance factor you are targeting, and the client's position within the training cycle. By the time you finish reading this book, you will know how to work all of these factors to maximize your client's gains.

The last two factors associated with biomechanical specificity are contractile specificity and movement pattern specificity. The type of muscle contraction that is used to perform a task is termed *contractile specificity.* The two most common muscle contractions associated with daily activities are isometric and isoinertial contractions (also called *dynamic constant load* and *isotonic contractions,* respectively). The term *isometric* is taken from the Greek roots *iso,* meaning "the same," and *metric,* meaning "length." This means that the muscle is producing force without changing length (e.g., gripping a coffee mug). *Isoinertial* means "the same load." This indicates that the muscle is moving an object of a certain weight through a specific ROM. Most daily activities incorporate both types of muscle contraction. For example, when you remove a gallon of milk from the refrigerator, you use isometric contractions of the hand and finger muscles to grip the handle

and isoinertial contractions of the arm and trunk muscles to move the jug. Therefore, the exercises prescribed to improve ADL performance should incorporate both of these actions.

The last principle of biomechanical specificity is movement pattern specificity. Although this principle is often ignored, it is one of the most important in training prescription. Physical performance factors such as strength and cardiovascular endurance do not translate directly into improved ADL performance. In the final chapter of this book, I present evidence that we can improve the transfer from overload-based training to ADL performance by using drills and games that incorporate motor patterns (patterns of movement) similar to those used in the ADLs we are attempting to improve. Motor pattern specificity is supported by scientific studies that show that using exercises that simulate daily activities results in increases superior to those produced by training designed to simply improve physical performance variables (de Vreede et al., 2005). If you stop to think about it, coaches have recognized this principle for years. It's the reason why their athletes spend more time on the field or court than they do in the weight room.

SUMMARY

By applying the principles of overload, adaptation, and specificity, including bioenergetic and biomechanical specificity, you can design effective, individualized exercise interventions for your clients. The principles presented in this chapter are used throughout this text for designing prescriptions to address specific ADL, balance, or mobility deficits affecting the daily performance of older clients. It is the use of these principles that separates exercise from exercise prescription.

Topical Bibliography

Biomechanical Specificity

Panariello, R.A. (1991). The closed kinetic chain in strength training. *NSCA Journal* 13:29-33

Exercise Specificity

Hewson, D.J., & Hopkins, W.G. (1996). Specificity of training and its relation to the performance of distance runners. *International Journal of Sports Medicine* 17:199-204.

Izquierdo, M., Hakkinen, K., Gonzalez-Badillo, J.J., Ibanez, J., & Gorostiaga, E.M. (2002). Effects of long-term training specificity on maximal strength and power of the upper and lower extremities in athletes from different sports. *European Journal of Applied Physiology* 87:264-271.

McCafferty, W.B., Horvath, S.M. (1977). Specificity of exercise and specificity of training: a subcellular review. *Res Q* 48:358-371.

Morrissey, M.C., Harman, E.A., & Johnson, M.J. (1995). Resistance training modes: Specificity and effectiveness. *Medicine and Science in Sports and Exercise* 27:648-660.

Pereira, M.I.R., & Gomes, P.S.C. (2003). Movement velocity in resistance training. *Sports Med* 33:427-438.

Overload and Adaptation

Fox, E.L., Bowers, R.W., & Foss M.L. (1989). *The Physiological Basis of Physical Education and Athletics*. Dubuque, Iowa: William C. Brown Publishers.

References

Behm, D.G. & Sale, D.G. (1993). Velocity specificity of resistance training. *Sports Med* 15:374-388.

Campos, G.E., Luecke, T.J., Wendeln, H.K., Toma, K., Hagerman, F.C., Murray, T.F., Ragg, K.E., Ratamess, N.A., Krarmer, W.J., & Staron, R.S. (2002). Muscular adaptations in response to three different resistance-training regimens: specificity of repetition maximum training zones. *Eur J Appl Physiol* 88:50-60.

de Vos, N.J., Singh, N.A., Ross, D.A., Stavrinos, T.M., Orr, R., Fiatarone Singh, M.A. (2005). Optimal load for increasing muscle power during explosive resistance training in older adults. *J Gerontol A Biol Sci Med Sci* 60:638-647.

de Vreede, P.L., Samson, M.M., van Meeteren, N.L., Duursma, S.A., Verhaar, H.J. (2005). Functional-task exercise versus resistance strength exercise to improve daily function in older women: a randomized, controlled trial. *J Am Geriatr Soc* 53:2-10.

Mow, S., Roos, B.A., Serravite, D.H., and Signorile, J.F. (2008). Optimal loading for power in older men. *Medicine and Science in Sports and Exercise* 40(5): S472.

Noble, D. (2008). Claude Bernard, the first systems biologist, and the future of physiology. *Exp Physiol* 93:16-26.

Poehlman, E.T. (1992). Energy expenditure and requirements in aging humans. J Nutr 122:2057-2065.

Plowman, S.A., & Smith, D.L. (1996). *Exercise Physiology for Health, Fitness, and Performance*. Boston: Allyn & Bacon.

Voight, M.L., & Cook, G. (1996). Clinical application of closed kinetic chain exercise. *J Sport Rehab* 5:25-44.

Training Exercises: From Theory to Practice

If the vegetarians among us will excuse the analogy, part II is the meat and potatoes of the book. Each chapter addresses a distinct physical attribute and presents the importance of that attribute to your clients' independence and personal well-being. Each chapter also describes the diagnostic tests used in evaluating the physical attribute and the training tools that have been shown to be most effective at bending that specific aging curve. Part II takes the concept of an exercise-based diagnostic and prescription model and shows you how to apply it in your daily interactions with your older clients.

Body Composition

lthough most body tissues and systems decline with age, body fat unfortunately doesn't follow that same blueprint. Instead, body fat increases from the late teens to the 70s and then demonstrates a slight, albeit undesirable, decrease thereafter (see figure 4.1). The age-associated condition of having small muscles with high body fat is known as *sarcopenic obesity*. The most commonly reported consequences of increased body fat are metabolic syndrome and a higher probability of cardiovascular disease. However, combined sarcopenia and obesity present additional problems. Our muscles are the engines that allow us to move our bodies and maintain our balance. If our engines grow smaller and weaker while our bodies grow heavier, mobility and balance problems are the inevitable result. In his commentary on sarcopenic obesity, Ronenn Roubenoff of the Jean Mayer USDA Human Nutrition Research Center on Aging at Tufts University notes that "the 'fat frail' have the worst of both worlds as they age—increased weakness due to sarcopenia and a need to carry greater weight due to obesity" (2004, p. 887).

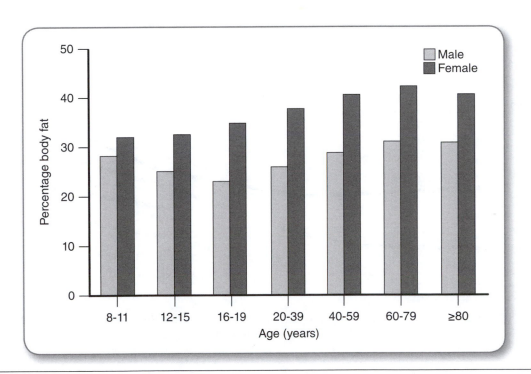

Figure 4.1 Mean percentage of body fat by age group and gender.

Based on data from CDC.

THE PREVALENCE OF OBESITY AND ITS CONSEQUENCES

So how prevalent is obesity among older persons? The increase in the incidence of overweight and obesity in the U.S. population reached a high enough level from the 1960s to 2004 to be called *epidemic*. Figure 4.2 shows that a similar exponential increase occurred for men and women aged 65 through 74 years. When the data are presented by U.S. state, the picture is no prettier. In 1995 the percentage of obese persons was less than 20% for every state in the union, but by 2005 every state except three showed an obesity level of 20% or more.

One of the most common methods for assessing obesity is body mass index (BMI), which is a person's ratio of weight (in kilograms) to height (in meters squared). Although this measurement has obvious limitations, since it does not distinguish between fat mass and FFM, it is nonetheless a good screening tool to evaluate population trends. It has been estimated that the number of persons older than 60 years with a BMI of more than 30 kg/m² increased from 14,600,000 (32%)

in 2000 to 20,900,000 (37.4%) in 2010 (Arterburn, Crane, & Sullivan, 2004). Additionally, statistics show that obesity among newly admitted nursing home residents rose from 15% in 1992 to more than 25% in 2002 (Lapane & Resnik, 2005).

Given these data, it should be no surprise that the American public shows an ever-increasing incidence of diabetes mellitus, hypertension, osteoarthritis, depression, and heart failure. Additionally, older Americans are requiring increasingly greater assistance to perform ADLs such as bathing, dressing, transferring, and making it to the bathroom.

APPLICATION POINT The loss of muscle mass and the increase in body weight commonly associated with aging reduce independence and increase the probability of falling among older individuals.

THE OBESITY PARADOX

Before we discuss the benefits of weight loss for older individuals, let's examine the so-called *obesity paradox*. Numerous studies and clinical observations have shown that elderly patients

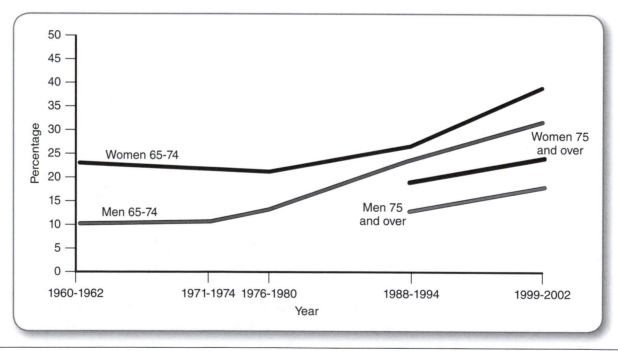

Figure 4.2   Percentage of people aged 65 and over who were obese from 1960 to 2002, arranged by gender and age group.

Based on data from Administration on Aging.

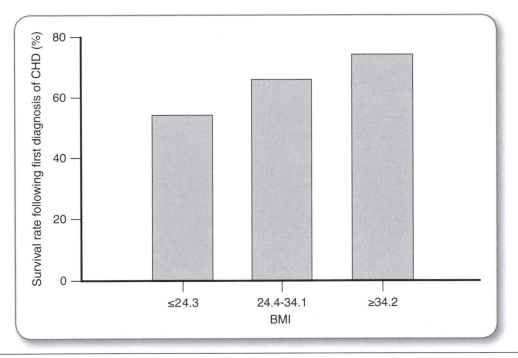

Figure 4.3   Relationship between body mass index and survival rates following the first diagnosis of congestive heart disease (CHD).

Data from Curtis et al. 2005.

who are overweight (BMI of 24.3-34.2 kg/m²) or obese (BMI of > 34.2 kg/m²) and have known heart failure have a reduced risk of mortality compared with underweight patients (BMI of < 24.3 kg/m²; see figure 4.3). But before we get too excited about the possibility of gaining weight to improve health, let's consider the issues that Shrinivas Habbu and colleagues have raised about these data. They pose the following questions about the results supporting the obesity paradox (Habbu, Lakkis, & Dokainish, 2006):

1. Was the clinical diagnosis of heart failure in obese patients accurate, or were the obese patients in these studies actually healthier than their nonobese counterparts?

2. Are the negative effects of muscle wasting, rather than the positive effects of obesity, the reason for the inverse relationship between BMI and mortality after heart failure?

3. What about the studies that have looked at severely obese populations (BMI of > 35 kg/m²) and suggested that severely obese patients may have worse outcomes than patients with normal weights or mild obesity?

Given these questions, Habbu and colleagues suggest that the relationship between mortality and obesity follows a U-shaped curve, where individuals with low (< 17.5 kg/m²) or high (> 35 kg/m²) BMI values are at greater risk for death, while individuals in the middle ranges are at less risk. However, research supporting the obesity paradox continues to emerge in the literature.

SARCOPENIC OBESITY AND ACTIVITIES OF DAILY LIVING

Given the increase in obesity between 2000 and 2010 and the decline in muscle mass that accompanies age, we can project a dramatic rise in sarcopenic obesity between now and 2020 as the baby boomers continue to age. This increase in body weight and decrease in muscle tissue will greatly increase the levels of disability in this population unless we as trainers intercede.

The substantial effect that sarcopenic obesity can have on independence is illustrated in figure 4.4. The figure compares perceived declines in the IADL performance of four different groups: a nonsarcopenic and nonobese group, a nonsarcopenic and obese group, a sarcopenic and nonobese group, and a sarcopenic and obese group. The IADLs include using the telephone, accessing transportation, getting groceries, making meals, doing housework, doing handyman work, doing laundry, taking medications, and managing money. As you can see from figure 4.4, the individuals with sarcopenic obesity were 2 to 3 times more likely to report losses in their IADL performance compared with lean persons with sarcopenia or obese persons without sarcopenia. In other words, it was the combined effects of sarcopenia and obesity that hindered independence. In fact, frail older persons with decrements in muscular endurance, walking speed, and grip strength can be easily identified by a combination of high fat mass, low muscle mass, and low muscle density. The take-home message is that greater fat mass combined with reduced muscle quality decreases quality of life in obese individuals with sarcope-

nia. But there is some good news. Physical activity can increase fitness and promote weight loss in middle age and may prevent mobility limitation and subsequent disability in old age. Additionally, the training techniques presented in this chapter can suppress and even reverse sarcopenic obesity in your older clients.

SARCOPENIC OBESITY AND FALL PROBABILITY

While there is limited information concerning falls and sarcopenic obesity, there is anecdotal evidence linking the two. For example, using data from a sample of 42,304 noninstitutionalized individuals, Eric Finkelstein and coworkers reported that slightly more than 20% of the adults examined had at least one injury each year that required medical treatment (Finkelstein, Chen,

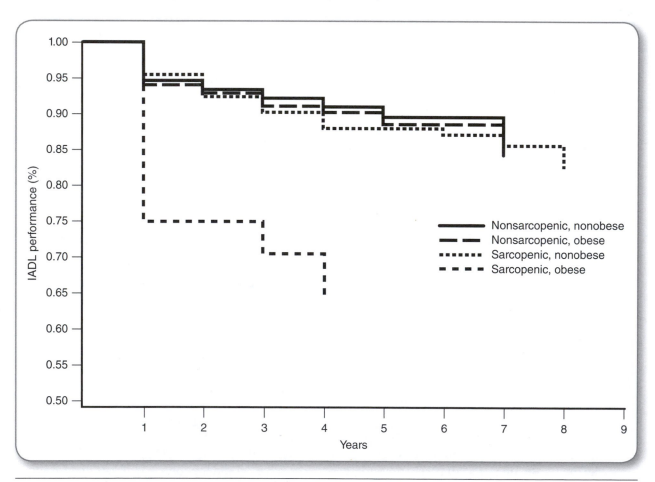

Figure 4.4   The combined effects of sarcopenia and obesity on IADL performance. Note the enormous effect exerted by the combination of these two conditions.

Reprinted by permission from Baumgartner et al. 2004.

Prabhu, Trogdon, & Corso, 2007). They also noted that the probabilities of sustaining an injury were 15% for persons who were overweight and 48% for patients with class III obesity (BMI of > 40 kg/m²). In fact, in a somewhat visionary statement these researchers noted the following: "If increasing BMI is causing the rise in injury rates, then the incidence of injuries, including those related to falls, sprains/strains, lower extremity fractures, and joint dislocations, are likely to increase as the prevalence of obesity increases" (Finkelstein, Chen, Prabhu, Trogdon, & Corso, 2007, p. 460).

APPLICATION POINT By increasing the activity levels of your clients you will not only improve their metabolism but also enhance their quality of life and reduce their likelihood of sustaining fall-related injury.

TESTING BODY COMPOSITION

There are a number of tools you can use to assess your client's body composition. The most common include the following:

- Dual-energy X-ray absorptiometry (DXA)
- Hydrostatic (underwater) weighing
- Air displacement plethysmography
- Bioimpedance
- Near-infrared spectroscopy
- Skinfold thickness and anthropometric measures

DXA, hydrostatic weighing, and air displacement plethysmography, while well-accepted methods for assessing body composition, are too expensive and require far too much space to be feasible for the typical fitness facility. Bioimpedance and infrared instruments are portable and can provide valid results when the correct formulas are used but are highly specialized pieces of equipment. Therefore we will examine the most accessible and effective methods available for body composition analysis: skinfold and anthropometric measurements.

Skinfold Measurements

There is a strong relationship between subcutaneous adiposity (fatty tissue under the skin) and whole-body adiposity and between direct skinfold depth measures and whole-body adiposity. Therefore, skinfold measurements are a good predictor of adiposity; however, the predictive value is better in men than it is in women. Of course, if you have a client who doesn't like to be pinched and prodded, you can take comfort in the fact that the BMI and waist circumference measurements presented in this chapter are also excellent indicators of adiposity and are highly correlated with cardiovascular risk.

Before we examine each of the skinfold measurements and the formulas used to predict adiposity, I suggest that you learn and follow these general principles presented by Jason Norcross (2002) on taking skinfold measurements:

- Make all measurements on the same side of the body.
- Place the calipers about 0.5 inches (1 cm) from where you pinch with the thumb and finger, perpendicular to the skinfold.
- Hold the pinch for 1 to 2 seconds before reading the calipers.
- Move from one site to another to give the skin adequate time to return to normal.
- Take at least three measurements at each site and average them to get a final number.

I would like to add that once you record a measurement, you should try to forget it so you will not prejudice your other readings.

In order to take skinfold measurements, you will need the following pieces of equipment:

- A cloth measuring tape
- A pair of quality skinfold calipers
- A marker to mark skinfold position (if desired)

Now that we have these basic tenets in place and our equipment is ready to go, let's look at the procedures used to measure each of the seven skinfolds:

1. Chest Skinfold Measurement

- Visualize a line from the axilla (armpit) to the nipple.
- Take a diagonal fold as close to the axilla as possible (figure 4.5).
- Make your measurement approximately 1 centimeter below your fingers along the diagonal fold line.

2. Midaxillary Skinfold Measurement

- Visualize a line descending vertically from the armpit (the midaxillary line).
- At a level just above the tip of the xiphoid process, draw a horizontal line across the rib cage.
- At the junction between these two lines, take a vertical skinfold and make your measurement (figure 4.6).
- To make this measurement easier, have the individual extend the arm up and slightly back to expose the midaxillary area.

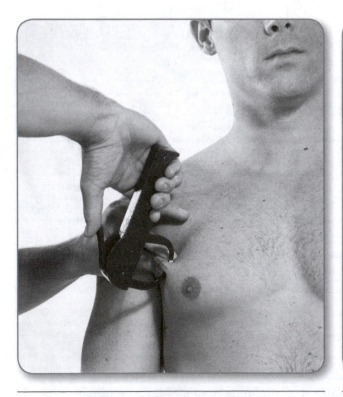

Figure 4.5   Chest skinfold measurement.

Reprinted by permission from Harman and Garhammer 2008.

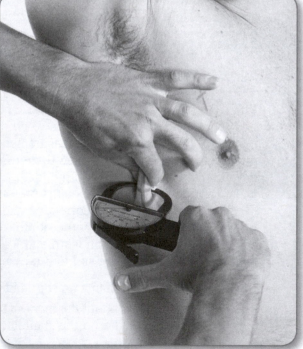

Figure 4.6   Midaxillary skinfold measurement.

Reprinted by permission from Harman and Garhammer 2008.

3. Suprailiac Skinfold Measurement

- Follow the midaxillary line down to the point of the hip bone, which is known as the *iliac crest.*
- At a point just above the iliac crest, take a diagonal skinfold in line with the natural fold of the skin in that location (figure 4.7).
- Take the measurement 1 centimeter below your fingers.

4. Abdominal Skinfold Measurement

- Draw a line 3 centimeters lateral to and 1 centimeter below the umbilicus (belly button).
- Take a vertical fold (figure 4.8).
- Make your measurement just to the side of your fingers closest to the umbilicus.

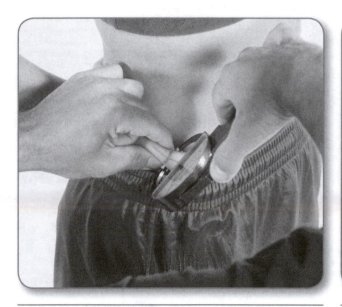

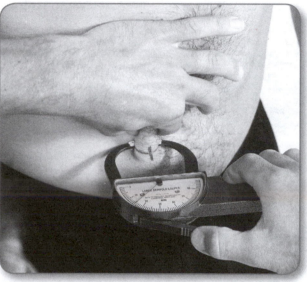

Figure 4.7   Suprailiac skinfold measurement (figure 4.7).

Reprinted by permission from Harman and Garhammer 2008.

Figure 4.8   Abdominal skinfold measurement.

Reprinted by permission from Harman and Garhammer 2008.

5. Thigh Skinfold Measurement

- Have the individual stand and shift the body weight away from the side being measured.
- Draw a line down the middle of the thigh from the inguinal crease (the crease between the leg and the trunk) to the proximal (top) border of the patella.
- Lift a vertical fold at the midpoint along this line.
- Take the measurement just below the pinch (figure 4.9).

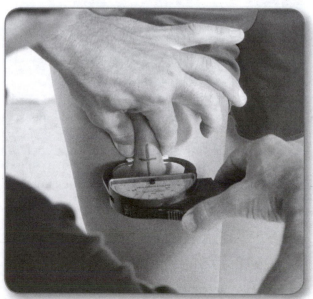

Figure 4.9   Thigh skinfold measurement.

Reprinted by permission from Harman and Garhammer 2008.

6. Triceps Skinfold Measurement

- Draw an imaginary line along the back of the arm from the olecranon process (the elbow) to the acromion process (the bony protrusion on top of the shoulder).
- Locate the midway point along this line.
- Take a vertical pinch (perpendicular to the midline) (figure 4.10).
- Make the measurement 1 centimeter above the midway point.

7. Subscapular Skinfold Measurement

- Locate the lower angle of the scapula (shoulder blade).
- Find the natural fold along this line, approximately 1-3 centimeters down.
- Take a diagonal fold (figure 4.11).
- Make the measurement approximately 1 centimeter below your fingers.

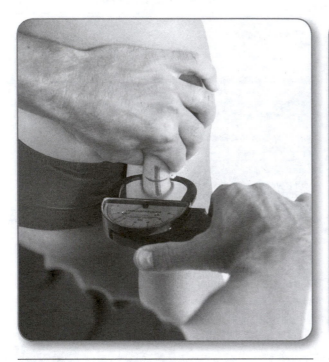

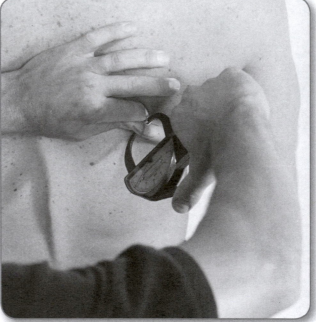

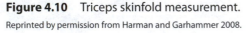

Figure 4.10   Triceps skinfold measurement.
Reprinted by permission from Harman and Garhammer 2008.

Figure 4.11   Subscapular skinfold measurement.
Reprinted by permission from Harman and Garhammer 2008.

The following are equations you'll need for computing the percentage of body adiposity from the sum of the seven skinfold measurements. These equations suffer from a number of shortcomings, and my suggestion is simply to use the sum of the seven skinfold measurements as an indicator of your client's body composition. However, knowing human nature, you and your client will want to have a tangible number indicating body adiposity; to get that, you'll need to use the equations.

Calculating Body Density

To calculate body density (BD) for men, use the following equation (Jackson & Pollack, 1978):

$$BD = 1.112 - 0.00043499(\text{sum of 7 skinfolds}) + 0.00000055(\text{sum of 7 skinfolds})^2 - 0.00028826(\text{age}).$$

To calculate BD for women, use this equation (Jackson, Pollack, & Ward, 1980):

$$BD = 1.097 - 0.00046971(\text{sum of 7 skinfolds}) + 0.00000056(\text{sum of 7 skinfolds})^2 - 0.00012828(\text{age}).$$

Once BD is known, you can calculate the percent body fat (%BF) from the following Siri formula (Siri, 1961):

$$\%BF = [(4.95 / BD) - 4.5] \times 100.$$

Calculating Body Mass Index

BMI is one of the most commonly used measures of body adiposity; however, you should consider it an inexact diagnostic tool for measuring obesity since it doesn't tell the relative contributions of FFM and fat mass to the client's weight. This problem is illustrated by the findings that both BMI and waist circumference are affected by fitness level. Moderately fit individuals who have the same BMI as unfit individuals have lower levels of total fat mass and abdominal subcutaneous and visceral fat.

Body Mass	
fat mass (FM)	The total mass of fatty tissue in your body.
fat free mass (FFM)	The mass of the body that includes everything but fat (e.g., bone, muscle, connective tissue, skin).

The rationale behind using BMI is its ease of measurement, its conventional use, and, most notably, its association with metabolic syndrome and coronary artery disease, especially when used in concert with waist circumference. In fact, the National Institutes of Health (NIH) has proposed that the relative risk factors associated with BMI should be greater for men and women with larger waist circumferences as opposed to smaller waist circumferences (National Institutes of Health et al., 2000). The following equation is used to compute BMI:

$$BMI = \frac{\text{weight (kg)}}{\text{height (m}^2)}$$

Measuring Waist Circumference and Calculating Waist-to-Hip Ratio

Waist circumference and waist-to-hip ratio are two measures of regional fat distribution, or, more simply, the location of your adipose tissue. The location of adipose tissue stores is of paramount importance because abdominal visceral adipose tissue (the fat surrounding the organs near your waist) is associated with cardiovascular disease and metabolic syndrome. Waist circumference is a great predictor of visceral adiposity when used alone or in concert with BMI. Increased waist circumference and BMI also have been shown to correlate directly to increased health costs. These measures are especially important for older clients, since older individuals are known to have more visceral adipose tissue than younger people have, and a high waist-to-hip ratio is an important independent predictor of cardiovascular risk. The National Institute of Diabetes and Digestive and Kidney Diseases has reported that women with waist-to-hip ratios greater than 0.8 and men with waist-to-hip ratios greater than 1.0 are at increased risk for cardiovascular disease. Why the difference

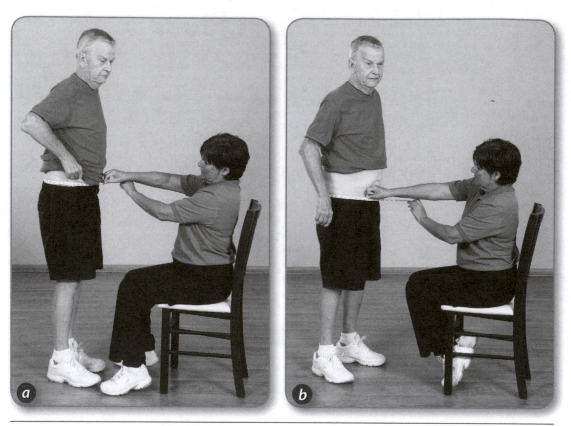

Figure 4.12   Measuring *(a)* waist circumference and *(b)* hip circumference.

between men and women? Typically women have wider hips and are pear shaped, while men have more central obesity and are more apple shaped. Figure 4.12 shows how to measure the waist circumference and hip circumference.

Equipment Needed

- A spring-loaded cloth measuring tape
- A marker to mark measurement position (if desired)

Protocol

- Ask the person being measured to stand straight but remain relaxed.
- Use a spring-loaded tape measure (to reduce tissue compression) to take the waist measurement at the narrowest part of the person's upper body. This position is usually at or slightly above the navel.
- Be sure that the person does not hold his breath or suck in the stomach during the measurement.
- While the individual remains standing, locate the widest point of his hips and buttocks.
- Place the spring-loaded tape measure horizontally around the hips at this position.

APPLICATION POINT   Using skinfolds to assess body composition provides a more accurate picture of body fat and lean body mass than BMI provides. The spreadsheet included on the DVD that accompanies this book will perform all these computations for you when you enter the skinfold values in the appropriate places. In addition, the diagnostic testing battery program will provide age- and gender-specific norms automatically.

- Write down the value to the nearest quarter of an inch (half of a centimeter).
- Be sure to keep the tape measure horizontal.
- Make at least three measurements to confirm your accuracy.

TRAINING INTERVENTIONS FOR SARCOPENIC OBESITY

There are two major goals in prescribing exercise to deal with sarcopenic obesity. The first is to increase the client's lean body mass (muscle, connective tissue, and bone), and the second is to reduce both subcutaneous fat and visceral fat.

When attempting to get rid of excess body fat, most people focus on a single concept: cutting calories. But using a calorie-restrictive diet as the only tool to reduce body weight can lead to a substantial loss of lean body mass that in turn can negatively affect performance and quality of life. The good news is that adding exercise to dieting can counteract some of these losses and help eliminate fat by burning extra calories. Overall we can be confident that

- aerobic exercise without dieting has limited weight loss potential and little or no effect on lean body mass,
- resistance exercise has little effect on weight loss but can increase FFM,
- weight loss due to dietary changes alone results in a loss of 25% to 30% of overall body mass,
- combining diet and exercise can increase weight loss, and
- an exercise protocol that includes resistance training helps to maintain lean body mass and performance.

Now let's look at the potential of exercise as a treatment for sarcopenic obesity.

Evaluating the Effectiveness of an Exercise

When trainers talk about exercise and weight loss, three questions predominate: "What kind of exercise burns the most calories?" "How long will it take to produce a meaningful training effect?" "Will the exercise burn fat?" The first question is easily answered. Since all fuel used in the body is ultimately processed by the aerobic energy pathways, we can use the amount of oxygen consumed during and after exercise to quantify caloric burn, or caloric output, resulting from exercise. But why do we measure oxygen consumption *after* the exercise is completed? The oxygen used after exercise is called *excess postexercise oxygen consumption*, or *EPOC*. Figure 4.13 shows patterns of EPOC following low-intensity (figure 4.13*a*) and high-intensity (figure 4.13*b*) exercise bouts. You can see that both the intensity and the duration of EPOC increase as the exercise session grows longer and more intense. So the answer to question one is that the exercise that produces the greatest increase in your oxygen consumption will burn the most calories.

The answer to the second question of how long it will take to produce a meaningful training effect is a bit more complex. For long-duration work, such as mall walking, the answer is not too difficult. The longer you exercise, the more calories you burn, as long as your pace is fairly constant. When it comes to EPOC, the number of calories burned is significantly higher when the exercise lasts 1 hour or longer. For interval training, however, which is an exercise routine that alternates bursts of work and recovery, the most effective duration of training depends on the intensity of the work cycle. We'll cover this in more detail later in this chapter. Finally, the length of any training session will depend on where your client is within the periodization scheme. Confused? Don't worry! I cover all of these concepts in this and subsequent chapters. Finding the best training duration is not quite as complex as it seems.

The final question of whether an exercise will burn fat is much easier to answer than most of us think it is. The answer is *yes!* By now most researchers and practitioners who deal with exercise and weight loss recognize that the key is caloric output. That's not to say that there is no such thing as a fat burning zone. There is. It's just that the zone is not that important. If low-intensity

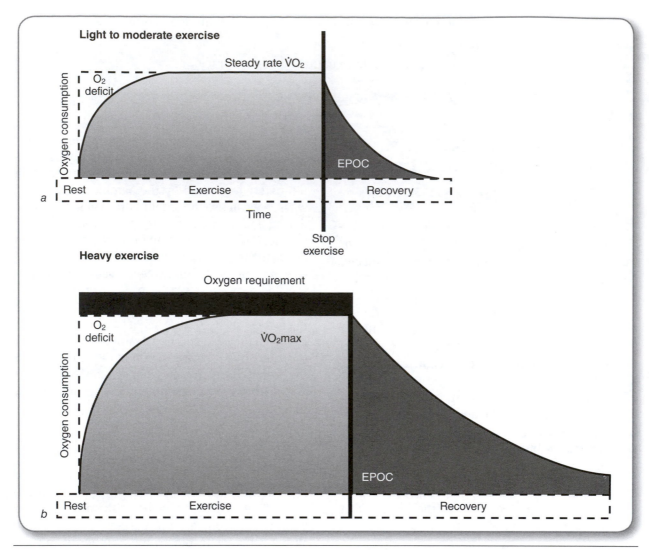

Figure 4.13   Illustration of EPOC following (a) short duration, low-intensity and (b) longer duration, high-intensity exercise bouts.

exercise targeting the fat burning zone was so effective, then exercise interventions such as weight training and interval training would not be as effective as they are in modifying body composition. Now that we have these basic concepts under our belts, let's look at the best way for you to reduce what's under your clients' belts.

> **APPLICATION POINT**   Higher-intensity exercise not only increases the number of calories burned during training but also extends the caloric burn following exercise.

Resistance Training

Although many of us have been taught that resistance training is not an effective tool for changing

body composition, nothing can be further from the truth, especially when you consider your older clients. Resistance training—whether using machine weights, free weights, bands and tubes, or the pool—gives your client a training "double whammy." While the intensity of the exercise increases your client's metabolic rate, the load stimulates muscle growth. Now let's look at the best ways to resistance train when the training goal is changes in body composition.

Effects on Metabolic Rate and Body Composition

One of the best pieces of advice to come down the pike from entertainers, orators, and writers is to save the best for last. Given my limited talents in all these areas, I will ignore this advice and give you the best first. In chapter 7, you'll see just how effective resistance training can be at increasing muscle mass while improving muscular strength, power, and endurance. But for now, let's look at how effective it can be at reducing the body fat that has developed a clinging fondness for our aging anatomy.

Resistance training increases resting metabolic rate (RMR) in your older clients just as it does in younger persons, and this increase in RMR is usually accompanied by an increase in FFM. Additionally, resistance training can significantly boost 24-hour energy expenditure and fat utilization.

These increases in energy expenditure and fat metabolism translate into changes in body composition when weight training is used as a long-term intervention. Reported changes include increases in FFM and strength. In older persons with type 2 diabetes, increases in energy expenditure are accompanied by reduced visceral and subcutaneous abdominal fat, increased leg and arm strength, increased insulin sensitivity, and decreased fasting blood glucose levels.

The effectiveness of resistance training in improving body composition and increasing metabolic rate does not appear to be limited to formalized equipment-dependent techniques. Tsuzuku and coworkers (2007) showed that 12 weeks of resistance training using rubber tubing decreased waist circumference, visceral fat thickness, and thigh fat thickness while increasing thigh muscle thickness in men and women aged 65 to 82 years.

Finally, when compared with aerobic training of the same intensity and duration, resistance training produces significantly higher EPOC, heart rate, ventilation, lactate concentration, and rating of perceived exertion. So it appears that the physiological responses to resistance training that cause such notable changes in body composition are not simply the consequences of high-intensity work. Resistance training appears to have its own unique place in your exercise toolbox when it comes to changing your client's body composition.

Effective Resistance Training Protocols

You can control a number of factors when designing a resistance training program for your client. These factors include resistance level, number of sets and sessions per week, equipment used, training patterns, and movement speeds.

As you will see in chapter 7, you can manipulate load to target strength, hypertrophy, power, and muscular endurance. Additionally, while single sets may be highly effective at the beginning of training, multiple sets appear necessary to produce significant improvements in trained individuals. The number of sessions per week will vary across any training cycle, but for your older clients, the optimal number appears to be 2 to 3 per week depending on the client's fitness level. Likewise, the most effective equipment depends on the training status and skill level of the client and the goal of the training.

When you talk about resistance training with your friends and colleagues (and I'm sure this is a hot topic at most backyard barbecues and parties), usually the discussion is framed in the context of a typical multiset system in which 2 to 3 sets of one exercise are repeated before a new exercise is begun. However, you are probably familiar with circuit training, in which single sets of various exercises are performed in succession until a circuit (a series of exercises) is completed. In circuit training the number of sets performed is increased by increasing the number of circuits performed. Given these possibilities for resistance training, what is the most effective intervention for improving your client's body composition?

In investigating the number of sets necessary to significantly affect caloric output both during and after exercise, Wayne Phillips and Joana Ziuraitis (2004) found that performing one 15-repetition set of eight different exercises could cause a moderate increase in caloric output. They noted that "additional sets, repetitions, and/or exercises appear to be necessary to achieve the minimum absolute volume of 150 kcal reported as eliciting health benefits with endurance-type physical activities" (p. 608). Concerning EPOC, as few as 16 sets of resistance training exercises performed at 75% of 1-repetition maximum (1RM) can increase caloric output for 24 hours after exercise. Though the number of calories burned during EPOC will be small (50-60 calories), these calories will still add up across weeks of training. It appears that during controlled speed training using hypertrophy-based loading (75% 1RM), 2 to 3 sets of 8 to 10 exercises will improve your client's body composition. But there are several other little tricks that you and I can use to improve these numbers.

The two most common patterns utilized during resistance training are multiset training and circuit training. Let's take a look at their effects on caloric output. When a typical three-set hypertrophy program (80% 1RM with a 120-second recovery) is compared with a typical circuit training program (50% 1RM with a 30-second recovery), the circuit training program is expected to produce significantly higher EPOC values for about 15 to 20 minutes after the end of the program even though both programs produce similar work volumes. One other advantage to the circuit training program is that due to the shorter recovery times, the same amount of work can be accomplished in less than half the time. So what's the downside of circuit training? As you'll see in chapter 7, the levels of hypertrophy achieved by circuit training are considerably lower.

So is it the shorter recovery time that makes the difference between a standard hypertrophy workout and a circuit training workout? Possibly, but let's not get into the mind-set of the less recovery, the better. Ronald Haltom and colleagues (1999) showed that when the loads, sets, and repetitions are held constant, the total energy expenditure is greater when recovery is allotted 60 seconds rather than 20 seconds (see figure 4.14). However, if your client is pressed for time, the 20-second recovery still works even if the 60-second recovery has the edge. This information will be very helpful when you learn (in chapter 9) how to plan the periodized programs that can maximize your clients' gains.

Another factor that can be manipulated to increase caloric burn during resistance training is movement speed. In chapter 7, we'll see that increasing movement speed during lifting is the most effective way to improve power output in older persons. However, that's not the end of the story. Increasing movement speed is also one of the most effective methods of increasing the number of calories burned during lifting. Giving up a little resistance in order to increase speed seems to be the way to go. Figure 4.15 shows the calories burned during three different squatting protocols: a slow protocol using four sets of eight repetitions at 80% of 1RM, a fast explosive protocol using four sets of eight repetitions at 60% of 1RM, and a fast explosive protocol using six sets of eight repetitions at 80% of 1RM. As you can see from the graph, the high-speed explosive training using 60% of 1RM burned more calories than the low-speed condition or the 80% of 1RM high-speed explosive condition burned. These results have strong implications for our discussion of improving ADL performance and reducing fall probability among older persons with sarcopenic obesity since high-speed training with moderate resistance is also one of the most effective ways to improve power in older persons. Therefore, high-speed, moderate-resistance training cycles appear to be a two-for-one special on your training menu. As you'll see in chapter 9, the ability

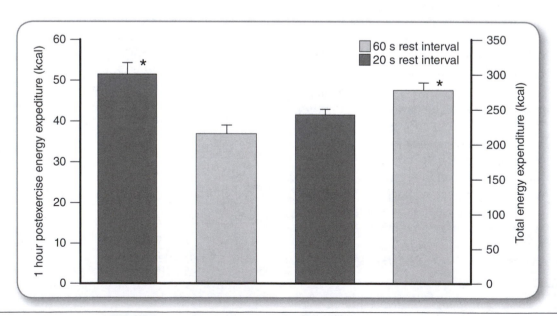

Figure 4.14 Postexercise and total energy expenditures resulting from circuit training protocols using recovery times of 20 seconds (dark gray) and 60 seconds (light gray).
* Indicates greater energy expenditure than the other rest interval.
Data from Haltom et al. 1999.

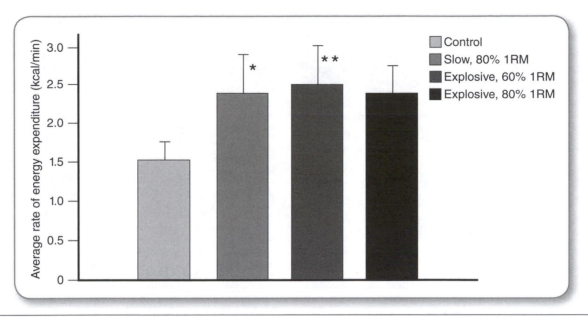

Figure 4.15   Rate of energy expenditure during squatting exercises using slow movement and heavy weight, explosive movement and moderate weight, and explosive movement and heavy weight.
* Indicates greater energy expenditure than the explosive, 80% 1RM group. ** Indicates that the explosive, moderate weight lifting pattern had a significantly higher energy expenditure than the other two lifting patterns.
Data from Mazzetti et al. 2007.

to manipulate load, speed, and volume during a resistance training cycle is the key to an effective periodized training program.

> **APPLICATION POINT**   You can use a number of resistance training tools to increase hypertrophy and decrease body fat selectively at different times during a training cycle. Heavier loads (~80% 1RM) increase muscle hypertrophy, while lighter loads (~50 to 60% 1RM) coupled with faster lifting speeds more effectively increase caloric output.

Aerobic Training Techniques: Interval Training

You're probably familiar with the numerous health benefits associated with moderate-duration or long-duration aerobic training, but this chapter is about body composition, so let's examine the most effective aerobic training method for making positive changes in fat and lean tissue. And the winner is . . . interval training. Interval training derives its benefits from a number of factors, including the following:

- It allows more work to be done per unit of time. Typical interval training programs weave

bouts of supramaximal (above $\dot{V}O_2$max but not superhuman) effort with periods of submaximal effort, allowing a higher average work intensity per unit of workout time.

- It is metabolically inefficient. The literature clearly indicates that the higher the work rate during any specific exercise modality, the less efficient the work becomes and the greater the number of calories burned per unit of time.

- It increases the level and duration of EPOC.

In fact, interval training can produce caloric outputs similar to those achieved through steady-state programs that take much longer to complete and require a substantially higher volume of work.

One of the most impressive studies to examine interval training as a modality for weight loss was performed by E.G. Trapp and colleagues (Trapp, Chisholm, Freund, & Boutcher, 2008). They compared a steady-state group training at approximately 60% of $\dot{V}O_2$max for 40 minutes to an interval group performing repeated intervals of 8 seconds of sprinting followed by 12 seconds of easy riding for a maximum of 20 minutes. Both groups improved their cardiovascular fitness; however, only the interval training group showed a significant decrease in total body mass and fat mass. And equally as important, the losses in fat mass came from the critical areas on the trunk and thighs (see figure 4.16). This may be especially important when considering the argument made by these researchers that "most exercise programs designed for weight loss have focused on steady-state exercise of around 30 minutes at a moderate intensity on most days of the week. Disappointingly, these kinds of exercise programs have led to little or no fat loss" (Trapp et al., 2008, p. 684). Given the findings of this study, there is a strong argument for using interval training to reduce body mass and fat mass in older individuals.

Now let's look at EPOC after aerobic training. EPOC may occur for 3 to 24 hours after steady-state training sessions performed for 50 minutes or more at an intensity of 70% of $\dot{V}O_2$max. Similar durations of EPOC are seen after training incorporating supramaximal intervals totaling 12 minutes (three 2-minute work periods with each separated by 3-minute recovery periods) or more at intensity levels of 105% of $\dot{V}O_2$max or more. While it is doubtful that your older clients will be able to reach these intensity levels at the beginning of their training, they may achieve or even surpass these levels once their fitness improves. Even though EPOC contributes, at most, 15% to

the total energy expenditure resulting from interval training, the combination of the increased energy expenditures during the training session and during EPOC clearly exceeds what may be expected from an equal duration of steady-state training.

APPLICATION POINT   Both steady-state training and interval training can be used at various times in a training cycle to make the most of their inherent differences in intensity and volume. Remember this when you read about periodized training in chapter 9.

Mixed Training Techniques

For years scientists and practitioners have debated the practicality of combining aerobic training and resistance training within the same training cycle. The argument against the concurrent use of these training techniques is that doing so causes an interference effect that reduces the effectiveness of at least one of the modalities. But the purpose of this chapter is not to examine possible interference due to concurrent muscular strength and cardiovascular endurance training; rather, the goal is to examine the potential for using these two

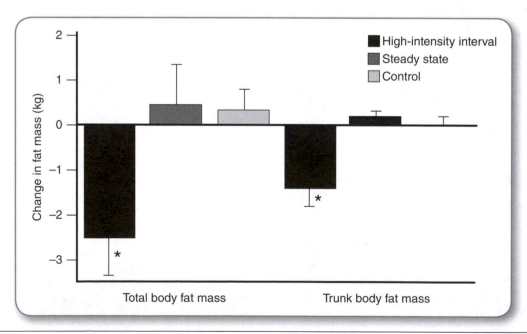

Figure 4.16   Changes in total-body fat mass and trunk fat mass due to high-intensity interval training and steady-state training over a 15-week period.
* Indicates greater decreases than the steady state and control groups.
Data from Trapp 2008.

training methods concurrently to improve body composition. So let's do just that.

We know that combining aerobic dance movements and resistance circuit training can significantly reduce body fat in older individuals. In addition, we can expect conservative increases in both strength and aerobic fitness as well as increases in high-density lipoprotein (HDL) levels. In an interesting study comparing standard resistance training to cardiovascular endurance training and to a combination of resistance training and cardiovascular endurance training, Dolezal and Potteiger (1998) provided a practical example of exercise specificity. In this study, aerobic capacity improved only in the cardiovascular endurance group, while the greatest gains in strength were seen in the resistance group. In addition, basal metabolic rate increased in the resistance and combined groups but not in the cardiovascular endurance group. We can conclude from this study that resistance training increases basal metabolic rate and muscular strength while cardiovascular endurance training increases aerobic power. Combining endurance and resistance training provides all of these benefits (albeit at a lesser magnitude) and may have a greater effect on improving body composition than either modality may have alone. Examples of specific changes across training cycles designed to improve body composition are provided in chapter 9 and on the DVD included with this book.

APPLICATION POINT   Although data suggest there is an interference effect when mixing cardiovascular endurance and resistance training, combined training is an effective strategy when considering changes in body composition, especially when you understand how to modify the training protocols.

SUMMARY

Exercise can have a positive effect on sarcopenic obesity. It is clear, however, that cardiovascular endurance exercise and resistance training and the combination of the two have different outcomes on body composition. Additionally, the intensity of the exercise intervention can affect the calories burned both during and after exercise. The diversity of the available training protocols and the capacity of these protocols to manipulate body fat and lean body tissue in different ways provide a wonderful menu from which you can choose when designing periodized training programs for your clients.

Topical Bibliography

The Prevalence of Obesity and Its Consequences

Arterburn, D.E., Crane, P.K., & Sullivan, S.D. (2004). The coming epidemic of obesity in elderly Americans. *J Am Geriatr Soc* 52:1907-1912.

Lapane, K.L., & Resnik, L. (2005). Obesity in nursing homes: An escalating problem. *J Am Geriatr Soc* 53:1386-1391.

Roubenoff, R. (2004). Sarcopenic obesity: The confluence of two epidemics. *Obes Res* 12:887-888.

The Obesity Paradox

Curtis, J.P., Selter, J.G., Wang, Y., Rathore, S.S., Jovin, I.S., Jadbabaie, F., Kosiborod, M., Portnay, E.L., Sokol, S.I., Bader, F., & Krumholz, H.M. (2005). The obesity paradox: Body mass index and outcomes in patients with heart failure. *Arch Intern Med* 165:55-61.

Flodin, L., Svensson, S., & Cederholm, T. (2000). Body mass index as a predictor of 1 year mortality in geriatric patients. *Clin Nutr* 19:121-125.

Fonarow, G.C. (2007). The relationship between body mass index and mortality in patients hospitalized with acute decompensated heart failure. *Am Heart J* 154:e21.

McAuley, P., Myers, J., Abella, J., Oliveira, R., Hsu, L., & Froelicher, V.F. (2007). Obesity: Experimental and clinical abstract 3600: An obesity paradox among apparently healthy male veterans. *Circulation* 116:815.

Habbu, A., Lakkis, N.M., & Dokainish, H. (2006). The obesity paradox: Fact or fiction? *Am J Cardiol* 98:944-948.

Sarcopenic Obesity and Activities of Daily Living

Baumgartner, R.N., Wayne, S.J., Waters, D.L., Janssen, I., Gallagher, D., & Morley, J.E. (2004). Sarcopenic obesity predicts instrumental activities of daily living disability in the elderly. *Obes Res* 12:1995-2004.

Bouchard, D.R., Beliaeff, S., Dionne, I.J., & Brochu, M. (2007). Fat mass but not fat-free mass is related to physical capacity in well-functioning older individuals: Nutrition as a determinant of successful aging (NuAge)—the Quebec Longitudinal Study. *J Gerontol A Biol Sci Med Sci* 62:1382-1388.

Cesari, M., Leeuwenburgh, C., Lauretani, F., Onder, G., Bandinelli, S., Maraldi, C., Guralnik, J.M., Pahor, M., & Ferrucci, L. (2006). Frailty syndrome and skeletal muscle: Results from the Invecchiare in Chianti study. *Am J Clin Nutr* 83:1142-1148.

Stenholm, S., Sainio, P., Rantanen, T., Koskinen, S., Jula, A., Heliövaara, M., & Aromaa, A. (2007). High body mass index and physical impairments as predictors of walking limitation 22 years later in adult Finns. *J Gerontol A Biol Sci Med Sci* 62:859-865.

Villareal, D.T., Banks, M., Siener, C., Sinacore, D.R., & Klein, S. (2004). Physical frailty and body composition in obese elderly men and women. *Obes Res* 12:913-920.

Sarcopenic Obesity and Fall Probability

Finkelstein, E.A., Chen, H., Prabhu, M., Trogdon, J.G., & Corso, P.S. (2007). The relationship between obesity and injuries among U.S. adults. *Am J Health Promot* 21:460-468.

Matter, K.C., Sinclair, S.A., Hostetler, S.G., & Xiang, H. (2007). A comparison of the characteristics of injuries between obese and non-obese inpatients. *Obesity (Silver Spring)* 15:2384-2390.

Testing Body Composition

Chan, J.M., Rimm, E.B., Colditz, G.A., Stampfer, M.J., & Willett, W.C. (1994). Obesity, fat distribution, and weight gain as risk factors for clinical diabetes in men. *Diabetes Care* 17:961-969.

Clarys, J.P., Provyn, S., & Marfell-Jones, M.J. (2005). Cadaver studies and their impact on the understanding of human adiposity. *Ergonomics* 48:1445-1461.

Cornier, M.A., Tate, C.W., Grunwald, G.K., & Bessesen, D.H. (2002). Relationship between waist circumference, body mass index, and medical care costs. *Obes Res* 10:1167-1172.

Daniel, J.A., Sizer, P.S., & Latman, N.S. (2007). Evaluation of body composition methods for accuracy. *Biomed Instrum Technol* 39:397-405.

De Michele, M., Panico, S., Iannuzzi, A., Celentano, E., Ciardullo, A.V., Galasso, R., Sacchetti, L., Zarrilli, F., Bond, M.G., & Rubba, P. (2003). Association of obesity and central fat distribution with carotid artery wall thickening in middle-aged women. *Stroke* 33:2923-2928.

Despres, J.P., Couillard, C., Gagnon, J., Bergeron, J., Leon, A.S., Rao, D.C., Skinner, J.S., Wilmore, J.H., & Bouchard, C. (2000). Race, visceral adipose tissue, plasma lipids, and lipoprotein lipase activity in men and women: The Health, Risk Factors, Exercise Training, and Genetics (HERITAGE) family study. *Arterioscler Thromb Vasc Biol* 20:1932-1938.

Després, J.P., & Lemieux, I. (2006). Abdominal obesity and metabolic syndrome. *Nature* 444:881-887.

Heymsfield, S.B., & Lichtman, S. (1990). New approaches to body composition research: A reexamination of two-compartment model assumptions. *Infusionstherapie* 17:4-8.

Jackson, A.S., & Pollack, M.L. (1978). Generalized equations for predicting body density for men. *Br J Nutr* 40:497-504.

Jackson, A.S., Pollack, M.L., & Ward, A. (1980). Generalized equations for predicting body density of women. *Med Sci Sport Exerc* 12:175-182.

Janssen, I., Heymsfield, S.B., Allison, D.B., Kotler, D.P., & Ross, R. (2002). Body mass index and waist circumference independently contribute to prediction of nonabdominal, abdominal subcutaneous, and visceral fat. *Am J Clin Nutr* 75:683-688.

Janssen, I., Katzmarzyk, P.T., Ross, R., Leon, A.S., Skinner, J.S., Rao, D.C., Wilmore, J.H., Rankinen, T., & Bouchard, C. (2004). Fitness alters the association of BMI and waist circumference with total and abdominal fat. *Obes Res* 12:525-537.

Kuk, J.L., Lee, S., Heymsfield, S.B., & Ross, R. (2005). Waist circumference and abdominal adipose tissue distribution: Influence of age and sex. *Am J Clin Nutr* 81:1330-1334.

Ledoux, M., Lambert, J., Reeder, B.A., & Despres, J.P. (1997a). A comparative analysis of weight to height and waist to hip circumference indices as indicators of the presence of cardiovascular disease risk factors. Canadian Heart Health Surveys Research Group. *CMAJ* 157:S32-S38.

Ledoux, M., Lambert, J., Reeder, B.A., & Despres, J.P. (1997b). Correlation between cardiovascular disease risk factors and simple anthropometric measures. Canadian Heart Health Surveys Research Group. *CMAJ* 157:S46-S53.

Lohman, T.G., & Going, S.B. (1993). Multicomponent models in body composition research: Opportunities and pitfalls. *Basic Life Sci* 60:53-58.

Mazariegos, M., Heymsfield, S.B., Wang, Z.M., Wang, J., Yasumura, S., Dilmanian, F.A., & Pierson, R.N. (1993). Aging affects body composition: Young versus elderly women pair-matched by body mass index. In K.J. Ellis & J.D. Eastman (Eds.), *Human body composition* (pp. 245-249). New York: Plenum Press.

Mazariegos, M., Wang, Z.M., Gallagher, D., Baumgartner, R.N., Allison, D.B., Wang, J., Pierson, R.N., & Heymsfield, S.B. (1994). Differences between young and old females in the five levels of body composition and their relevance to the two-compartment chemical model. *Journal of Gerontology* 49:M201-M208.

Nieves, D.J., Cnop, M., Retzlaff, B., Walden, C.E., Brunzell, J.D., Knopp, R.H., & Kahn, S.E. (2003). The atherogenic lipoprotein profile associated with obesity and insulin resistance is largely attributable to intra-abdominal fat. *Diabetes* 52:172-179.

Norcross, J. (2002). Body composition for beginners, part 2. www.tmuscle.com/free_online_article/sports_body_training_performance_science/body_comp_for_beginners_part_2.

Ohlson, L.O., Larsson, B., Svardsudd, K., Welin, L., Eriksson, H., Wilhelmsen, L., Bjorntorp, P., & Tibblin, G. (1985). The influence of body fat distribution on the incidence of diabetes mellitus. 13.5 years of follow-up of the participants in the study of men born in 1913. *Diabetes* 34:1055-1058.

Peterson, M.J., Czerwinski, S.A., & Siervogel, R.M. (2003). Development and validation of skinfold-thickness prediction equations with a 4-compartment model. *Am J Clin Nutr* 77:1186-1191.

Reeder, B.A., Senthilselvan, A., Despres, J.P., Angel, A., Liu, L., Wang, H., & Rabkin, S.W. (1997). The association of cardiovascular disease risk factors with abdominal obesity in Canada. Canadian Heart Health Surveys Research Group. CMAJ 157:S39-S45.

Wellens, R.I., Roche, A.F., Khamis, H.J., Jackson, A.S., Pollack, M.L., & Siervogel, R.M. (1996). Relationships between the body mass index and body composition. *Obes Res* 4:35-44.

Withers, R.T., LaForgia, J., Pillans, R.K., Shipp, N.J., Chatterton, B.E., Schultz, C.G., & Leaney, F. (1998). Comparisons of two-, three-, and four-compartment models of body composition analysis in men and women. *J Appl Physiol* 85:238-245.

Zhu, S., Heshka, S., Wang, Z., Shen, W., Allison, D.B., Ross, R., & Heymsfield, S.B. (2004). Combination of BMI and waist circumference for identifying cardiovascular risk factors in whites. *Obes Res* 12:633-645.

Training Interventions for Sarcopenic Obesity

Sedlock, D.A., Fissinger, J.A., & Melby, C.L. (1989). Effect of exercise intensity and duration on postexercise energy expenditure. *Medicine and Science in Sports and Exercise* 21:662-666.

Quinn, T.J., Vroman, N.B., & Kertzer, R. (1994). Postexercise oxygen consumption in trained females: Effects of exercise duration. *Medicine and Science in Sports and Exercise* 26:908-913.

Treuth, M.S., Hunter, G.R., & Williams, M. (1996). Effects of exercise intensity on 24-h energy expenditure and substrate oxidation. *Medicine and Science in Sports and Exercise* 28:1138-1143.

Resistance Training

Ades, P.A., Savage, P.D., Brochu, M., Tischler, M.D., Lee, N.M., & Poehlman, E.T. (2005). Resistance training increases total daily energy expenditure in disabled older women with coronary heart disease. *J Appl Physiol* 98:1280-1285.

Ballor, D.L., Harvey-Berino, J.R., Ades, P.A., Cryan, J., & Calles-Escandon, J. (1996). Contrasting effects of resistance and aerobic training on body composition and metabolism after diet-induced weight loss. *Metabolism* 45:179-183.

Binder, E.F., Yarasheski, K.E., Steger-May, K., Sinacore, D.R., Brown, M., Schechtman, K.B., & Holloszy, J.O. (2005). Effects of progressive resistance training on body composition in frail older adults: Results of a randomized, controlled trial. *J Gerontol A Biol Sci Med Sci* 60:1425-1431.

Burleson, J.M.A., O'Bryant, H.S., Stone, M.H., Collins, M.A., & Triplett-McBride, T. (1998). Effect of weight training exercise and treadmill exercise on post-exercise oxygen consumption. *Medicine and Science in Sports and Exercise* 30:518-522.

Campbell, W.W., Crim, M.C., Young, V.R., & Evans, W.J. (1994). Increased energy requirements and changes in body composition with resistance training in older adults. *Am J.Clin Nutr* 60:167-175.

Haltom, R.W., Kraemer, R.P., Sloan, R.A., Hebert, E.P., Frank, K., & Tryniecki, J.L. (1999). Circuit weight training and its effects on excess postexercise oxygen consumption. *Medicine and Science in Sports and Exercise* 31:1613-1618.

Ibañez, J., Izquierdo, M., Argüelles, I., Forga, L., Larrión, J.L., García-Unciti, M., Idoate, F., & Gorostiaga, E.M. (2005). Twice-weekly progressive resistance training decreases abdominal fat and improves insulin sensitivity in older men with type 2 diabetes. *Diabetes Care* 28:662-667.

Hurley, B.F., & Roth, S.M. (2000). Strength training in the elderly effects on risk factors for age-related diseases. *Sports Med* 30:249-268.

Mazzetti, S., Douglass, M., Yocum, A., & Harber, M. (2007). Effect of explosive versus slow contractions and exercise intensity on energy expenditure. *Medicine and Science in Sports and Exercise* 39:1291-1301.

Murphy, E., & Schwarzkopf, R. (1992). Effects of standard set and circuit weight-training on excess post-exercise oxygen consumption. *J Appl Sport Sci Res* 6:88-91.

Melby, C., Scholl, C., Edwards, G., & Bullough, R. (1993). Effect of acute resistance exercise on postexercise energy expenditure and resting metabolic rate. *Journal of Applied Physiology* 75:1847-1853.

Nemoto, K., Gen-no, H., Masuki, S., Okazaki, K., & Nose, H. (2007). Effects of high-intensity interval walking training on physical fitness and blood pressure in middle-aged and older people. *Mayo Clin Proc* 82:803-811.

Phillips, W.T., & Ziuraitis, J.R. (2004). Energy cost of single-set resistance training in older adults. *J Strength Cond Res* 18:606-609.

Pratley, R., Nicklas, B., Rubin, M., Miller, J., Smith, A., Smith, M., Hurley, B., & Goldberg, A. (1994). Strength training increases resting metabolic rate and norepinephrine levels in healthy 50- to 65-yr-old men. *Journal of Applied Physiology* 76:133-137.

Ryan, A., Pratley, R.E., Elahi, D., & Goldberg, A.P. (1995). Resistive training increases fat-free mass and maintains RMR despite weight loss in postmenopausal women. *J Appl Physiol* 79:818-823.

Short, K.R., Wiest, J.M., & Sedlock, D.A. (1996). The effect of upper body exercise intensity and duration on post-exercise oxygen consumption.. *Int J Sports Med* 17:559-563.

Treuth, M.S., Hunter, G.R., Weinsier, R.L., & Kell, S.H. (1995). Energy expenditure and substrate utilization in older women after strength training: 24-h calorimeter results. *J Appl Physiol* 78:2140-2146.

Tsuzuku, S., Kajioka, T., Endo, H., Abbott, R.D., Curb, J.D., & Yano, K. (2007). Favorable effects of non-instrumental resistance training on fat distribution and metabolic profiles in healthy elderly people. *Eur J Appl Physiol* 99:549-555.

Williamson, D.L., & Kirwan, J.P. (1997). A single bout of concentric resistance exercise increases basal metabolic rate 48 hours after exercise in healthy 59-77-year-old men. *Journal of Gerontology: Medical Sciences* 52A: M352-M355.

Aerobic Training Techniques: Interval Training

Burgomaster, K.A., Howarth, K.R., Phillips, S.M., Rakobowchukl, M., McDonald, M.J., McGee, S.L., & Gibala, M.J. (2008). Similar metabolic adaptations during exercise after low volume sprint interval and traditional endurance training in humans. *J Physiol* 586:151-160.

Daussin, F.N., Ponsot, E., Dufour, S.P., Lonsdorfer-Wolf, E., Doutreleau, S., Geny, B., Piquard, F., & Richard, R. (2007). Improvement of VO$_2$max by cardiac output and oxygen extraction adaptation during intermittent versus continuous endurance training. *Eur J Appl Physiol* 101:377-383.

LaForgia, J., Withers, R.T., & Gore, C.J. (2006). Effects of exercise intensity and duration on the excess post-exercise oxygen consumption. *J Sports Sci* 24:1247-1264.

Talanian, J.L., Galloway, S.D., Heigenhauser, G.J., Bonen, A., & Spriet, L.L. (2007). Two weeks of high-intensity aerobic interval training increases the capacity for fat oxidation during exercise in women. *J Appl Physiol* 102:1439-1447.

Trapp, E.G., Chisholm, D.J., Freund, J., & Boutcher, S.H. (2008). The effects of high-intensity intermittent exercise training on fat loss and fasting insulin levels of young women. *Int J Obes (Lond)* 32:684-691.

Mixed Training Techniques

Dolezal, B.A., & Potteiger, J.A. (1998). Concurrent resistance and endurance training influence basal metabolic rate in non-dieting individuals. *J Appl Physiol* 85:695-700.

Dudley, G.A., & Djamil, R. (1985). Incompatibility of endurance- and strength-training modes of exercise. *Journal of Applied Physiology* 59:1446-1451.

Glowacki, S.P., Martin, S.E., Mauer, A., Baek, W., Green, J.S., & Crouse, S.F. (2004). Effects of resistance, endurance, and concurrent exercise on training outcomes in men. *Medicine and Science in Sports and Exercise* 36:2119-2127.

Hakkinen, K., Alen, M., Kraemer, W.J., Gorostiaga, E.M., Izquierdo, M., Rusko, H., Mikkola, J., Hakkinen, A., Valkeinen, H., Kaarakainen, E., Romu, S., Erola, V., Ahtiainen, J., & Paavolainen, L. (2003). Neuromuscular adaptations during concurrent strength and endurance training versus strength training. *Eur J Appl Physiol* 89:52.

Hickson, R.C. (1980). Interference of strength development by simultaneously training for strength and endurance. *European Journal of Applied Physiology* 45:255-263.

Kraemer, W.J., Vescovi, J.D., Volek, J.S., Nindl, B.C., Newton, R.U., Patton, J.F., Dziados, J.E., French, D.N., & Häkkinen, K. (2004). Effects of concurrent resistance and aerobic training on load-bearing performance and the army physical fitness test. *Mil Med* 169:994-999.

Leveritt, M., Abernathy, P., Barry, B., & Logan, P.A. (2003). Concurrent strength and endurance training: The influence of dependent variable selection. *J Str Cond Res* 17:503-508.

Sale, D.G., MacDougall, J.D., Jacobs, I., & Garner, S. (1990). Interaction between concurrent strength and endurance training. *J Appl Physiol* 68:260-270.

Sale, D.G., Jacobs, I., MacDougall, J.D., & Garner, S. (1990). Comparison of two regimens of concurrent strength and endurance training. *Medicine and Science in Sports and Exercise* 22:348-356.

Takeshima, N., Rogers, M.E., Islam, M.M., Yamauchi, T., Watanabe, E., & Okada, A. (2004). Effect of concurrent aerobic and resistance circuit exercise training on fitness in older adults. *Eur J Appl Physiol* 93:173-182.

Walberg, J.L. (1989). Aerobic exercise and resistance weight-training during weight reduction. Implications for obese persons and athletes. *Sports Med* 7:343-356.

References

Arterburn, D.E., Crane, P.K., & Sullivan, S.D. (2004). The coming epidemic of obesity in elderly Americans. *J Am Geriatr Soc* 52:1907-1912.

Dolezal, B.A., & Potteiger, J.A. (1998). Concurrent resistance and endurance training influence basal metabolic rate in non-dieting individuals. *J Appl Physiol* 85:695-700.

Finkelstein, E.A., Chen, H., Prabhu, M., Trogdon, J.G., & Corso, P.S. (2007). The relationship between obesity and injuries among U.S. adults. *Am J Health Promot* 21:460-468.

Habbu, A., Lakkis, N.M., & Dokainish, H. (2006). The obesity paradox: Fact or fiction? *Am J Cardiol* 98:944-948.

Haltom, R.W., Kraemer, R.P., Sloan, R.A., Hebert, E.P., Frank, K., & Tryniecki, J.L. (1999). Circuit weight training and its effects on excess postexercise oxygen consumption. *Medicine and Science in Sports and Exercise* 31:1613-1618.

Jackson, A.S., & Pollack, M.L. (1978). Generalized equations for predicting body density for men. *Br J Nutr* 40:497-504.

Jackson, A.S., Pollack, M.L., & Ward, A. (1980). Generalized equations for predicting body density of women. *Med Sci Sport Exerc* 12:175-182.

Lapane, K.L., & Resnik, L. (2005). Obesity in nursing homes: An escalating problem. *J Am Geriatr Soc* 53:1386-1391.

National Institutes of Health, National Heart, Lung, and Blood Institute, North American Association for the Study of Obesity. (2000) The Practical Guide: Identification, Evaluation, and Treatment of Overweight and Obesity in Adults. NIH Publication Number 00–4084. National Institutes of Health Rockville, MD.

Norcross, J. (2002). Body composition for beginners, part 2. www.tmuscle.com/free_online_article/sports_body_training_performance_science/body_comp_for_beginners_part_2.

Phillips, W.T., & Ziuraitis, J.R. (2004). Energy cost of single-set resistance training in older adults. *J Strength Cond Res* 18:606-609.

Roubenoff, R. (2004). Sarcopenic obesity: The confluence of two epidemics. *Obes Res* 12:887-888.

Siri, W. E. (1961). Body composition from fluid space and density. In J. Brozek & A. Hanschel (Eds.), *Techniques for measuring body composition* (pp. 223-244). Washington, DC: National Academy of Science.

Trapp, E.G., Chisholm, D.J., Freund, J., & Boutcher, S.H. (2008). The effects of high-intensity intermittent exercise training on fat loss and fasting insulin levels of young women. *Int J Obes (Lond)* 32:684-691.

Tsuzuku, S., Kajioka, T., Endo, H., Abbott, R.D., Curb, J.D., & Yano, K. (2007). Favorable effects of non-instrumental resistance training on fat distribution and metabolic profiles in healthy elderly people. *Eur J Appl Physiol* 99:549-555.

5

Flexibility

Although flexibility is a major factor affecting functional performance, it seems to hold the position of helpful sidekick in most studies examining exercise interventions in older persons. For example, numerous studies have included a flexibility component as a supplement to strength or cardiovascular training, while several others have reported increased flexibility as a result of resistance or aerobic training. This chapter looks at the helpful sidekick of strength and cardiovascular training in a new light, examining not only the importance of flexibility in promoting healthy aging but also the flexibility modalities that are most successful in addressing the needs of older clients.

DEFINING FLEXIBILITY AND THE STRAIN–STRESS CURVE

Flexibility can be either static or dynamic. Static flexibility is the maximum end ROM of a specific joint or series of joints. In practical terms it is a measure of how far a client can stretch while moving slowly to the end of his ROM and then maintaining that position for a specified time (usually a few seconds). Typically static flexibility is assessed with tests such as the chair sit-and-reach

test (which is described later in this chapter). Dynamic flexibility, in contrast, is a measure of how far a client can stretch while moving at a moderate to fast speed to the end of her ROM.

It is possible to evaluate flexibility at any point in a person's ROM by examining how much a muscle and its connective tissue will stretch (show strain or deformation) when a load (stress) is applied (see figure 5.1). There are two areas within the curve in figure 5.1. The first is the elastic area, where the muscle and connective tissue stretch and then rebound back. The second is the plastic area, where all or a portion of the deformation remains for a time after the stress is removed. We will examine how to target the elastic area of the curve when we look at power and speed training in chapters 7 and 10. In this chapter we are focusing on flexibility training, so let's look at exercise interventions that increase deformation in the plastic area of the curve in order to increase the lengths of the connective tissue and muscle. But don't concern yourself with trying to target the plastic area, since most stretches are designed to apply the greatest stretch at the end ROM, which, as you can see from figure 5.1, is the plastic area.

In the literature there are two responses to stretching: an immediate, or acute, response to a single bout and a delayed, or chronic, response due to repeated bouts across a prolonged (greater

Types of Flexibility

static flexibility	The ability to slowly move a specific joint or series of joints to the end range of motions and maintain that position without moving.
dynamic flexibility	The ability to actively move through the full range of motion of a joint or series of joints at a specific movement speed, transitioning through each position.

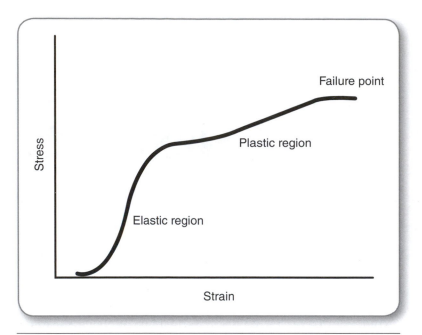

Figure 5.1   The strain–stress curve for flexibility.

than 4 weeks) period. For clarity, this text uses the terms *stretching* to describe the acute act of stretching and *flexibility training* to describe a program of stretches performed on a regular basis to increase flexibility.

POSSIBLE CAUSES OF DECLINING FLEXIBILITY WITH AGING

Declines in ROM may result from age-related connective tissue restructuring, trauma from mechanical stress, diseases such as arthritis, and, most importantly within the context of this book, reduced activity levels. As you learned in chapter 1, aging is associated with increasing levels of the stiffer type I collagen and decreasing levels of type III collagen; in addition the elastin, which gives spring to tissues, degenerates. The reasons for the increased stiffness of collagen include a greater fiber diameter, a greater number of the cross-linkages that give stiffness to the collagen fibers, and a reduction in fluid content. It has been suggested that mechanical stress decreases ROM through continued microscopic damage that may lead to changes in the structure of cartilage, causing reduced tensile strength and increased potential for osteoarthritis. Finally, there is a clear positive association between activity levels

and joint ROM. The more active the client is, the better the joint ROM, and vice versa. This is because active individuals have increased connective tissue compliancy and higher sarcomere numbers.

WHY TRAIN FOR FLEXIBILITY?

While the benefits derived from lifting weights or distance walking are easy to understand, for most clients something as passive as holding a stretch for 30 seconds just doesn't feel like exercise. Therefore, if you would like to generate enthusiasm for stretching, you should know its benefits so that you can share this knowledge with your clients. Although clients may not recognize it, declines in flexibility are associated with reduced ability to perform ADLs and increased probability of falls. If we provide flexibility training, we can help clients to bend the aging curves and take one more step toward maintaining independence and reducing falls.

Flexibility Declines and Performance of Activities of Daily Living

Age-related declines in flexibility (ROM) are associated with declines in mobility and ADL performance. In fact, ROM seems to be the key to improving the ability to perform functional movements. As ROM declines, people slowly lose their ability to walk, bend down, handle objects, bend their arms, and reach above their heads. This loss of movement not only increases the consequences of certain diseases such as arthritis but also affects an otherwise healthy older client. In fact, declines in ROM are among the strongest predictors of declines in activity levels and ADL performance.

Flexibility Declines and Fall Probability

Reduced flexibility increases the probability of falls. Notably, reduced ankle dorsiflexion has been linked to an increased likelihood of falling, and correlations have been reported between ankle ROM and balance. Reduced hip ROM has also been linked to an increased likelihood of falling. You've probably noticed that older people walk differently than younger people walk. Researchers who examine gait (walking) patterns have observed lower peak hip extension, increased anterior pelvic tilt, and lower hip extensor flexibility in older adults. Also, when compared with their younger and more flexible counterparts, older adults adopt a rigid movement strategy to prevent falling. This shouldn't surprise us. Picture in your mind a young person trying to avoid a fall or reduce the consequences of a fall. Young people tend to lower their center of gravity by bending at the knees and to make large, rapid upper-body and lower-body movements to counteract the momentum of the fall and adjust their base of support. In contrast, older individuals adopt a stiffer strategy in an attempt to brace themselves against the fall by straightening their legs and tightening their muscles in anticipation of falling. Similar differences in strategy occur once a fall has reached the point of no return. Younger persons, especially trained ones, allow themselves to fall while bending or tucking to reduce potential injury. Older persons, who lack the flexibility and confidence to do this, often adopt a stiffer, avoid-the-ground approach that leads to a higher incidence of serious and even catastrophic injuries. Flexibility training has been shown to have a positive influence on ankle, hip, and other joint ROMs, giving older adults an increased capacity to engage these joints when dealing with falling hazards and subsequent losses of balance. It's not much of a stretch (sorry, couldn't help myself) to hypothesize that increases in flexibility translate into a positive effect on falls, although no studies have examined the relationship directly.

APPLICATION POINT Interventions to increase flexibility help older adults to maintain their ability to perform ADLs and to reduce their probability of falling.

TYPES OF STRETCHING

Before we look at the effectiveness of various stretching protocols, we need to discuss the types of stretching. Just as there are two types of flexibility, there are two basic types of stretching techniques: static and dynamic. Other terms synonymous with *static stretching* are *isometric, slow,* or *controlled stretching.* Although there are a number of very exact definitions associated with the terms *static stretching* and *dynamic stretching,* it's not my intention to stretch out the discussion here. For our discussion, we will use the following definitions.

Static stretching is using little or no velocity while stretching a muscle or a group of muscles to the farthest comfortable position and maintaining that position for some time. This type of stretching can be performed either actively or passively. An active stretch is one in which a person assumes and then holds a position with no outside assistance. A passive stretch is when a person relaxes while some outside agent (a weight, a cable, or another person) provides the stretching force. In this text, when we talk about static stretching, we will discuss only active stretching.

Dynamic stretching is moving the body in a set pattern while gradually increasing ROM. There are two ways of performing dynamic stretches. The first, controlled dynamic stretching, uses flowing movements at controlled speeds. The second method, called *ballistic stretching,* uses movements such as bouncing to stretch the muscles and connective tissues beyond their normal ROM. Although considerable data indicate the success of ballistic stretching in increasing flexibility, there is even greater concern about the negative consequences of ballistic stretching, especially injury. Since aging muscle and connective tissue are more susceptible to injury, we will limit our discussion to controlled dynamic stretching.

A final stretching technique is proprioceptive neuromuscular facilitation (PNF), which can be thought of as a static stretching technique that uses your nervous system as a sort of "set-up" mechanism. PNF stretches use neuromuscular responses to prepare a muscle for stretching. There are a number of ways to incorporate neuromuscular responses into stretches. The most common is the contract–relax (CR) technique. The preparatory movement uses a maximal concentric contraction followed by an isometric contraction of the antagonist muscle, or reciprocal muscle, at the end ROM. Then there is a short time of relaxation and a passive (usually partner-assisted) stretch of the antagonist. The concept is that contracting the muscle before the stretch activates the Golgi tendon organ (GTO), which senses tension and sends an inhibitory message to the muscle's motor nerve, thereby relaxing the muscle (see figure 5.2). Since this inhibitory message lasts about 5 seconds, the stretch should occur immediately after the contraction.

A related technique is the contract–relax with agonist contract (CRAC) technique, which begins exactly as the CR technique begins. The only difference is that following the relaxation phase there is a concentric contraction of the agonist. This technique uses reciprocal inhibition to increase the stretch. Reciprocal inhibition is a reflex that begins with the muscle spindle. The reflex that is most commonly associated with the muscle spindle is the stretch reflex, in which a muscle contracts when it is stretched quickly (such as when the doctor hits your patellar tendon with a hammer). But there is another important reflex associated with the muscle spindle in which the spindle sends a second signal to the antagonist muscle to relax (see figure 5.3). CRAC stretching takes advantage of this reflex to facilitate stretching of the antagonist muscle.

The use of reciprocal inhibition is also evident in the agonist contract–relax (ACR) technique, in which the agonist muscle is contracted to send the inhibitory message to the antagonist. The

antagonist is then relaxed and a person or a device is used to increase the stretch.

A PNF stretching method that has gained considerable favor in the past decade is active assisted stretching (AAS). This technique begins with a concentric contraction of the agonist muscle to send the reciprocal inhibition reflex to the antagonist being stretched. Once your client has reached end ROM, a rope, towel, or strap is used to assist and further increase the stretch.

DO STRETCHING AND FLEXIBILITY TRAINING INCREASE FLEXIBILITY?

Remember that in this chapter I distinguish between stretching and flexibility training. First let's look at stretching and whether acute bouts of stretching increase flexibility in the short term. Acute increases in ROM and decreases in passive muscle tension are known results of stretching. This acute change has been linked to viscoelastic stress relaxation, which is the decrease in tensile stress that occurs when a body is held under tension at a fixed length. For example, if a person stretches the hamstrings for 30 seconds, for a moment afterward the muscle group is more relaxed than it was before the stretch occurred.

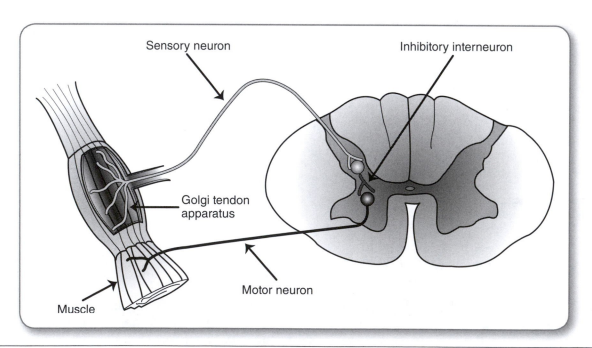

Figure 5.2 The negative (inhibitory) loop from the GTO to the spinal cord and back to the motor nerve. Notice the inhibitory interneuron that tells the motor nerve to reduce its activity and thereby reduce tension on the muscle.

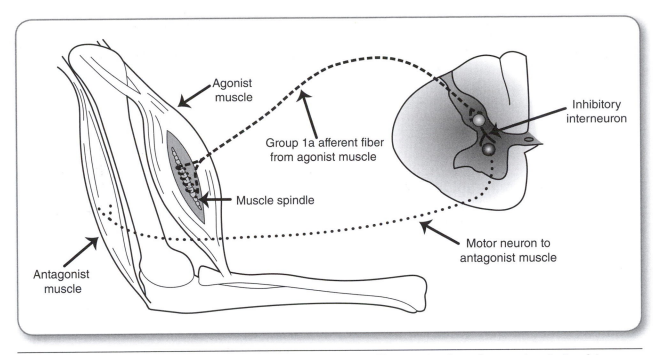

Figure 5.3   Reciprocal inhibition. Note the group 1a afferent nerve fiber running from the muscle spindle of the agonist muscle to the spinal cord (dashed line) and its connection (synapse) with the inhibitory interneuron (solid line), which in turn synapses with the motor neuron (dotted line) of the antagonist muscle. This means that contraction of the agonist muscle causes relaxation of the antagonist muscle. Also shown is the connection to the agonist motor neuron, which causes the stretch reflex.

The degree of relaxation is affected by gender, the temperature of the muscle tissue, and the muscle fiber type.

A lot of research on stretching is conducted with young subjects, but stretching in older people has also been examined, and the results are similar. Both groups demonstrate significant increases in immediate ROM as a result of stretching.

Numerous studies have reported the positive effects of *flexibility training,* whether offered alone or in concert with other modalities, on ROM in older individuals. Let's look at the results of these two approaches to training.

Flexibility Training Only

When performed alone as the only intervention in a study, both static and dynamic flexibility training improve flexibility in the majority of the muscles targeted. These results have been consistent for the ankle plantar flexors and dorsiflexors, spinal flexors and extensors, and knee flexors and extensors in programs ranging from 10 weeks to 7 months, although the results for the knee flexors and extensors are less consistent.

Because reduced ankle dorsiflexion has been linked to an increased likelihood of falling, several studies have evaluated the effects of static stretching on the ankle joint. Let's look at one of these studies and its revealing results. Johnson and coworkers (2007) examined the effects of a static stretching program on ankle dorsiflexion ROM. Women 76 to 91 years of age performed the program 5 days a week for 6 weeks. The authors reported a significant increase in ROM of 12.3° ± 4.4° and concluded that a 6-week stretching program can significantly increase ankle dorsiflexion ROM in elderly women. These results are promising!

External resistance can also be used to increase ROM in older individuals. Adding a modest weight of 1 to 3 pounds (0.45-1.35 kg) to a stretching exercise routine can produce greater improvements in ROM than unloaded stretching can produce in many joints. Additionally, the use of AAS, in which a rope or towel is used to apply external force, can significantly improve ROM in the knee extension, trunk rotation, back scratch, and sit-and-reach tests, even in a very old population.

I would be remiss if I left this topic without mentioning two of the oldest and most respected methods of increasing flexibility, yoga and tai chi. Iyengar yoga has been shown to increase peak hip extension in older adults, and it can also reduce pain intensity, functional disability, and pain medication usage in people with chronic low back pain. Tai chi repeatedly has been shown to improve spinal ROM and lower-body flexibility in older adults.

> **APPLICATION POINT** Flexibility training alone, without the addition of any other training modalities, can improve ROM and reduce passive resistance.

Flexibility Training and Other Modalities

We have seen that flexibility training often plays Robin to the Batman of other training modalities. The good news is that pairing flexibility training with strength and aerobic training consistently increases ROM in most joints. However, combining these modalities may not be without consequence, since combining flexibility training with other modalities can result in interference effects that reduce the effectiveness of the flexibility training component. Aquatic exercise programs commonly incorporate a flexibility component into each workout. These programs have been shown to increase flexibility significantly in healthy older persons. Additionally, several studies have examined the effects of aquatic training on flexibility of patients with arthritis and have observed positive results.

> **APPLICATION POINT** Flexibility can be improved even by programs that combine flexibility training with other training modalities; however, mixed programs may be less effective than programs concentrating solely on flexibility.

STRETCHING, FLEXIBILITY TRAINING, AND INJURY PREVENTION

It is not clear whether stretching can prevent injuries. Early review papers concluded that acute stretching before training or exercise does not reduce the incidence of injury; however, it has been suggested that engaging in flexibility training over an extended time might have a positive effect on injury prevention. A review article by Woods and coworkers (Woods et al., 2007) questioned the conclusions made in the earlier reviews. These authors argued that stretching can provide protection against injury if it is

- tailored to the needs of the individual,
- completed within 15 minutes of activity,
- done consistently and with proper form,
- accompanied by a warm-up that produces mild sweating, and
- involves three 30-second stretches targeting each muscle group at least once per week.

Thus, if long-term changes in muscle length, connective tissue compliance, and neuromuscular response are desired, regular flexibility training rather than acute stretching is the answer.

> **APPLICATION POINT** Regular flexibility training rather than acute stretching leads to long-term changes, including structural changes in muscle and connective tissue, that can protect against injury.

Numerous studies have examined the possibility of using stretching to reduce the delayed-onset muscle soreness (DOMS) that occurs following exercise or other physical activity. While a few studies have shown that stretching can reduce DOMS, the majority of the studies demonstrated little or no positive effect on DOMS.

STRETCHING, FLEXIBILITY TRAINING, AND PERFORMANCE

Does stretching affect performance? By performance, I mean the ability to perform activities, whether they are sport-related or everyday activities involving jumping, pushing, lifting, or walking. In general, the studies with younger men and women show that an acute bout of stretching either does not affect or reduces both power and strength. Results with older persons show the same trend—there is no improvement in gait performance and there is a significant decline in strength following acute stretching.

Studies examining the ability of *flexibility training* to increase muscular performance have produced more positive results, especially in older persons. In a review article looking at nine studies on the effects of flexibility training on performance, Ian Shrier (2004) noted that seven of the studies reported positive responses and none reported negative effects on performance. And the results for older persons are equally impressive.

As you read earlier in this chapter, there is an undeniable correlation between flexibility and ADL performance and fall prevention. However, the number of studies that have examined flexibility training as an independent intervention for successful aging is nominal. Those that have examined flexibility training with older persons have shown that flexibility training improves gait speed, the ability to rise from a chair, lower-body power, object transfer, and cardiovascular performance. Although yoga is more than a simple stretching modality, its effect on flexibility is paramount. Studies examining yoga performed by older persons have shown positive results for both gait and quality of life.

PRACTICAL ASPECTS OF FLEXIBILITY TRAINING

Now that we have examined the benefits of flexibility training, let's answer two fundamental questions: "What is the best way to stretch?" and "How long should a stretch be held?" These questions can't be answered in isolation since the type of stretch dictates the duration for which it is held. So let's look at each question separately and then summarize how the two parameters interact.

What Is the Best Way to Stretch?

Most of the studies comparing static, ballistic, and PNF stretching have reported greater increases in ROM with PNF stretching than with static or ballistic stretching. They have also reported that the increase in ROM resulting from PNF stretching lasts for a longer time. When PNF stretching is used during flexibility training, the greatest improvements occur with techniques incorporating reciprocal inhibition, such as ACR and CRAC. For that reason, the exercise section at the end of this chapter provides many stretches using PNF or AAS. However, care should be taken when applying PNF techniques to older individuals due to age-related alterations in muscle elasticity. This is especially true when partner stretches are used. I advise using the rope or towel methods provided in this chapter since they allow clients to dictate their end ROM based on their personal perception. This carries a much lower probability of acute injury than assisted methods in which you attempt to stretch the client using feedback as you go. Remember that feedback is provided only after discomfort has been felt and the feeling can be relayed to you.

How Long Should a Stretch Be Held?

The question that most of us hear when we talk to our patients about stretching is, "How long should I hold a stretch?" The answer to this question, like the answers to most questions, is not as simple as it seems. The answer depends on two factors: the type of stretch employed and the age of the client. Since these two factors interact with each other, my response to the question includes both factors. With regard to static stretching, the old adage of "Longer is better" appears to need some adjustment for age. In younger persons 30 seconds seems to be optimal, and prolonging the stretch for 60 seconds produces no additional benefit. In older individuals, however, this is not the case. Extending a static stretch from 15 or 30 seconds to 60 seconds during a flexibility training program not only increases improvements in ROM but also increases the length of time those improvements last.

When we examine PNF stretches, especially those that use reciprocal inhibition, it appears advantageous to use shorter durations and per-form a number of repetitions. This is due to the limited amount of time, approximately 30 milliseconds, that reciprocal inhibition lasts. However, in the case of longer contractions, this duration may be prolonged. It has been shown that prolonging a PNF hamstring stretch for 10 rather than 5 seconds produces significantly better results, although some practitioners have suggested limiting the duration of active isolated stretches to 2 or 3 seconds.

TESTING FLEXIBILITY

As you are no doubt aware, before you can give a true exercise prescription, you must diagnose your client's needs. This section provides four tests to evaluate flexibility: the chair sit-and-reach test, the back scratch test, the modified trunk rotation test, and the ankle flexibility test. These tests evaluate flexibility of the hamstrings, shoulder, trunk, and ankle, respectively.

Comparing your client's test results to age- and gender-specific norms for older adults (see the appendix, p. 299) allows you to establish the need for flexibility training at each joint. Also, remember to ask the client what types of movements are difficult to do. For example, clients who have trouble bending over to reach things on the floor or to put on their shoes may have ROM limitations in their back and hamstrings. On the other hand, if transfer of objects from one counter to another is the problem, the client may be experiencing reduced trunk flexibility. Remember that losses in flexibility most likely will not be consistent across all joints, so assessment for a targeted training prescription is imperative.

Chair Sit-and-Reach Test

The chair sit-and-reach test (figure 5.4) is an accurate and reliable modification of the standard sit-and-reach test and is a safe and well-accepted method for measuring flexibility of the hamstrings and lower back in older adults (Jones, Rikli, Max, & Noffal, 1998). The client performs the test while seated in a straight-back chair with a seat height of about 17 inches (43 cm). Unlike in the original test, your client doesn't have to go to the floor to be assessed. You should record the distance reached along a ruler of at least 18 inches (45.7 cm) in length centered on the client's big toe. Normative values for this test are taken from a study by Rikli and Jones (1999b).

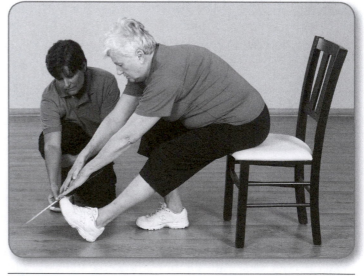

Figure 5.4 The chair sit-and-reach test evaluates flexibility in the low back and hamstrings.

Equipment Needed

• A standard straight-back chair with a seat height of 17 inches (43 cm)

- A ruler of sufficient length (about 18 in. or 45.7 cm) to measure the client's reach

Protocol

- Have the client sit on the chair with the front edge of the chair seat in the crease between the lower leg and the buttocks.
- Demonstrate the proper position and form to be used during the testing.
- Ask the client to keep the left leg bent with the foot flat on the floor and extend the right leg completely so that the knee is straight and the heel is in contact with the floor with the ankle flexed to 90°.
- Have the client place the dominant hand on top of the nondominant hand and with a straight arm and extended fingers lean as far forward as possible, sliding both hands down the ruler while keeping the head up and the spine as straight as possible.
- The client should reach with the fingertips and attempt to reach past the toe.
- Remind the client to exhale during the attempt, to move slowly, and to never bounce into the stretch.
- The knee must remain straight throughout the test; if the knee bends, ask the client to sit back until the knee is straight.
- For a reach to be counted, it must be maintained for at least 2 seconds.
- The client should perform two practice trials followed by two test trials.
- Repeat for the left leg.
- Record the reach distance from the fingertips to the toe. Give a negative or minus score if the reach does not pass the toe and a positive or plus score if the reach passes the toe. Take the best score.

▦ Back Scratch Test ▦

Shoulder flexibility is one of the flexibility measures displaying the closest association with the ability to perform IADLs. The back scratch test (see figure 5.5) is a simple test that uses the distance a person can reach down the back as an assessment of shoulder flexibility. The only measuring device used is an 18-inch (45.7 cm) ruler.

Equipment Needed

- A ruler of sufficient length to measure the client's reach (approximately 18 in. or 45.7 cm)

Protocol

- Demonstrate this test before having the client begin.
- Begin with the client standing with the back straight.
- Have the client reach behind with the right hand and place it over the right shoulder with the palm facing the back. Then have the client reach behind with the left hand and place it on the lower back with the palm facing away from the back.

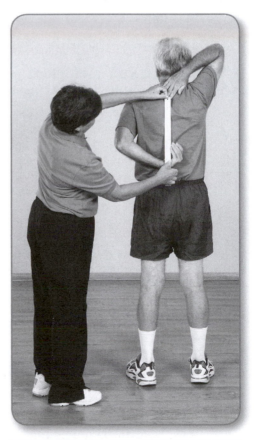

Figure 5.5 The back scratch test assesses shoulder flexibility.

- The client should attempt to touch or overlap the fingers of each hand by reaching as far as possible along the spine.
- For a reach to be counted, it must be maintained for at least 2 seconds.
- The client should perform two practice trials followed by two test trials.
- Repeat the test for the left side switching hand positions.
- Use the 18-inch (45.7 cm) ruler to record reach distance. Assign a minus score when the fingers don't touch and a plus score when the fingers overlap. Use the best score.

Modified Trunk Rotation Test

This test is a modified version of the test designed by Hoeger (1998) to measure the rotational flexibility of the trunk. This modified version (see figure 5.6) is more suitable for older persons because it involves forward rather than backward full-body rotation. I have included this test since it assesses the core muscles that are so important for the transfer of strength and power from the lower body to the upper body in most daily activities.

Equipment Needed

- A yardstick or meterstick
- Velcro or tape to hold the measuring stick to the wall
- Tape or some type of marker to indicate foot position

Protocol

- Demonstrate the proper position and form before the test begins.
- Have the client start the test standing with the shoulders perpendicular to the wall. The client's toes should touch a vertical tape line that is aligned with the 12-inch mark on a yardstick (30.5 cm mark on a meter stick) mounted horizontally to the wall (by masking tape or Velcro) at the height of the client's shoulders.

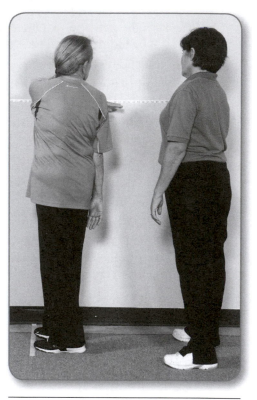

Figure 5.6 The modified trunk rotation test assesses core ROM.

- Have the client rotate forward and reach as far along the measuring stick as possible.
- Evaluate the client's performance by measuring how far the client is able to extend the fingertips along the measuring stick. The distance reached is relative to the 12-inch (30.5 cm) mark on the measuring stick. So if the client reaches the 23-inch (58.4 cm) mark, the reach is 23 inches minus 12 inches, which equals 11 inches. For metric, it would be 58.4 centimeters minus 30.5 centimeters, which equals 27.9 centimeters.
- The client should perform three trials on each side. Use the best score for the analysis.

Ankle Flexibility Testing

For assessing dorsiflexion and plantar flexion, I have provided tests that use a standard goniometer (see figure 5.7). While there are no norms for older clients performing these tests, we can use norms produced using more sophisticated testing techniques to provide reasonable assessments of flexibility. Given the important contribution of ankle ROM to independence, gait, and dynamic balance, I felt that failure to provide norms for flexibil-

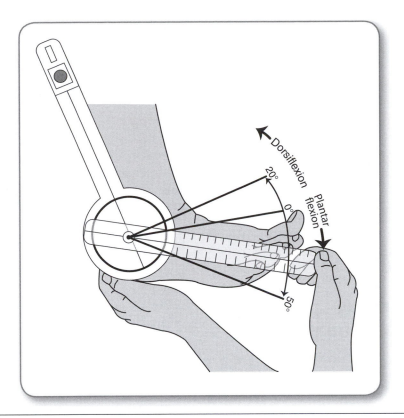

Figure 5.7   Testing for plantar flexion and dorsiflexion.

ity of this joint would severely limit the usefulness of its assessment. The norms I have extrapolated for these tests are presented in the appendix (p. 299).

Equipment Needed

- A chair or training table
- A goniometer

Protocol

- Start with your client sitting on a tall chair or the end of a training table. The feet should be at least 1 foot (0.3 m) off the ground.
- Kneel on the side you intend to measure and use your goniometer to make sure the client's knee is at 90°. This is important since one of the muscles that crosses the ankle, the gastrocnemius, also crosses the knee joint.
- While making sure that the client maintains the 90° angle at the knee, align your goniometer with the outside of the ankle joint (the lateral aspect of the malleolus for you biomechanists!). One arm of the goniometer should be lined up with the middle of the fibula (feel for it) and the other should be lined up with the outside of the foot just below the toe joint.
- Ask the client to dorsiflex (point toward the sky with the toes) and take your dorsiflexion measurement. Then ask the client to point the toes toward an imaginary spot on the floor 10 feet (3 m) behind the chair and take your plantar flexion measurement.
- Make three measurements on each side to ensure consistency and use the best score for the analysis.

FLEXIBILITY PROGRAM DESIGN

It is clear that flexibility training can help your clients maintain their ability to function independently and to prevent injuries, including those due to falls. So how should you incorporate flexibility training into a client's overall exercise program? The simple answer is that you should diagnose the client's needs using the tests provided in this chapter, apply a targeted program, incorporate the training into a logical pattern of work and recovery, provide motor training for transfer to everyday tasks, and evaluate the client's progress to make necessary changes in order to maximize gains.

Flexibility Training and Other Exercise Modalities

One question that might be on your mind is how to combine flexibility training with other training modalities. First of all, you do not need to worry about major interference effects, especially when working with your older clients. Problems like reduced explosive power when jumping or performing a maximal lift, while important to athletes, are of minimal importance to your older clients, especially once their training has increased their physical reserves. Second, you don't have to decide what other modalities to combine with the flexibility training; your diagnostic analysis will tell you what modalities should predominate in any training cycle. For example, low scores on the 30-second chair stand or modified ramp power tests would dictate that strength and power training should be the predominant factor in the training cycle, while low scores on the 6-minute walk test point to the need for cardiovascular training. Of course, flexibility training can be the major target of a training cycle if the client's scores on the chair sit-and-reach, back scratch, or modified trunk rotation tests are the client's lowest ones. Regardless of the dominant need revealed by the diagnostic battery, flexibility training should always make up some part of your exercise prescription. And third, many training modalities, such as tai chi and yoga, can address multiple needs, although their effects may not be as impressive as those produced by programs with a specific targeted goal. In part III of this book, we will discuss how to blend modalities to maximize

benefits and explain how flexibility can be added as the major ingredient, or spice, to create the most effective exercise prescription.

Periodizing Flexibility Training

As you will learn in chapter 9, training cycles last 4 to 8 weeks depending on the targeted outcome. These cycles are modulated by changes in training intensity and volume. Additionally, they end with reduced periods of activity, called *tapers*, that maximize the fitness benefits of the training period. Although you may feel that stretching is a low-intensity exercise, for many of your clients it can be extremely challenging, even more so than other exercises such as walking or calisthenics that they perform on a more regular basis. The good news is that flexibility training can be periodized during a cycle targeting flexibility, during a cycle targeting another goal such as muscular strength or cardiovascular conditioning, or during a taper. Incorporating flexibility training is especially effortless during the translational tapers presented in this text since these tapers feature ADL-specific exercises that can be done with increasing ROM as a primary goal. You will see how simple it is to incorporate flexibility into both the training and translational periods when you read part III, but for now let me give you some concrete examples of periodized flexibility training.

Applying periodized flexibility training during a cycle that has increased flexibility as its primary objective might look like this: Low-intensity, low-volume flexibility training slowly progresses across the first week. Alternating increases in volume (the number of stretches and the frequency of training) and intensity (the difficulty of the stretch and the amount of ROM targeted) are added across the next week and a half. A decline in volume with increasing intensity defines the last part of the third week and the beginning of the fourth week, and a continued decline in both parameters occurs during the taper at the end of the fourth week.

When a training cycle has strength or cardiovascular training as a primary goal, flexibility training can be added in a complementary pattern, increasing in intensity and volume on days when the primary goal is showing a decline in intensity and volume, and vice versa. Finally, the recovery or translational cycle can use motor learning exercises that simulate real-life ADL activities designed to increase ROM.

Translational Cycles and Flexibility

As their name indicates, translational cycles translate improvements in a particular physical parameter into meaningful changes in ADL and IADL performance. They accomplish this by using motor pattern training exercises that are highly dependent on the particular physical parameter. In other words, if a training cycle has as a primary goal of increasing flexibility, then translational exercises should be prescribed that require clients to reach for objects beyond their normal ROM or mobility drills that concentrate on increasing stride length. Additionally, if flexibility is a secondary goal of the training cycle, the motor training pattern should incorporate an aspect that addresses flexibility. For example, if the primary goal is strength, activities such as lifting weighted objects or body weight can include extending the ROM of the operational joints. Picture moving a pot from a somewhat uncomfortably high or low shelf or rising from a bed or chair of lower-than-normal height. A word to the wise, however—approach these combined skills cautiously, using gradual progressions, and remember that adding a reaching challenge to a lifting challenge creates a skill that may be considerably more intense than perceived. Keep in mind the old adage about the whole being greater than the sum of its parts.

FLEXIBILITY TRAINING EXERCISES

Now that I have covered the rationale for flexibility training and you have learned how to incorporate flexibility training into an overall training program, let's look at exercises that you can incorporate into a flexibility training cycle for your client. The exercises presented in this section provide a number of options for increasing joint ROMs. Improving the ROM of joints and the elasticity of muscles and tendons will most likely have a positive effect on ADL performance, mobility, and fall prevention. These exercises can be incorporated into training cycles as well as translational cycles, and flexibility may become the principal goal of a training cycle if the results of your diagnostic tests indicate that it should be so.

Like the exercises in the resistance training chapter (chapter 7), the exercises in this chapter are organized by the muscles and joints they target. When possible, the primary exercise presented for a given joint or muscle involves PNF stretching or AAS. Other stretches, including static stretches and stretches performed in the pool, are presented as variations.

You will recall that AAS is a type of PNF stretching in which your client begins each exercise by using the muscle on one side of a joint to stretch the muscle on the other side of that joint. AAS tells the muscle being stretched to relax via reciprocal inhibition. Once the active portion of the stretch is completed, your client uses a hand, a towel, or a rope to extend the stretch even further. We have shown the positive effect of these stretches on ADL performance and flexibility in our laboratory.

For all AAS, the duration of the stretch is between 2 to 3 seconds and increases in ROM come from completing multiple repetitions. The next logical question is how many. If your client is beginning a flexibility training program dictated by a diagnostic profile, I suggest beginning with two or three repetitions per side and increasing to about ten repetitions during the first 6 weeks of the 8-week training cycle. During the last 2 weeks you can then provide a taper and begin to incorporate translational drills that increase stride length and step height to allow your client's increases in flexibility to be "translated" into patterns used in daily activities. These drills are presented in chapter 10 and on the accompanying DVD. For a general program that accompanies other training modalities (the Robin program!), 3 to 5 repetitions per side is sufficient.

If you are using static stretches, the minimum duration of the stretch should be 20 to 30 seconds; however, extending the stretch to 60 seconds has been shown to have greater benefits in older persons. Once again, 3 to 5 repetitions seem to be optimal.

Regardless of the technique you use, remember to target all the important joints and train for symmetry (in other words, always train both sides). Remember, however, that we're using a diagnosis–prescription model here, so if a particular joint or side needs more attention, provide it, and symmetry will be improved.

Safety Precautions for Active Assisted Stretching

Before we look at the various flexibility exercises, let's consider the basic safety precautions for stretching:

→ Do not allow your client to begin stretching before the tissues are warmed up. Remember that warm muscle, like warm taffy, has a higher level of compliance.

→ Remember that your older clients, especially women older than 65 and men older than 80, may have osteopenia (preliminary losses in bone strength) or even osteoporosis (high levels of bone loss), in which case the application of any stretching, especially active partner-assisted or self-assisted stretching, should be done with extreme caution.

→ If your client has a hip replacement, do not use stretches that require the leg to cross the midline of the body, and do not allow the hip joint to be brought beyond a right angle.

→ Caution your client to avoid pain. Stretching is a progressive process and pain should never be part of that process.

→ Never allow your client to use ballistic movements or momentum to increase the end point of the stretch. These actions can result in microscopic or even gross muscle damage. Soreness experienced the day after stretching is most likely due to DOMS and should be dealt with using the typical strategy of rest, ice, compression, and elevation. But remember what your grandmother told you: An ounce of prevention is worth a pound of cure.

→ Remind your client to exhale during the stretch and to never hold the breath. Especially for older persons, stretching may require significant levels of muscle tension and can result in extreme changes in blood pressure if the breath is held.

The instructions for the following exercises speak directly to the client. You may read the instructions to your client if desired.

Lower-Body Stretches 83

Hip and Thigh 83

    Quadriceps Stretches 83

    Hamstring Stretches 84

    Leg Adductor Stretches 85

    Leg Abductor Stretches 86

    Hip Extensor Stretches 87

Lower Leg 88

    Calf Stretches 88

    Dorsiflexor Stretches 89

Upper-Body Stretches 91

Neck 91

    Forward, Backward, and Side Stretches 91

Shoulder 92

    Rotator Cuff Stretches 92

    Internal Rotator Stretches 92

    External Rotator Stretches 93

    Anterior Rotator Stretches 93

    Downward Rotator Stretches 94

Core Stretches 96

Low Back, Sides, and Abdominal Muscles 96

    Low Back Stretches 96

    Stretches for the Obliques and Other Abdominal Muscles 97

LOWER-BODY STRETCHES
HIP AND THIGH
Quadriceps Stretches

Application   The quadriceps muscles make up the largest muscle group of the lower body. They are responsible for locomotion, lifting objects, rising from a chair, and a myriad of other activities. Quadriceps flexibility contributes to hip ROM, and decreases in hip ROM are associated with reduced stride length and gait speed and increased likelihood of falling.

Position   Stand up straight behind a sturdy chair with the knees slightly bent and the feet hip-width apart. Hold onto the back of the chair for support and place a loop fashioned at one end of a rope or towel around the right ankle. Grasp the free end with the other hand.

Execution   Start the *active assisted standing quadriceps stretch* by bending the right knee and bringing the right foot toward the buttocks without the help of a towel or rope. This contraction of the hamstrings initiates the reciprocal inhibition of the quadriceps. Then assist the stretch by using the towel or rope to pull the foot further upward (see figure 5.8).

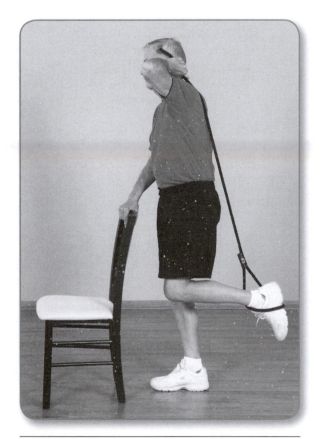

Figure 5.8   Active assisted standing quadriceps stretch.

Variations

- The active assisted standing quadriceps stretch can be performed while lying on one side to create a *side-lying quadriceps stretch*. The procedure of first contracting the hamstrings and then aiding the stretch with a rope or towel is the same.

- A static version of this stretch that does not use a rope or towel can be performed in these same standing and lying positions. In the static quadriceps stretch, there is no emphasis on using the agonist muscle to stretch the antagonist muscle, as there is with the active assisted stretch.

- The standing versions of the stretch can be performed in the pool with or without using the wall for support.

Safety   The general rules governing safety during stretching (presented earlier) should be followed at all times. In addition, during the standing stretch you must be careful to maintain balance throughout the stretch. It is better to sacrifice those last few degrees of motion than to experience a fall and its consequences. Finally, remember that these stretches target the quadriceps group, and so using trunk flexion or extension to increase the degree of stretch does little to increase hip ROM and may cause acute or chronic back injury.

Hamstring Stretches

Application   Hamstring stretches hold an important place in the hearts of all athletes, trainers, and therapists. As the antagonist muscles to the quadriceps, the hamstrings are in a unique position for control and potential damage. In fact, it has been argued that increasing the flexibility of the hamstrings can increase stride length and gait speed by reducing coactivation.

Position   For the *active assisted seated hamstring stretch,* sit up straight in a chair and place both feet flat on the floor. Place the middle of a towel or rope around the instep of one foot and extend that leg straight out so the heel is on the floor and the toe is pointed toward the ceiling (see figure 5.9). Keep the other knee bent with the feet on the floor and grasp the ends of the rope or towel with both hands.

Execution   Initiate the stretch by slowly leaning forward as far as feels comfortable. Then assist the stretch by pulling on the rope or towel. Relax and return to the upright sitting position. Aim for a deeper stretch with each repetition.

Variations   Given the attention the hamstrings have received in the literature, it's no surprise that there are a number of variations for us to examine.

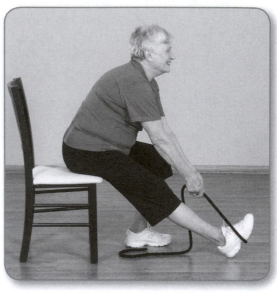

Figure 5.9   Active assisted seated hamstring stretch.

- The *active assisted seated hamstring stretch* can be performed while seated on the floor.
- When this stretch is performed as a static stretch, without the use of a stretching aid, it becomes the famous *hurdler's stretch.*
- A stretch that isolates the hamstrings to a greater extent is the *lying leg extension.* To perform this exercise, lie down on your back with the right leg bent and the right foot flat on the floor. Bend the left leg at the knee and bring it in toward the chest. Loop a towel or rope over the left foot and grasp the ends of the towel or rope with both hands. Fully extend the left leg and initiate the stretch by lifting the left leg as far as possible. Assist the stretch by pulling on the towel or rope. Then repeat the stretch on the opposite side. Keep the back flat on the floor throughout the stretch. This exercise can also be done as a static stretch while lying on the floor.
- The leg extension stretch can also be performed while your client stands with his or her back to the wall, holding onto the overflow or side. The stretch can be performed without assistance, or a flotation device may be used to aid the stretch.

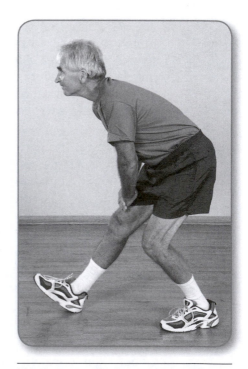

Figure 5.10   The bent-over hamstring stretch is a variation of the standing hamstring stretch.

- Another variation is a more subtle *bent-over hamstring stretch* (see figure 5.10). Assume the position shown in figure 5.10. Rest the hands on the thighs and bend at the waist. While keeping the forward leg extended and bending the rear leg, let the pelvis slip back into a somewhat seated position.

Leg Adductor Stretches

Application The capacity to adjust lateral position when navigating around an object or when recovering from a trip is an important factor in maintaining independence and preventing fall-related injuries. Increasing leg adductor flexibility enhances a person's ability to make lateral movements.

Position The *active assisted leg adductor stretch* is an active assisted stretch. Lie on your back with the right leg bent and the right foot flat on the floor. This is the beginning position that allows you to stabilize your body and set the rope or towel properly. Bend the left leg at the knee and bring it in toward the chest. Place a loop fashioned at one end of a rope or towel over the left foot, wrap the rope or towel around the inside of the ankle, and grasp the other end with the left hand.

Execution Extend the left leg so that it is lying straight on the floor. The right leg may be bent with the sole of the foot on the floor or be extended straight out as shown in figure 5.11. Many clients will find it more comfortable to have both legs straight. Keeping the left knee straight, initiate the stretch by sliding the left leg along the floor in an outward arc as far as feels comfortable. Assist the stretch by pulling on the rope and hold the stretch for 2 to 3 seconds. Relax by returning the leg to the starting position. Then repeat the movement, increasing the arc for a deeper stretch with each repetition. Repeat this stretch for the opposite side.

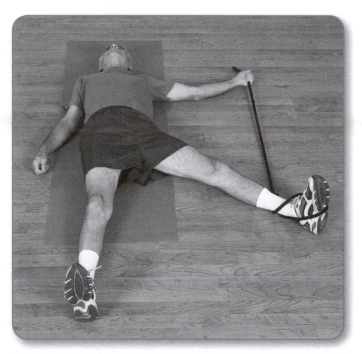

Figure 5.11 Active assisted leg adductor stretch.

Variations

- One of the most common static adductor stretches is the *side lunge*. Stand with the feet about twice shoulder-width apart. Keeping one leg straight with the toes facing forward, bend the other leg, squatting down until the stretch is felt along the inner thigh. The side lunge can also be performed on a support surface such as a stability ball or while holding onto the back of a chair for support. When using the stability ball, place it in front of you so that you can extend your arms forward and use the ball to maintain your balance as you lunge to the side. Obviously the ball will roll slightly to accommodate the shift in your upper-body position as you perform the exercise.
- The leg adductors can also be stretched with one of two techniques used to perform the *butterfly stretch*. One technique is done while sitting on the floor and the other is

done while lying on the floor. Begin the sitting stretch, often called the *seated lotus,* with the knees bent and the soles of the feet touching each other. Grasp the ankles to hold the feet together and then apply pressure to the inner thighs and push the knees toward the floor. Hold the stretch for 30 to 60 seconds and then return the knees to the starting position. For the lying stretch, called the *back lotus,* lie on your back with the knees bent and the soles of the feet together. Slowly lower both knees toward the floor to begin the stretch. Increase the ROM of the stretch by pushing downward on the inner thighs.

- The adductors can also be stretched in the pool. In this case the stairs, an ankle flotation device, or a noodle can be used to assist in the lifting motion of the leg.

Leg Abductor Stretches

Application   Leg abductor ROM can affect the length of an older person's lateral stepping and ability to crossover step. Since recovery from a stumble often requires stepping and since most falls that result in hip fracture occur to the side and back, the flexibility of the leg abductors should be considered an important factor when training older clients.

Position   Start by lying on your back with the right leg extended. Bend the left leg at the knee and bring it up toward the chest. Place a loop fashioned at one end of a rope or towel over the left foot, wrap the rope or towel around the outside of the ankle, grasp the other end with the right hand, and straighten the left leg while adjusting the length of the towel or rope (see figure 5.12).

Execution   Keeping the back flat on the floor, cross the left leg across the right leg as far as feels comfortable and then assist the stretch by pulling on the rope. Hold the stretch for 2 to 3 seconds. Relax by returning the leg to the starting position. Repeat the movement, increasing the arc for a deeper stretch with each repetition. Then repeat the stretch for the opposite side.

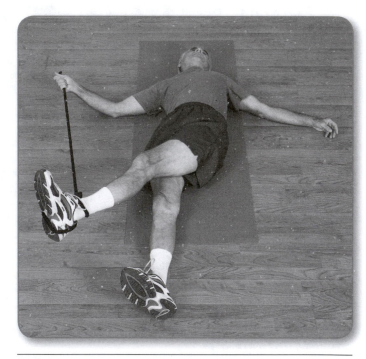

Figure 5.12   Active assisted leg abductor stretch.

Variations

- The same stretch can be performed as a static stretch on land.
- The shoulder–hip counterrotation stretch can be used in the pool. Begin by standing in water that is chest deep to shoulder deep and lean against the wall of the pool to increase stability. Cross the leg closest to the wall across the midline of the body, being sure that the hips rotate away from the wall. At the same time lean and rotate the upper body toward the pool wall. Repeat the stretch on the other side. You should feel the stretch in the hip and waist.

Safety   From a safety point of view, these exercises offer little concern. However, they may not be appropriate if you have had a hip replacement. Also, forcing a stretch beyond ROM can cause a rotation at the waist that may place undue stresses on the lower back.

Hip Extensor Stretches

Low flexibility in the hip extensors can disrupt gait and balance. The stretches described here are designed to increase flexibility in the gluteal muscles. These muscles make up one of the largest muscle groups in the body.

Position   Begin the *seated gluteal stretch* in a seated upright position. First, extend the left leg and flex the right leg, bringing it up toward the chest. Grab the right ankle with the left hand and block the right leg with the right forearm and elbow (see figure 5.13).

Execution   Pull the right foot toward the left shoulder and hold for 30 to 60 seconds. Change sides and repeat the exercise.

Variations

- The seated gluteal stretch can also be performed while in a lying position or while seated in a chair (see figure 5.14).
- One of the most common gluteal stretches and a stretch that also works the oblique muscles is the *seated twist*. To perform the stretch, sit on the floor with the left leg extended forward. Bend the right leg and place the right foot outside the left knee.

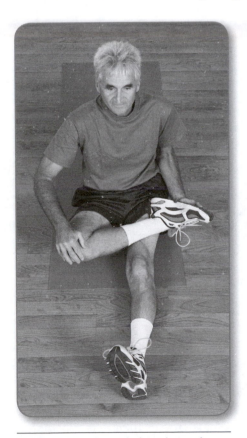

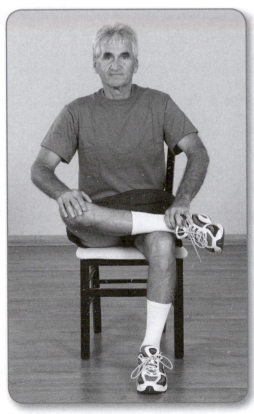

Figure 5.13   Seated gluteal stretch.

Figure 5.14   Seated gluteal stretch performed in an armless chair.

Using the right arm for support, rotate the upper body to the right, using the left hand or elbow to increase the stretch. Then perform the stretch on the other side.

- A variation that can be used in the pool is the *hip flexion gluteal stretch*. Perform the exercise in water that is chest to shoulder deep and hold onto the overflow gutter with one hand. Bring the knee that is farthest from the wall up toward the chest and use the hand farthest from the wall to grab the knee. Push the knee across the body and hold the stretch before returning to the starting position. Then turn around and repeat the stretch on the other leg.

Safety   The gluteal muscles are very large muscles and are an integral part of the kinetic chain that forms a direct link with the musculature of the lower back. It should go without saying that pushing these stretches beyond your comfort zone can cause connective tissue and muscle damage or injuries anywhere along that kinetic chain.

LOWER LEG

Calf Stretches

Application   There is a direct relationship between ankle flexibility and gait speed and physical activity. Additionally, the Achilles tendon is highly susceptible to injury, especially injury due to explosive movements made by athletes. It is also especially prone to injury due to the connective tissue changes that occur with age.

Position   The *active assisted seated calf stretch* is the active assisted stretch that targets the gastrocnemius and soleus muscles. To perform the stretch, sit up straight with the left leg fully extended forward and the left heel in contact with the floor. The right leg should be bent at the knee with the right foot flat on the floor. Place the middle of a rope or towel around the ball of the foot and grasp the ends with both hands (see figure 5.15).

Execution   Initiate the movement by pointing the toes of the foot toward the shin. Assist the stretch by pulling on the rope or towel and hold the stretch for 2 to 3 seconds. Then switch positions and repeat this stretch on the opposite side.

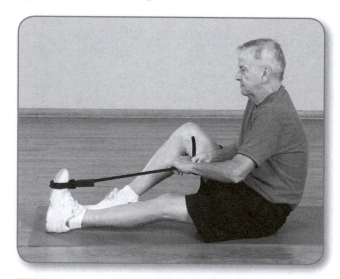

Figure 5.15   The active assisted seated calf stretch.

Variations   The *standing calf stretch* is one of the best known calf stretches, especially among runners. To begin the stretch, stand facing a wall or other stable object and place the hands on the wall at a height slightly above shoulder level and a width slightly wider than shoulder width. Bring the right foot back until it is difficult to keep it on the ground. Keeping the rear heel on the ground, push forward slowly, controlling the tension with the arms (see figure 5.16*a*). Since the gastrocnemius crosses the knee and ankle joints, straightening the knee stretches the gastrocnemius. If the knee is bent, however, the soleus will be the target of the stretch (see figure 5.16*b*).

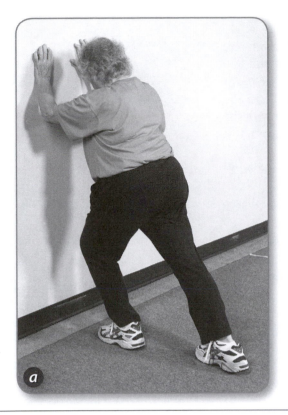 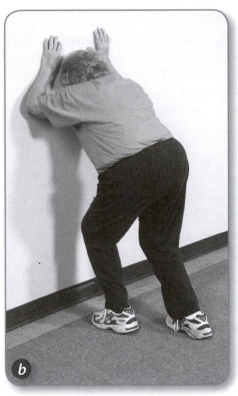

Figure 5.16   Standing calf stretch with *(a)* straight leg to target the gastrocnemius muscle and *(b)* bent knee to target the soleus muscle.

Dorsiflexor Stretches

Application   Dorsiflexion ROM is an important factor affecting gait and stair descent in older persons. It is a major predictor of disability in this population; fortunately, it can be improved through flexibility training.

Position   The *active assisted dorsiflexor stretch* presented here begins with sitting upright in a chair or on the floor with one leg crossed over the opposite knee. Grasp the ankle with one hand and the underside of the toes and ball of the foot with the other (see figure 5.17).

Execution   To start the action, exhale and pull the toes toward the shin (extend the toes). Hold the stretch and then relax. The stretch should be felt in the sole of the raised foot. From the same position, switch the grip to the top of the foot and push the toes toward the calf to stretch the shin muscles.

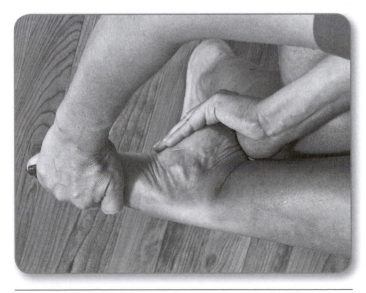

Figure 5.17   Active assisted dorsiflexor stretch.

Variations

- One of the simplest variations of the dorsiflexor stretch is a *full plantar flexion* or toe point.
- A second alternative is a *standing dorsiflexor stretch.* To perform the stretch, stand with the leg to be stretched positioned backward with the top of the foot against the floor (see figure 5.18). Stretch the dorsiflexors by pressing the front of the foot closer to the floor. The stretch should be felt across the front of the foot and shin.
- The *standing quadriceps stretch* also applies a stretch on the dorsiflexors.

Safety   The concern for injuries when using these stretches is first and foremost related to the small size of the muscles. Care should be taken, especially during the standing dorsiflexor stretch, to not injure this muscle group.

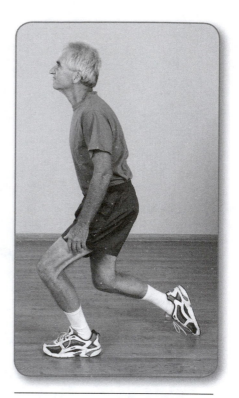

Figure 5.18   A standing dorsiflexor stretch.

UPPER-BODY STRETCHES
NECK

Forward, Backward, and Side Stretches

Application   The neck musculature is often tight and sore due to the accumulation of both physical and psychological stresses. These muscles have enough work to do holding the combined masses of the head and brain in a position that is well forward of their own location. Add in the fact that people today spend hours in front of computers, books, and other media in an even greater head-forward position and that these media usually create intellectual and psychological stresses that further tighten these muscle groups, and you have a clear argument for the need to stretch these muscles. If you need a more practical example of the benefits of neck flexibility, think about turning to look over your shoulder when you're backing up the car!

Position   Begin with the head in a neutral position. This position is often described as having a string attached to the middle of the top of the head so the head is hanging in balance like a plumb bob.

Execution   Start this series of exercises by lowering the chin to the chest to stretch the back of the neck (see figure 5.19*a*). Then point the chin toward the ceiling, stretching the muscles on the front of the neck (see figure 5.19*b*). Next, tip the head to one side and attempt to touch the ear to the shoulder. Then switch to the other side, so that both sides of the neck are stretched (see figure 5.19*c*). These exercises stretch the neck muscles in the major planes of motion. Because these are static stretches they should be held for 30 to 60 seconds.

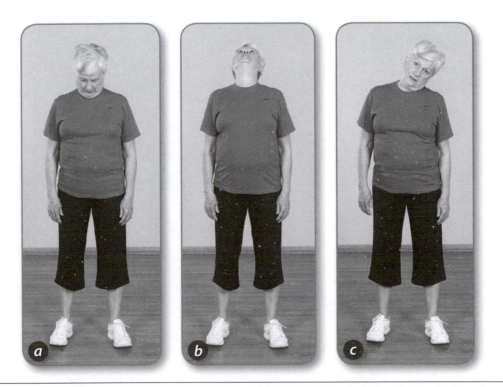

Figure 5.19   The *(a)* forward, *(b)* backward, and *(c)* side positions for stretching the neck musculature.

Variations

- The neck stretches can be performed in the pool at any water level.
- The neck stretches can be performed as PNF stretches by pushing the head against the hands in each plane of action and using controlled pressure to aid the stretch.

Safety   The major safety consideration when stretching the neck musculature is to squelch the temptation to rotate the head around the neck since doing so increases the potential for injuries to the cervical spine. Also remember that this is the neck we're working with here, so don't get too enthusiastic when performing an assisted stretch.

SHOULDER

Rotator Cuff Stretches

Application   The incidence of rotator cuff injuries in men and women older than age 50 is surprising. Additionally, shoulder ROM has a direct effect on independence in older persons.

Internal Rotator Stretches

Position   To begin the exercise, sit in a chair with the right arm in front of the body and bent to 90°. Reach across under the right arm with the left hand and grab the right wrist (see figure 5.20).

Execution   Push outward to stretch the rotator cuff musculature and hold the stretch for 30 to 60 seconds. Then switch arms and repeat the exercise on the left side.

Variation   This exercise can also be performed while standing in the pool.

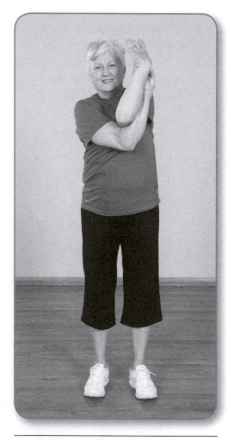

Figure 5.20   Internal rotator stretch.

External Rotator Stretches

Position   The first stretch is the *active assisted cross-body shoulder stretch.* Begin this stretch by actively reaching across the body with the left arm at shoulder level.

Execution   Grasp the right elbow with the left hand and pull the right arm across the body until a sufficient stretch is felt in the left rear deltoid and back muscles (see figure 5.21). Then, switch sides.

Variations

- This exercise can be performed while standing in the pool.
- Another variation of this exercise is to intertwine the hands and roll the shoulders forward while extending the arms. This stretch can be performed in a standing or seated position.

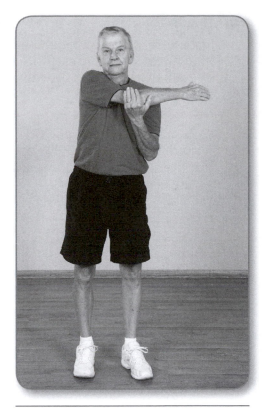

Figure 5.21   The active assisted cross-body shoulder stretch.

Anterior Rotator Stretches

Position   Let's begin with an active assisted stretch called the *active assisted back arm stretch.* Stand up straight and grasp the end of a towel or rope with the right hand and extend the right arm back. Reach behind the hips with the left hand and grasp the free end of the towel or rope. Move the hands shoulder-width apart and get rid of any slack in the rope or towel. With the palms facing downward, extend both arms back behind the hips (see figure 5.22).

Execution   Keep the arms straight and use the muscles of the upper back to initiate the movement by pressing the arms upward until a stretch is felt in the chest and the fronts of the arms. Increase the stretch by pulling outward on the towel or rope. Given that this is an AAS, it should be held for 2 to 3 seconds and the arms should be relaxed before repeating the movement. Aim for a deeper stretch with each repetition.

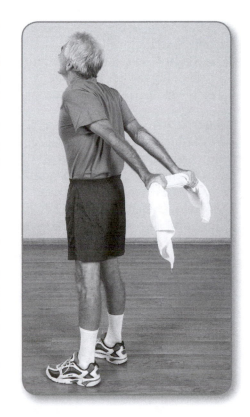

Figure 5.22   The active assisted back arm stretch for the anterior of the rotator cuff.

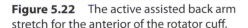

Variations

- To perform the first variation, the *behind-the-back stretch,* keep the right arm straight and bring it across the back. Then reach behind the back with the left arm and grab the right elbow with the left hand. Pull the right arm across the body. Switch arms and repeat the exercise.

- This stretch can also be performed while standing in the pool.

- The second variation is the *doorway stretch.* Stand in a doorway with the upper arms at shoulder height or slightly higher. Place the forearms along each side of the doorway and take a step forward while leaning through the doorway to stretch the chest and the fronts of the shoulders. To perform this stretch in the pool, stand in chest-deep water and place the hands on either wall at the corner of the pool.

- Another variation is an active assisted stretch called the *overhead back stretch.* To prepare for the stretch, stand up straight, extend the arms overhead, and grasp a towel or rope at a distance slightly greater than shoulder width. To start the movement, press the arms backward, using the muscles of the upper back to stretch the fronts of the shoulders, the chest, the rib cage, and the abdominal muscles. Then relax the arms and repeat the movement for a deeper stretch.

- A final stretch is the *kneeling chest and shoulder stretch.* Start the stretch by getting down on hands and knees. Sit back on the heels, and then slowly stretch both arms forward to full extension. Keep both palms on the floor and press the chest down to the floor. This stretch can also be performed in shallow water. To begin, kneel or stand while holding onto the overflow or wall, then sit backward, stretching the chest and shoulders.

Downward Rotator Stretches

Position   To begin the *active assisted back scratch stretch,* stand straight with one end of a towel or rope in the right hand. Point the right elbow toward the ceiling so that the right hand is positioned behind the right shoulder and the towel or rope is dangling behind the back. Reach behind the back with the left hand and grasp the other end of the rope or towel near the hips (see figure 5.23).

Execution   Initiate the stretch by reaching the right hand as far down the back as feels comfortable. Assist the stretch by using the left hand to pull down on the rope or towel. Hold the stretch for 2 to 3 seconds. Then return the arms to a relaxed position. Repeat the movement, aiming for a deeper stretch with each repetition. Repeat the stretch on the opposite side. Remember the number of repetitions is dependent on whether flexibility is a priority given the client's diagnostic profile, the existing flexibility of the client, and, of course, the week of the training cycle (if the stretch is being used as part of a targeted periodization cycle).

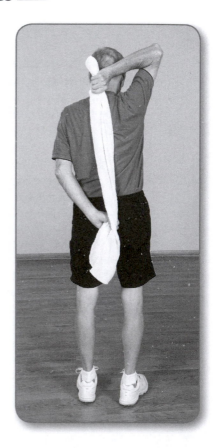

Figure 5.23   The active assisted back scratch stretch for the downward rotators.

Variations   The back scratch stretch can also be performed without the rope or towel as a static or self-assisted stretch. Reach down the middle of the back with the right hand so that the right elbow is pointed toward the ceiling. Reach the left hand over the head and grasp the right elbow with the left hand. Now apply pressure on the right elbow down, back, and toward the midline of the body (see figure 5.24). Then switch sides and repeat the exercise. This stretch can be performed in the pool.

Safety   Remember that out of all the joints in the body, the rotator cuff of the shoulder has the greatest number of degrees of freedom for movement. So what's the cost of all this freedom? The rotator cuff is also one of the most vulnerable joints when it comes to injury. The rotator cuff will do its best to accommodate each stretch, and it's best to return the favor by not taking too much advantage of its friendly nature and causing it injury. In other words, remain under control when performing all shoulder stretches and remember to listen to your body when it tells you it's at the end of its comfort zone.

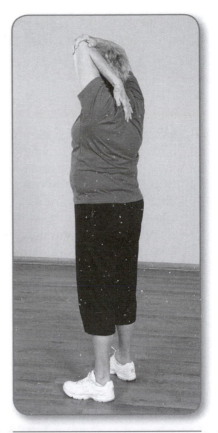

Figure 5.24   The back scratch stretch performed without the rope or towel as a static or self-assisted stretch.

CORE STRETCHES
LOW BACK, SIDES, AND ABDOMINAL MUSCLES
Low Back Stretches

Application One of the hottest catchphrases in the fitness industry is *core*. The core body muscles are the links that transfer power and force from the lower body to the upper body and vice versa. In fact, preliminary data from our laboratory show that core flexibility correlates to every measure of ADL performance examined. Among the most vulnerable of the muscles in the core are the muscles of the lower back. In the United States, tightness and pain in these muscles cost billions of dollars per year in treatment expenses and lost productivity and are among the most debilitating musculoskeletal problems. To give you an example of the prevalence of low back pain, in 2010 the term *lower back pain* in the NIH PubMed search engine found 19,200 references on the subject. The same search on Google produced 23,500,000 hits.

Position Let's begin with an active assisted stretch called the *active assisted seated cat stretch*. You'll probably recognize the stretch because it is nearly identical to the sit-and-reach test. To begin the stretch, sit up straight and lean slightly forward in an armless chair. Grasp one end of a towel or rope in the left hand and the other end in the right hand. Keeping the feet close together, step on the middle of the rope or towel, making sure to keep both feet firmly planted against the floor (see figure 5.25).

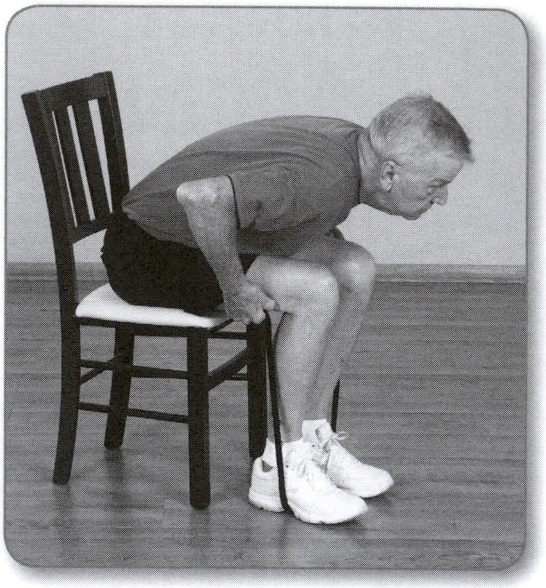

Execution Lean forward while slowly rounding the back like a cat; assist the stretch by pulling upward on the rope. Hold the stretch for 2 to 3 seconds.

Figure 5.25 The active assisted seated cat stretch.

Variations

• The first variation, the *cat stretch*, brings you closer (literally) to the canine and feline companions with whom you may share your home. Get down on the hands and knees. Start the stretch by dropping the stomach toward the floor and curling the back, bringing the back of the head toward the buttocks (see figure 5.26*a*). Then arch the back upward by moving the chin toward the thighs (see figure 5.26*b*). Hold each position for 30 to 60 seconds.

• The sit-and-reach stretch can be performed as both an active assisted (see figure 5.27) and a static (see figure 5.28) stretch. In addition to stretching the hamstrings, it is also a low back stretch.

• To perform the *cross-legged forward stretch*, start in a sitting position with the legs crossed and the arms folded across the chest or relaxed at the sides. Tuck the chin into the chest and roll forward, attempting to touch the forehead to the floor. Hold the stretch for 30 to 60 seconds and then return to the starting position. This stretch can also be performed in a chair while using the arms to assist the stretch.

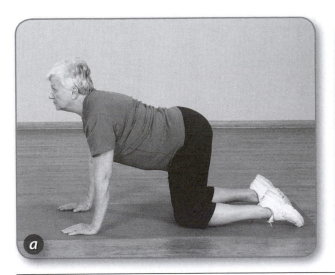 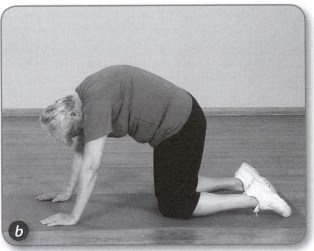

Figure 5.26   The cat stretch arching *(a)* upward and *(b)* downward.

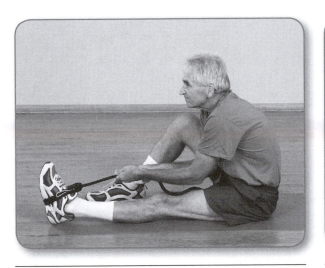 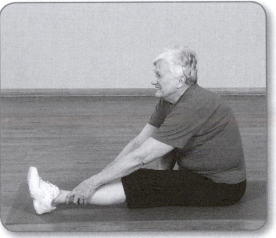

Figure 5.27   The active assisted sit-and-reach stretch.   **Figure 5.28**   The static sit-and-reach stretch.

• For the *lying tuck,* lie on your back and bring both knees to the chest. Grab under both knees and pull the knees toward the armpits. Hold the stretch for 30 to 60 seconds and return to the starting position.

Stretches for the Obliques and Other Abdominal Muscles

Application   The muscles of the core are often viewed as stability muscles, and I provide a number of strengthening exercises for these muscles. Our bodies use the rotation of the shoulder girdle around the hips to produce power and perform the majority of daily activities. Since ROM is one of the major tools used to generate power, the flexibility of the core muscles is an integral component of core function.

Position   Let's begin with the *active assisted seated overhead trunk twist,* an active assisted stretch. Sit upright on an armless chair and extend both arms completely overhead, grasping a towel or rope with the hands slightly greater than shoulder-width apart.

Execution   Initiate the stretch by turning to one side and using the waist muscles to stretch the muscles on the other side. Assist the stretch by pulling out, around, and forward on the rope or towel with one hand and out, around, and backward on the rope or towel with the other hand (see figure 5.29). Hold the stretch for 2 to 3 seconds. Repeat this stretch on the opposite side.

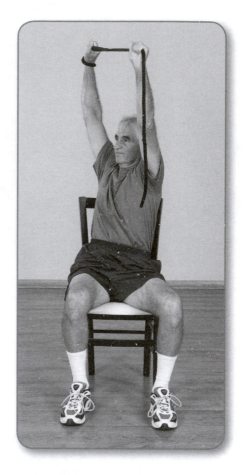

Figure 5.29   The active assisted seated overhead trunk twist for the obliques.

Variations

- The *seated twist* variation can be performed on the floor. Place the right leg over the left, keeping the right knee bent to about 90°. Then put the left elbow behind the right knee and rotate, using the obliques (side muscles) for the movement and the elbow for leverage (see figure 5.30). Change sides and repeat the exercise.

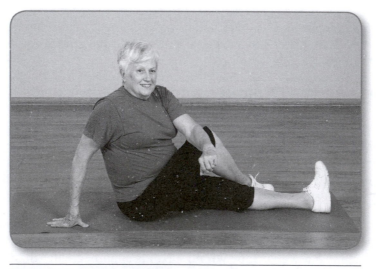

Figure 5.30   The seated twist.

- The obliques can also be stretched with *active assisted lateral reaches* (see figure 5.31). To perform the lateral reach as an active assisted stretch, stand with both arms completely extended overhead and grasp a towel or rope with the hands slightly greater than shoulder-width apart. Perform a side bend to the right using the obliques to initiate the movement. Assist the stretch by pulling the rope or towel with the right hand. This stretch increases the flexibility of all the trunk muscles on the opposite side of the direction of the lean. Since this is an active assisted stretch, perform it a number of times and use short holds lasting 2 to 3 seconds. Attempt to bend deeper into the stretch with each repetition. As with all unilateral stretches, repeat this stretch for the opposite side.

- The lateral reach can also be performed as a static stretch. Place one hand on the corresponding hip and raise the other hand overhead so that the arm points upward and the elbow is slightly flexed. Next, reach farther across and over the head. Hold the stretch for approximately 30 seconds before returning to the starting position. Then repeat the stretch on the same side or alternate sides. Feel the stretch along the sides, along the back, and in the abdominal muscles. The same exercise can be performed in chest-deep to waist-deep water in the pool.

- Like the seated twist, the *knee crossover* is another stretch targeting the rotational ROM at the waist (see figure 5.32). Begin by lying on your back and bringing the left knee to the stomach. Grasp the left knee with the right hand and pull it across the body while keeping the body facing upward. Hold the position for 2 to 3 seconds and then repeat the stretch. Remember to switch legs to perform the exercise on the other side.

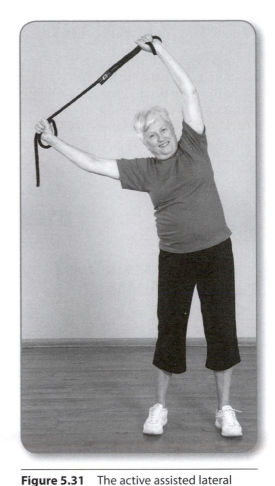

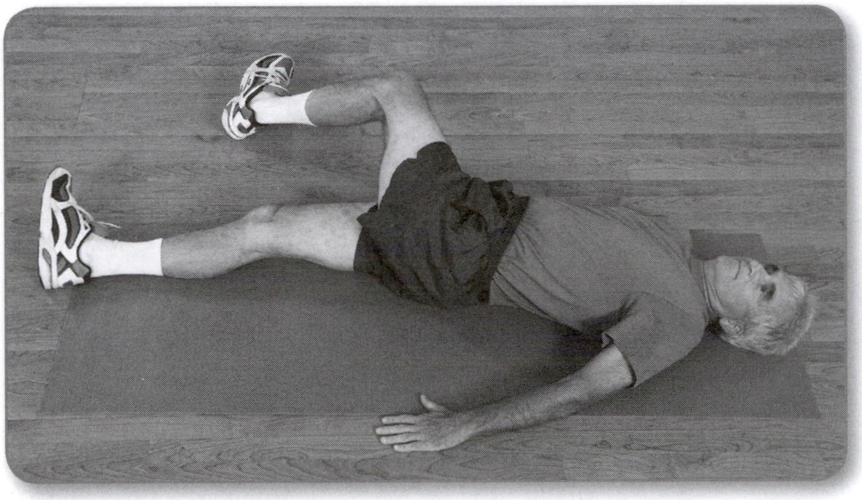

Figure 5.31 The active assisted lateral stretch.

Figure 5.32 The knee crossover stretch.

SUMMARY

For me, there is something very in sync in bending to stretch and bending the flexibility aging curve. Though when discussing flexibility I seem to find an analogy at every bend in the road (sorry!), there are two very clear messages to take away from this chapter. The first is that flexibility, which is often treated as a second-rate training modality in the fitness environment, is one of the most important factors dictating independence, mobility, and reduced fall probability among older adults. The second—and perhaps the more gratifying—is that you can use the simple training tools presented in this chapter to improve clients' flexibility and produce these beneficial improvements.

Topical Bibliography

Possible Causes of Declining Flexibility With Aging

Alnaqeeb, M.A., Al-Zaid, N.S., & Goldspink, G. (1984). Connective tissue changes and physical properties of developing and aging skeletal muscle. *Journal of Anatomy* 139:677-689.

Anderson, B., Burke, E., & Burke, B.S. (1991). Scientific, medical, and practical aspects of stretching. *Clinics in Sports Medicine* 10:63-86.

Brown, D.A., & Miller, W.C. (1998). Normative data for strength and flexibility of women throughout life. *European Journal of Applied Physiology* 78:77-82.

Goldspink, G., Williams, P., & Simpson, H. (2002). Gene expression in response to muscle stretch. *Clinical Orthopaedics and Related Research* 403S:S146-S152.

Holland, G.J., Tanaka, K., Shigematsu, R., & Nakagaichi, M. (2002). Flexibility and physical functions of older adults: A review. *J Aging Phys Act* 10:169-206.

Kempson, G.E. (1991). Age-related changes in the tensile properties of human articular cartilage: A comparative study between the femoral head of the hip joint and the talus of the ankle joint. *Biochim Biophys Acta* 1075:223-230.

Noyes, F.R., & Grood, E.S. (1976). The strength of anterior cruciate ligament in humans and rhesus monkeys: Age-related and species-related changes. *J Bone Joint Surg* 58A:1074-1082.

Raab, D.M., Agre, J.C., McAdam, M., & Smith, E.L. (1988). Light resistance and stretching exercise in elderly women: Effect upon flexibility. *Archives of Physical Medicine and Rehabilitation* 69:268-272.

Ronsky, J.L., Nigg, B.M., & Fisher, V. (1995). Correlation between physical activity and the gait characteristics and ankle joint flexibility of the elderly. *Clinical Biomechanics* 10:41-49.

Why Train for Flexibility?

Allander, E., Bjornsson, O.J., Olafsson, O., Sigfusson, N., & Thorsteinsson, J. (1974). Normal range of joint movements in shoulder, hip, wrist and thumb with special reference to side: A comparison between two populations. *International Journal of Epidemiology* 3:253-261.

Badley, E.M., Wagstaff, S., & Wood, P.H. (1986). Measures of functional ability (disability) in arthritis in relation to impairment of range of joint movement. *Ann Rheum Dis* 43:563-569.

Beissner, K.L., Collins, J.E., & Holmes, H. (2000). Muscle force and range of motion as predictors of function in older adults. *Phys Ther* 80:556-563.

Benedetti, M.G., Berti, L., Maselli, S., Mariani, G., & Giannini, S. (2007). How do the elderly negotiate a step? A biomechanical assessment. *Clin Biomech (Bristol, Avon)* 22:567-573.

Bergstrom, G., Aniansson, A., Bjelle, A., Grimby, G., Lundgren-Lindquist, B., & Svanborg, A. (1985). Functional consequences of joint impairment at age 79. *Scand J Rehab Med* 17:183-190.

Boone, D.C., & Azen, S.P. (1979). Normal range of motion of joints in male subjects. *J Bone Joint Surg Am* 61:756-759.

Ge, W. (1998). Age-related differences in body segmental movement during perturbed stance in humans. *Clin Biomech (Bristol, Avon)* 13:300-307.

Gehlsen, G.M., & Whaley, M.H. (1990). Falls in the elderly: Part II. Balance, strength, and flexibility. *Archives of Physical Medicine and Rehabilitation* 71:739-741.

Germain, N.W., & Blair, S.N. (1983). Variability of shoulder flexion with age, activity and sex. *American Correctional Therapeutic Journal* 37:156-160.

Golding, L.A., & Lindsay, A. (2002). Flexibility and age. *Perspective* 15:28-30.

Holland, G.J., Tanaka, K., Shigematsu, R., & Nakagaichi, M. (2002). Flexibility and physical functions of older adults: A review. *J Aging Phys Act* 10:169-206.

Jette, A.M., Branch, L.G., & Berlin, J. (1990). Musculoskeletal impairments and physical disablement among the aged. *J Gerontol: Medical Science* 45:M203-M298.

Kemoun, G., Thoumie, P., Boisson, D., & Guieu, J.D. (2002). Ankle dorsiflexion delay can predict falls in the elderly. *Journal of Rehabilitative Medicine* 34:278-283.

Kerrigan, D.C., Lee, L.W., Collins, J.J., Reilly, P.O., & Lipsitz, L.A. (2001). Reduced hip extension during walking: Healthy elderly and fallers versus young adults. *Archives of Physical Medicine and Rehabilitation* 82:26-30.

Lee, L.W., Zavarei, K., Evans, J., Lelas, J.J., Riley, P.O., & Kerrigan, D.C. (2005). Reduced hip extension in the elderly: Dynamic or postural? *Arch Phys Med Rehabil* 86:1851-1854.

Means, K.M., O'Sullivan, P.S., & Rodell, D.E. (2000). Balance, mobility, and falls among elderly African American women. *Am J Phys Med Rehabil* 79:30-39.

Mecagni, C., Smith, J.P., Roberts, K.E., & O'Sullivan, S.B. (2000). Balance and ankle range of motion in community-dwelling women aged 64 to 87 years: A correlational study. *Phys Ther* 80:1004-1011.

Menz, H.B., Morris, M.E., & Lord, S.R. (2005). Foot and ankle characteristics associated with impaired balance and functional ability in older people. *J Gerontol A Biol Sci Med Sci* 60:1546-1552.

Menz, H.B., Morris, M.E., & Lord, S.R. (2006). Foot and ankle risk factors for falls in older people: A prospective study. *J Gerontol A Biol Sci Med Sci* 61:866-870.

Rider, R.A., & Daly, J. (1991). Effects of flexibility training on enhancing spinal mobility in older women. *Journal of Sports Medicine and Physical Fitness* 31:213-217.

Ronsky, J.L., Nigg, B.M., & Fisher, V. (1995). Correlation between physical activity and the gait characteristics and ankle joint flexibility of the elderly. *Clinical Biomechanics* 10:41-49.

Richardson, J., Bedard, M., & Weaver, B. (2001). Changes in physical functioning in institutionalized older adults. *Disabil Rehabil* 23:683-689.

Wada, N., Sohmiya, M., Shimizu, T., Okamoto, K., & Shirakura, K. (2007). Clinical analysis of risk factors for falls in home-living stroke patients using functional evaluation tools. *Arch Phys Med Rehabil* 88:1601-1605.

Types of Stretching

Alter, M.J. (1996). *Science of flexibility* (2nd ed.). Champaign, IL: Human Kinetics.

Appleton, B. (1998). Stretching and flexibility—types of stretching. www.cmcrossroads.com/bradapp/docs/rec/stretching.

Gleim, G.W., & McHugh, M.P. (1997). Flexibility and its effects on sports injury and performance. *Sports Med* 24:289-299.

Moore, M., & Kukulka, C. (1991). Depression of Hoffmann reflexes following voluntary contraction and implications for proprioceptive neuromuscular facilitation therapy. *Phys Ther* 71:321-333.

Do Stretching and Flexibility Training Increase Flexibility?

Brown, M., & Holloszy, J.O. (1991). Effects of low intensity exercise program on selected physical performance characteristics of 60- to 71-year olds. *Aging* 3:129-139.

Hughes, S.L., Seymour, R.B., Campbell, R.T., Huber, G., Pollak, N., Sharma, L., & Desai, P. (2006). Long-term impact of Fit and Strong! on older adults with osteoarthritis. *Gerontologist* 46:801-814.

Johnson, E., Bradley, B., Witkowski, K., McKee, R., Telesmanic, C., Chavez, A., Kennedy, K., & Zimmerman, G. (2007). Effect of a static calf muscle-tendon unit stretching program on ankle dorsiflexion range of motion of older women. *J Geriatr Phys Ther* 30(2):49-52.

Morey, M.C., Cowper, P.A., Feussner, J.R., DiPasqusale, R.C., Crowley, G.M., Samsa, G.P., & Sullivan, R.J. (1991). Two-year trends in physical performance following supervised exercise among community-dwelling older veterans. *JAGS* 39:986-992.

Raab, D.M., Agre, J.C., McAdam, M., & Smith, E.L. (1988). Light resistance and stretching exercise in elderly women: Effect upon flexibility. *Archives of Physical Medicine and Rehabilitation* 69:268-272.

Templeton, M.S., Booth, D.L., & O'Kelly, W.D. (1995). Effects of aquatic therapy on joint flexibility and functional ability in subjects with rheumatic disease. *J Orthop Sports Phys Ther* 23:376-381.

Tsourlou, T., Benik, A., Dipla, K., Zafeiridis, A., & Kellis, S. (2006). The effects of a twenty-four-week aquatic training program on muscular strength performance in healthy elderly women. *J Strength Cond Res* 20:811-818.

Wang, T.J., Belza, B., Elaine Thompson, F., Whitney, J.D., & Bennett, K. (2007). Effects of aquatic exercise on flexibility, strength and aerobic fitness in adults with osteoarthritis of the hip or knee. *J Adv Nurs* 57:141-152.

Wyatt, F.B., Milam, S., Manske, R.C., & Deere, R. (2001). The effects of aquatic and traditional exercise programs on persons with knee osteoarthritis. *J Strength Cond Res* 15:337-340.

Stretching, Flexibility Training, and Injury Prevention

Hart, L. (2005). Effect of stretching on sport injury risk: A review. *Clin J Sport Med* 15:113.

Herbert, R.D., & de Noronha, M. (2007). Stretching to prevent or reduce muscle soreness after exercise. *Cochrane Database Syst Rev* 17:CD0004577.

Rodenburg, J.B., Steenbeek, D., Schiereck, P., & Bär, P.R. (1994). Warm-up, stretching and massage diminish harmful effects of eccentric exercise. *Int J Sports Med* 15:414-419.

Woods, K., Bishop, P., & Jones, E. (2007). Warm-up and stretching in the prevention of muscular injury. *Sports Med* 37:1089-1099.

Stretching, Flexibility Training, and Performance

Alexander, N.B., Galecki, A.T., Grenier, M.L., Nyquist, L.V., Hofmeyer, M.R., Grunawalt, J,C,, Medell, J.L., & Fry-Welch, D. (2001). Task-specific resistance training to improve the ability of activities of daily living-impaired older adults to rise from a bed and from a chair. *Journal of the American Geriatric Society* 49:1418-1427.

Carmel, M.P., Czaja, S., Morgan, R.O., Asfour, S., Khalil, T., & Signorile, J.F. (2000). The effects of varying training speed on changes in functional performance in older women. *The Physiologist* 43(4): 321.

Cramer, J.T., Housh, T.J., Johnson, G.O., Miller, J.M., Coburn, J.W., & Beck, T.W. (2004). Acute effects of static stretching on peak torque in women. *J Str Cond Res* 18:236-241.

Cramer, J.T., Housh, T.J., Weir, J.P., Johnson, G.O., Coburn, J.W., & Beck, T.W. (2005). The acute effects of static stretching on peak torque, mean power output, electromyography, and mechanomyography. *Eur J Appl Physiol* 93:530-539.

DiBenedetto, M., Innes, K.E., Taylor, A.G., Rodeheaver, P.F., Boxer, J,A,, Wright, H.J., & Kerrigan, D.C.. (2005). Effects of a gentle Iyengar yoga program on gait in the elderly: An exploratory study. *Arch Phys Med Rehabil* 86:1830-1837.

Gurjão, A.L., Gonçalves, R., de Moura, R.F., & Gobbi, S. (2009). Acute effect of static stretching on rate of force development and maximal voluntary contraction in older women. *J Strength Cond Res* 23:2149-2154.

Hartmann, A., Murer, K., De Bie, R.A., & De Bruin, E.D. (2009). The effect of a foot gymnastic exercise programme on gait performance in older adults: A randomised controlled trial. *Disabil Rehabil* 21:1-10.

Kerrigan, D.C., Xenopoulos-Oddsson, A., Sullivan, M.J., Lelas, J.J., & Riley, P.O. (2003). Effect of a hip flexor-stretching program on gait in the elderly. *Arch Phys Med Rehabil* 84:1-6.

Kokkonen, J., Nelson, A.G., & Cornwell, A. (1998). Acute muscle stretching inhibits maximal strength performance. *Res Quar Exerc Sport* 69:411-415.

Nelson, A.G., Driscoll, N.M., Landin, D.K., Young, M.A., & Schexnayder, I.C. (2005). Acute effects of passive muscle stretching on sprint performance. *J Sports Sci* 23:449-454.

Oken, B.S., Zajdel, D., Kishiyama, S., Flegal, K., Dehen, C., Haas, M., Kraemer, D.F., Lawrence, J., & Leyva, J. (2006). Randomized, controlled, six-month trial of yoga in healthy seniors: Effects on cognition and quality of life. *Altern Ther Health Med* 12:40-47.

Reid, D.A., & McNair, P.J. (2010). Effects of an acute hamstring stretch in people with and without osteoarthritis of the knee. *Physiotherapy* 96:14-21.

Shrier, I. (2004). Does stretching improve performance? A systematic and critical review of the literature. *Clin J Sport Med* 14:267-273.

Stanziano, D., Roos, B., Perry, A.C., Lai, S., & Signorile, J.F. (2009). The effects of an active-assisted stretching program on measures of flexibility and functional performance in elderly persons. *Clin Interv Aging* 4:115-120.

Unick, J., Kieffer, H.S., Cheesman, W., & Feeney, A. (2005). The acute effects of static and ballistic stretching on vertical jump performance in trained women. *J Strength Cond Res* 19:206-212.

Young, W., & Elliot, S. (2001). Acute effects of static stretching, proprioceptive neuromuscular facilitation stretching and maximal voluntary contractions on explosive force production and jumping performance. *Res Q Exerc Sport* 72:273-279.

Testing Flexibility

Graf, A., Judge, J.O., Õunpuu, S., & Thelen, D.G. (2005). The effect of walking speed on lower-extremity joint powers among elderly adults who exhibit low physical performance. *Arch Phys Med Rehabil* 86:2177-2183.

Heyward, V.H. (1997). *Advanced fitness assessment and exercise prescription* (3rd ed.). Champaign, IL: Human Kinetics.

Hoeger, W.W.K., Hoeger, S.A. (1998). Muscular flexibility assessment and prescription. In: Hoeger WWK, Hoeger SA, editors. *Lifetime Physical Fitness and Wellness: A Personalized Program*. Englewood, CA: Brooks Cole; pp. 121–140.

Jones, C.J., Rikli, R.E., Max, J., & Noffal, G. (1998). The reliability and validity of a chair sit-and-reach test as a measure of hamstring flexibility in older adults. *Res Quar Exerc Sport* 69:338-344.

Moseley, A.M., Crosbie, J., & Adams, R. (2001). Normative data for passive ankle plantarflexion-dorsiflexion flexibility. *Clin Biomech* 16:514-521.

Osness, W.H., Adrian, M., Clark, B.A., Hoeger, W., Raab, D., & Wiswell, R. (1990). *Functional fitness assessment for adults over 60 years (a field based assessment)*. Reston, VA: American Alliance for Health, Physical Education, Recreation and Dance.

Rikli, R.E., & Jones, C.J. (1999a). Development and validation of a functional fitness test for community-residing older adults. *Journal of Aging and Physical Activity* 7:129-161.

Rikli, R.E., & Jones, C.J. (1999b). Functional fitness normative scores for community residing older adults, ages 60-94. *Journal of Aging and Physical Activity* 7:162-181.

Shepard, R.J. (1997). *Aging, physical activity, and health*. Champaign, IL: Human Kinetics.

Shepard, R.J., Berridge, J.M., & Montelpare, W. (1990). On the generality of the "sit and reach" test: An analysis of flexibility data for an aging population. *Research Quarterly for Exercise and Sport* 61:326-330.

Stanziano, D., Roos, B., Perry, A.C., Lai, S., & Signorile, J.F. (2009). The effects of an active-assisted stretching program on measures of flexibility and functional performance in elderly persons . *Clin Interv Aging* 4:115-120.

Flexibility Training Exercises

Aagaard, P., Simonsen, E.B., Andersen, J.L., Magnusson, S.P., Bojsen-Moller, F., & Dyhre-Poulsen, P. (2000). Antagonist muscle coactivation during isokinetic knee extension. *Scand J Med Sci Sports* 10:58-67.

Bassey, E.J., Morgan, K., Dallosso, H.M., & Ebrahim, B.J. (1989). Flexibility of the shoulder joint measured as range of abduction in a large representative sample of men and women over 65 years of age. *European Journal of Applied Physiology* 58(353): 360.

Carolan, B., & Cafarelli, E. (1992). Adaptations in coactivation after isometric resistance training. *Journal of Applied Physiology* 73(3): 911-917.

Christiansen, C.L. (2008). The effects of hip and ankle stretching on gait function of older people. *Arch Phys Med Rehabil* 89(8): 1421-1428.

Cunningham, D.A., Paterson, D.H., Himann, J.E., & Rechnitzer, P.A. (1993). Determinants of independence in the elderly. *Canadian Journal of Applied Physiology* 18(3): 243-254.

Gehlsen, G.M., & Whaley, M.H. (1990). Falls in the elderly: Part II. Balance, strength, and flexibility. *Archives of Physical Medicine and Rehabilitation* 71:739-741.

Hartmann, A., Murer, K., De Bie, R.A., & De Bruin, E.D. (2009). The effect of a foot gymnastic exercise programme on gait performance in older adults: A randomised controlled trial. *Disabil Rehabil* 21:1-10.

Kang, H.G., & Dingwell, J.B. (2007). Separating the effects of age and walking speed on gait variability. *Gait Posture* 27(4): 572-577.

Lee, L.W., Zavarei, K., Evans, J., Lelas, J.J., Riley, P.O., & Kerrigan, D.C. (2005). Reduced hip extension in the elderly: Dynamic or postural? *Arch Phys Med Rehabil* 86(9): 1851-1854.

Maffulli, N., Testa, V., & Capasso, G. (1991). Achilles tendon rupture in athletes: Histochemistry of the triceps surae muscle. *J Foot Surgery* 30(6): 529-532.

Reeves, N.D., Spanjaard, M., Mohagheghi, A.A., Baltzopoulos, V., & Maganaris, C.N. (2008). The demands of stair descent relative to maximum capacities in elderly and young adults. *J Electromyogr Kinesiol* 18(2): 218-227.

Ronsky, J.L., Nigg, B.M., & Fisher, V. (1995). Correlation between physical activity and the gait characteristics and ankle joint flexibility of the elderly. *Clinical Biomechanics* 10:41-49.

Smith, A.M. (1981). The coactivation of antagonist muscles. *Canadian Journal of Applied Physiology* 59:733-747.

Tainaka, K., Takizawa, T., Katamoto, S., & Aoki, J. (2009). Six-year prospective study of physical fitness and incidence of disability among community-dwelling Japanese elderly women. *Geriatr Gerontol Int* 9(1): 21-28.

Woo, J., Ho, S.C., & Yu, A.L.M. (1999). Walking speed and stride length predicts 36 months dependency, mortality, and institutionalization in Chinese aged 70 and older. *J Am Geriatr Soc* 47:1257-1260.

References

Hoeger, W.W.K., Hoeger, S.A. (1998). Muscular flexibility assessment and prescription. In: Hoeger WWK, Hoeger SA, editors. *Lifetime Physical Fitness and Wellness: A Personalized Program.* Englewood, CA: Brooks Cole; pp. 121–140.

Johnson, E., Bradley, B., Witkowski, K., McKee, R., Telesmanic, C., Chavez, A., Kennedy, K., & Zimmerman, G. (2007). Effect of a static calf muscle-tendon unit stretching program on ankle dorsiflexion range of motion of older women. *J Geriatr Phys Ther* 30(2):49-52.

Jones, C.J., Rikli, R.E., Max, J., & Noffal, G. (1998). The reliability and validity of a chair sit-and-reach test as a measure of hamstring flexibility in older adults. *Res Quar Exerc Sport* 69:338-344.

Rikli, R.E., & Jones, C.J. (1999b). Functional fitness normative scores for community residing older adults, ages 60-94. *Journal of Aging and Physical Activity* 7:162-181.

Shrier, I. (2004). Does stretching improve performance? A systematic and critical review of the literature. *Clin J Sport Med* 14:267-273.

Woods, K., Bishop, P., & Jones, E. (2007). Warm-up and stretching in the prevention of muscular injury. *Sports Med* 37:1089-1099.

chapter

6

Bone, Falls, and Fractures

Bones are the framework of our bodies. In fact, the skeleton is often used as an analogy for any basic structure around which the rest of a project is built. But these bones, our living levers, lose their strength and resilience with age and become more susceptible to fractures. Add to this the fact that balance declines with age, and you have the perfect storm. While no storm can be avoided, those of us who live in Florida know that it is possible to weather a storm if we hunker down and ride it out. This chapter teaches you how to prepare your clients to weather the perfect storm of fall and fracture and to reduce both the consequences and the fear they commonly associate with falling.

STRUCTURE OF BONE

Our skeletons are made up of two types of bone that differ considerably in their structure (see figure 6.1). The first type is cortical, or compact, bone. As the name implies, this bone is dense and is laid down in concentric rings (lamellae) that often surround a central canal containing blood vessels and nerves (see figure 6.2). The ringlike structure is called the *Haversian system* or *osteon*, and the central canal is called the *Haversian canal*. Lamellae also form near the outer surface of the bone and between the Haversian systems, where they are called *outer circumferential lamellae* and *interstitial lamellae,* respectively. Between the lamellae in small spaces, called *lacuna,* are bone cells called *osteocytes*. Osteocytes can communicate by sending electrical signals to each other through small canals called *canaliculi.* The

surface of cortical bone is covered by an outer layer called the *cortical layer* or *cortex.* The cortex is made up of two distinct layers: the outer layer, or periosteum, and the inner layer, or endosteum. There are also canals that run between all of these layers; these are called *Volkmann's canals.*

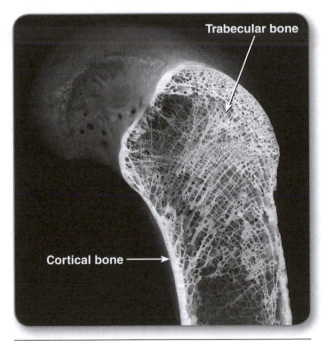

Figure 6.1 Illustration of two major types of bone: cortical and trabecular.

The second type of bone is trabecular bone, also known as *cancellous* or *spongy bone* (see figure 6.3). In contrast to compact bone, trabecular bone is extremely porous. It has a three-dimensional structure composed of bony rods and plates called

105

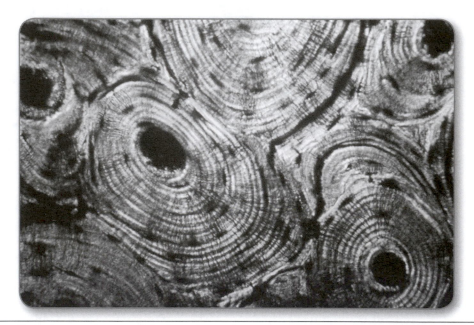

Figure 6.2   Detailed microscopic view of the lamellae in the Haversian system in cortical bone.

trabeculae. The spaces between the trabeculae are filled with bone marrow.

As might be expected given their names, cortical bone is found primarily on the surface of the bones and trabecular bone makes up the interior of the bones. The highest ratio of cortical bone to trabecular bone is seen in the appendicular skeleton (along the shafts of the long bones of the limbs), while the lowest ratio is found in the axial skeleton (spine). Additionally, the ratios in the different bones of the body and even within a single bone vary considerably.

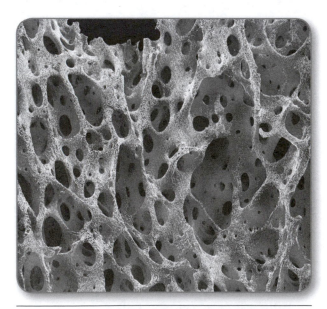

Figure 6.3   Microscopic view of trabecular (spongy) bone.

FACTORS AFFECTING BONE STRENGTH

The three major factors that affect bone strength are bone density, bone quality, and bone geometry. If we think of bone as the wooden frame of a building, bone density is akin to the wood studs and beams; bone quality is like the knotholes, splits, and other flaws that might weaken the wood; and geometry is like the architectural design of the building that allows the wood to provide structural strength. Let's look at how each of these qualities affects the bones of your clients.

Bone Density

The simplest definition of bone density is the mass of bone per unit volume. More specifically, we are concerned with the mineral density, or the level of mineralization, of bone. Of the three factors affecting bone strength, bone density has the greatest influence, accounting for 50% to 80% of a bone's resistance to fracture. The loss of bone density, which leads to a condition called *osteoporosis,* is a particular concern for older women. In women, the estimated rate of bone loss after menopause is between 1% and 2% per year for the first 10 years; this number eventually declines to 0.3% to 0.5% per year, which is similar to the premenopausal level of

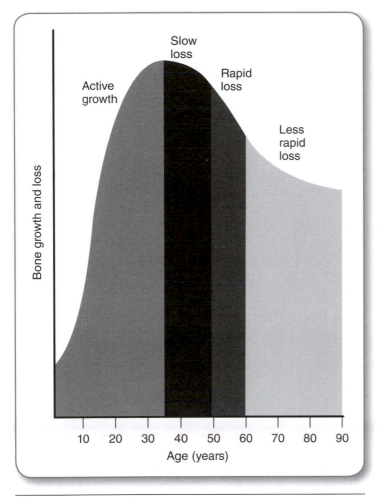

Figure 6.4 Changes in bone growth and bone loss in women from infancy to old age. Notice the rapid bone loss between the ages of 50 and 60 years, when menopause is most prevalent.

The major minerals in bone, in order of quantity, are calcium, magnesium, sodium, and potassium. These minerals provide hardness, rigidity, and strength. As we will see in the next section, bone mineral density is the most common way to assess osteoporosis and osteopenia.

Bone Geometry

The third factor, bone morphology, is simply the geometry of bone. One of the major features affecting bone geometry is bone growth. As we age, our bones increase in diameter. If you think of a bone as a cylinder, an increase in diameter becomes very important. Picture two pieces of plastic pipe with the same wall thickness but with different diameters. One has a 1-inch (2.5 cm) diameter and the second has a 3-inch (7.6 cm) diameter. Which pipe would be more difficult to bend? The answer is the 3-inch (7.6 cm) pipe—it is more difficult to bend because of its larger diameter (see figure 6.5). Material engineering tells us that the larger the diameter of a pipe, the more the pipe resists bending. This is important when we consider the changes in bone strength that occur during the aging process. As women lose bone density, they tend to experience compensatory increases in bone diameter through a process called *periosteal apposition*, which is the addition of tissue along the outer surface of the bone. In fact, postmenopausal women who lose tissue from the interior of a bone typically see increases in the diameter of that bone. Figure 6.6 shows the changes in internal and external diameters that occur across a typical life span. Unfortunately, these changes cannot completely compensate for the age-associated losses in bone density.

Bone strength is also affected by a bone's internal architecture. Just as the framework of a roof truss has a specific geometry that increases the structural integrity of the truss, trabecular bone has a specific geometry that maximizes the strength of the bone (see figure 6.7).

The geometry of trabecular bone can change, just as the structures of roof trusses can be changed, to adapt to the stresses the bone must resist. This reengineering occurs throughout our

bone loss. The pattern of bone loss in women, which is shown in figure 6.4, is well known and has been presented in both the scientific and popular literature. However, osteoporosis is also a concern for your older male clients.

Bone Quality

The second factor to consider when discussing bone strength is the structural material from which bone is constructed. The two major components that increase the structural integrity of bone are collagen and minerals. These two components add compliance and strength to bone.

Approximately 27% to 29% of bone is collagen. Collagen adds both strength and flexibility. However, both the content and quality of collagen decline with age, which in turn reduces both strength and compliance.

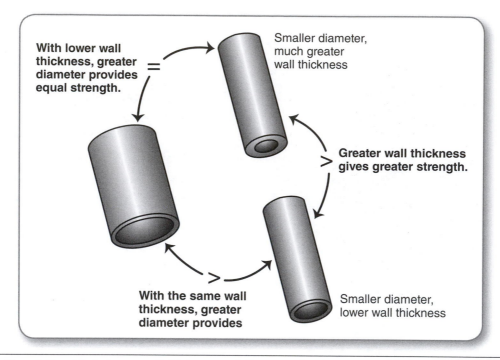

Figure 6.5   The relationship between wall thickness and diameter of a pipe as a model of changes in wall thickness and diameter of a bone.

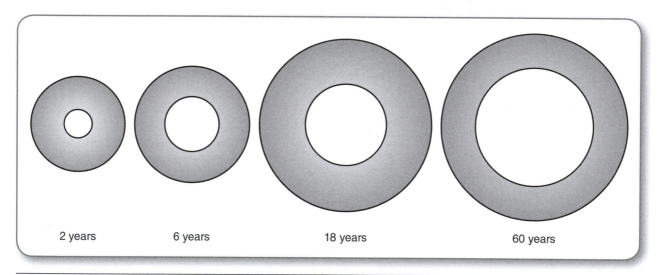

Figure 6.6   Internal and external bone diameters of 2-, 6-, 18-, and 60-year-olds.

Reprinted by permission from Van der Maulen, Beaupre, and Carter 1993.

lives. If the resorption (breaking down) of bone exceeds its rate of formation, both the longitudinal trabecular rods and the radial trabecular plates grow thinner. A resorption–formation mismatch not only decreases the strengths of these structures but also produces large resorption cavities that have a greater effect on bone strength than the reduction in trabecular bone itself has (see figure 6.7). The U.S. Surgeon General has likened the eating away of trabecular bone to a house having its frame eaten by termites, a description that fits very nicely with my analogy between trabecular bone and the framework of a roof truss.

The final aspect of bone geometry that affects bone strength is really an issue of structural integrity. Microfractures or cracks may develop in the

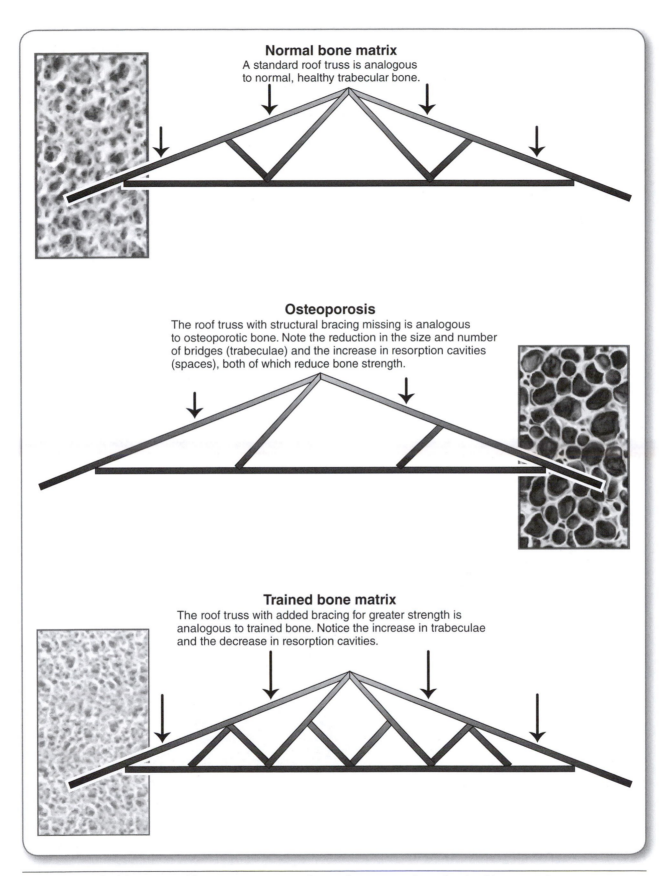

Figure 6.7 Of roof trusses and bone: a comparison of normal, osteoporotic, and trained bone matrix.

trabeculae, weakening the bone even more and heightening the risk of fracture. These cracks are analogous to the cracks that threaten the structural integrity of overpasses and bridges, causing nations throughout the world to struggle with maintaining their physical infrastructures. We can experience these same problems if we fail to attend to our own personal infrastructure through proper diet and exercise.

APPLICATION POINT   The strength of bone is affected by more than its density. It is also affected by the geometry and integrity of the bone's framework. Training can affect all three factors.

OSTEOPENIA AND OSTEOPOROSIS

There are two terms frequently used to describe bone loss. The first is *osteopenia* and the second and better known is *osteoporosis*. We can visualize osteopenia and osteoporosis as being part of a continuum of bone loss. A distribution curve of the bone density of healthy young individuals is used to define these two conditions (see figure

6.8). Osteopenia is a level of bone density that is between 1 and 2.5 standard deviations below the mean, while osteoporosis is defined by bone densities that are at least 2.5 standard deviations below the mean. While the distribution curve provides a nice visual representation of the two conditions and is meaningful to statisticians, it might be nice for the rest of us to have these descriptions put into terms that are a bit more tangible. Individuals with osteopenia have a lower bone density than that of 84% to 97% of healthy young adults. In comparison, individuals with osteoporosis have a lower bone density than that of 97% of the young reference population.

A definition of osteoporosis by the NIH Consensus Development Panel on Osteoporosis Prevention, Diagnosis, and Therapy concentrates more on structural strength than on bone density. The report states that osteoporosis is "a skeletal disorder characterized by compromised bone strength leading to an increased risk of fracture" (2001).

The National Osteoporosis Foundation (2008) offers this definition of osteoporosis:

> Osteoporosis, or porous bone, is a disease characterized by low bone mass and structural deterioration of bone tissue, leading to bone fragility and an

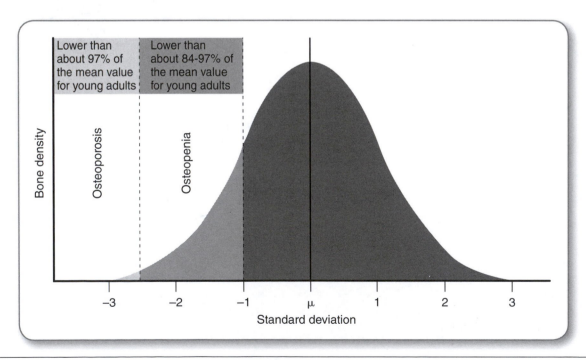

Figure 6.8   A bell-shaped curve showing the standard distribution of bone densities of healthy young adults. Individuals who have osteopenia have bone densities that are 1 to 2.5 standard deviations below the mean, while people with osteoporosis have bone densities that fall at least 2.5 standard deviations below the mean.

Bone Density	
osteopenia	A condition characterized by lower than normal bone density; may be the precursor for osteoporosis.
osteoporosis	A disease where bone mass and structure decline to a point where there is a significant increase in fragility and susceptibility to fracture.

increased susceptibility to fractures, especially of the hip, spine and wrist, although any bone can be affected. In simpler terms, osteoporosis is a condition in which the bones become weak and can break from a minor fall or, in serious cases, from a simple action such as a sneeze.

Whether osteopenia and osteoporosis are defined by bone density, bone quality, or bone architecture, the ultimate concern is the increased risk of serious fracture associated with these conditions. Fractures result in loss of independence, hospitalization, and even death and cost Americans more than 18 billion dollars per year.

APPLICATION POINT   Rather than considering osteopenia and osteoporosis as two distinct conditions, look at them as two points on a continuum of bone loss.

Prevalence and Consequences of Osteopenia and Osteoporosis

So just how prevalent are osteopenia and osteoporosis among older persons? Let's look at some of the available data and projections. *The 2004 Surgeon General's Report on Bone Health and Osteoporosis: What It Means to You* begins with a very bleak view of the future in the United States. It predicts that "by 2020 half of all Americans over 50 will have weak bones unless we make changes to our diet and lifestyle" (Surgeon General, 2004, p. 3).

The National Osteoporosis Foundation (2008) provides the following data on the prevalence of osteoporosis in the United States: 10 million people have osteoporosis and 34 million more have low bone mass. Of the 10 million people with osteoporosis, approximately 80% are women. Osteoporosis is responsible for more than 1.5

million fractures annually, including 300,000 hip fractures, 700,000 vertebral fractures, 250,000 wrist fractures, and more than 300,000 fractures at other sites.

Osteoporosis is not limited to Americans. If we look at the combined data for the United States, Europe, and Japan, the numbers are just as profound. Osteoporosis affects approximately 75 million people in Europe, the United States, and Japan. In the United Kingdom, 1 in 2 women and 1 in 5 men are expected to experience an osteoporosis-related fracture after the age of 50. In fact, estimates are that the rate of hip fractures in the United Kingdom will increase by nearly 150% between 1985 and 2016 and that associated costs will reach more than £2 billion by 2020. In Japan, there was a 170% increase in new hip fractures from 1987 to 1997, and estimates suggest that the total number of hip fractures will increase by more than 55% from 2010 to 2030. For Australia and New Zealand, the picture is just as bleak. More than 2.2 million Australians have osteoporosis, and it's been estimated that 42% of the women and 27% of the men over the age of 50 in Australia will experience an osteoporotic fracture. The costs associated with osteoporosis are approximately 7.4 billion U.S. dollars annually. These figures are similar to those reported for New Zealand, where the likelihood of osteoporotic fracture and associated health costs are expected to increase by 30% from 2007 to 2020.

Testing Bone Density

Bone density assessments are typically done by DXA. A DXA instrument is a very fancy scanning machine that shoots a high-energy and low-energy X-ray beam through the patient's bones. The two beams are absorbed to varying degrees. The instrument uses the difference in the absorption of these two beams to determine the density of the patient's bones. While you may not have the capacity to evaluate the bone density of an older client, you should encourage the client to be evaluated on a regular basis and you should require a report of the client's bone density before beginning a training program.

EXERCISE TRAINING TO PREVENT OSTEOPOROSIS

There are a number of factors placing older individuals at risk for osteoporotic fracture (see the sidebar). The typical interventions for preventing osteoporosis include diet, exercise, and medication. This section concentrates on exercise interventions; however, some information on diet and medication will, by necessity, be included in the information. In preparing to write about the topic of exercise and bone loss, I was fortunate enough to find a review paper by Katarina Borer (2005) that presented seven basic principles for maximizing the influence of exercise on bone. I will use these principles as the skeleton for the following discussion on exercise to prevent bone loss.

1. Bone adapts best to dynamic rather than static mechanical stimulation. The message that tells bone to grow in response to mechanical loading is most likely fluid flow through the canalicular channels and around the bone trabeculae. This fluid flow is caused by strain placed on the bone. Therefore, the cyclic changes in stress characteristic of dynamic exercise have a greater effect on bone restructuring than simple static loading has.

2. If a bone is to respond to training, the stimulus must be at a suprathreshold level. It appears that intensity is the name of the game for making positive physiological changes in bone (see figure 6.9). If we examine methods of increasing the intensity of loading on bone, two exercise modalities come to the forefront: high-impact aerobics and resistance training. High-impact exercise may not be appropriate for older individuals; this makes resistance training the intervention that holds the most promise for older clients. In fact, high-intensity resistance training has been shown to have positive effects on bone density at the spine and, to a limited extent, the femoral neck as long as sufficient training loads are provided. To further emphasize the necessity for external loading in order to generate exercise-associated changes in bone density, consider the

Risk Factors for Osteoporotic Fractures

Age

History of falls

First degree family history of hip fractures

Gender

Asian or White ethnic origin

Premature menopause

Primary amenorrhea or amenorrhea associated with low estrogen

Frailty or poor health

Low bone mineral density

Dementia

Low body mass index

Cigarette smoking

Excessive alcohol consumption

Low dietary calcium intake

Vitamin D deficiency

Glucocorticoid therapy

Impaired vision

Low physical activity levels or long-term immobilization

Neuromuscular disorders

conclusion reached by Harri Suominen (2006, p. 85) in a review article examining muscle training for bone strength:

> Although aerobic exercise is important in maintaining overall health, the resistance type of muscle training may be more applicable to the basic rules of bone adaptation and site-specific effects of exercise, have more favorable effects in maintaining or improving bone mass and architecture, and be safe and feasible for older people.

3. The response that any bone has to a mechanical stimulus such as exercise is proportional to the loading cycle, which is how frequently the stimulus is applied. There are two methods for loading a client's skeleton to increase bone density and improve architecture: (1) applying a continuous load, as is done in isometrics, or

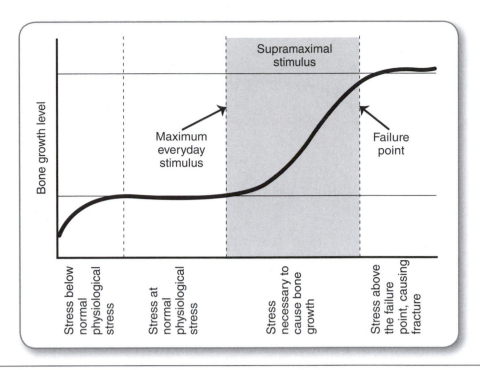

Figure 6.9   Levels of bone growth in response to various stress levels. The highlighted area of the graph shows stress levels above those associated with normal physiological daily functioning and below those causing damage to the bone.

(2) following a loading and unloading cycle, as is done when performing repetitions during weight training. Using a loading and unloading cycle is more effective for improving bone density. There are even some guidelines for using this cycle! Increasing the number of loading cycles appears to have a positive effect up to approximately 40 cycles per day. After that, adding more cycles has little additional effect (see figure 6.10). In other words, when using resistance training to increase bone density, you should limit the number of repetition and set combinations for a particular skeletal area to 40 per day. After that, you should increase the resistance to stimulate improvements. In addition, using multiple sets with sufficient recovery can further increase the osteogenic (bone creation) response.

We should not leave the discussion of loading frequency without looking at whole-body vibration (WBV). Animals with low bone density that are exposed to mechanical vibrations show significant increases in bone strength due to trabecular bone restructuring. These changes include increases in the number of trabecular rods as well as reductions in the spaces between rods. Additionally, the vibratory stimulus leads to a significant increase in the amount of surface actively producing bone mass. WBV interventions with human participants have demonstrated a positive effect on bone that may exceed responses seen with resistance training. One caution before exposing clients to vibratory training: Check the precautions provided by the manufacturers of these devices and be sure that you thoroughly understand the proper use of each device.

4. The response of bone to exercise is improved by brief but intermittent exercise. It appears that one of the reasons why intermittent stimuli work better than continuous stimuli is that the bone cells responsible for bone growth show the same desensitization that other receptors in the body demonstrate. For example, when you walk into a club where the music is blasting, the noise may seem unbearable at first, but soon your ears adjust and you can function almost normally. A similar situation occurs with the way bone responds to exercise. Thus performing two intense sessions on a single day appears to be more effective than performing a single session; however, adding a third session to the day does not appear to offer any advantage. For example, it has been shown that breaking 120 jumps into two 60-jump sessions per day improves the potential for improvements in bone structure by 50%;

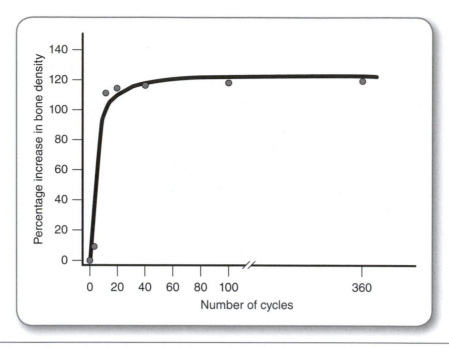

Figure 6.10   Changes in bone mass in response to the number of loading cycles. The rate of improvement plateaus when the number of loading cycles exceeds 40 per day.

however, dividing those 120 jumps into three sessions generates no additional improvements.

In addition, spreading the total volume of work performed per week across 5 days has a greater osteogenic effect than doing the same volume of work in fewer days. Robling and colleagues (2002) put it like this: "Human exercise programs aimed at maintaining or improving bone mass might achieve greater success if the daily exercise regime is broken down into smaller sessions separated by recovery periods" (p. 196).

> **APPLICATION POINT**   Short, intense exercise bouts build bone more effectively than longer sessions do. If the goal is to reduce exercise time, it's better to shorten each exercise session than to reduce the number of sessions performed.

5. Bone responds best when the exercise employs a pattern that differs from the usual loading pattern. Tissue adapts when it is faced with a challenge that is beyond those encountered in everyday life. This overload is the stimulus for tissue change. So when prescribing resistance training, you should consider varying the amount of resistance, the method used to provide that resistance, and the directions in which the force is applied. Fortunately, variations in load and volume are the bases of the periodization program described in chapter 9. In addition, this chapter as well as chapter 7 introduces a number of ways to apply resistance to bone and muscles, including everything from using free weights to performing aquatic exercises. The least addressed and most unique effects, however, may be achieved by varying the directions in which the load is applied. The benefits of applying novel loading patterns are obvious when examining bone architecture. Although many of the exercise interventions produce small changes in bone density, the resulting increases in bone strength are often impressive. This appears to be the result of increased structure in the planes of action in which the loads are applied. It's really quite simple: Our bones do what we do. Let me give you an example. Outside my front door is a wooden telephone pole that's taken repeated poundings from the hurricanes that make their way through Florida every summer. Instead of replacing the entire pole, the electric company strapped a 6-foot (2 m) metal plate to the side of the pole, strengthening the pole along the lines of greatest stress.

APPLICATION POINT The multidirectional drills that are used to translate physical improvements to ADL motor patterns (see chapter 10) incorporate low-level plyometrics across different planes of motion and so in addition to motor skill training give clients changes in force application that strengthen the bones along the structural lines that receive the greatest overloads in daily life.

6. For bone to adapt, it must have sufficient energy to rebuild itself. The development of new bone is an anabolic process. This means that it is a building process that requires the building blocks needed to build bone and the energy needed to get the work done. The two major dietary problems older clients may face when it comes to building bone are low energy intake (especially low protein intake) and low calcium intake. Ilich, Brownbill, and Tamborini (2003) examined the combined and independent effects of calcium and energy (calories from food) availability on total bone mineral density. They showed that postmenopausal women with calcium or energy intakes below the median intake amounts, 750 milligrams each day and 1,694 kilocalories each day, respectively, had lower bone mineral density than postmenopausal women who had calcium and energy intakes above the median amounts. Low energy intake and low protein levels are also associated with reduced circulating insulin-like growth factor 1 (IGF-1), thyroid hormone (T_3), and estradiol, all of which can contribute to bone loss.

7. For exercise to work there should be abundant calcium and vitamin D availability. Since I love analogies, let's use one to examine the associations between calcium and vitamin D intake and bone. Completing any kind of construction project requires raw materials to build the structure and vehicles to deliver those raw materials to the construction site. Only when the materials and the transport vehicles are both present can the construction project begin. Calcium is the major raw mineral used to build bone, along with phosphate and magnesium. These raw materials need to be delivered from the digestive system to the building sites in the bones. This is where vitamin D comes in. Vitamin D facilitates the absorption of calcium, phosphate, and magnesium ions through the intestinal wall and into the bloodstream. In their review entitled "Osteoporosis: Recommendations for Resistance Exercise and Supplementation with Calcium and Vitamin D to Promote Bone Health," Melissa Benton and Andrea White (2006) provide the following opinion:

> Although HRT [hormone replacement therapy] was once the cornerstone of clinical management, it is no longer an appropriate therapeutic alternative. Currently, resistance exercise is the most effective intervention for prevention of bone loss in both healthy and sick populations. However, adequate calcium and vitamin D intake are essential for bone health. Due to confounding factors that may modify the effectiveness of individual therapies, a combination of resistance exercise and supplementation with calcium and vitamin D is recommended for prevention of osteoporosis in women. (p. 208-209)

BETTER BALANCE AND AGILITY

If bone density is the problem, falls are the mechanism by which that problem is transformed into injury. In the beginning of this chapter, I discussed strengthening bone to reduce the potential for fractures resulting from a fall. This portion of the chapter continues that discussion by examining balance and agility. As you will see in chapter 10, balance and agility training fits perfectly into the recovery or translational cycles of a periodized workout.

Frequency of Falls

In the United States, one adult over the age of 65 is treated in the emergency room for a fall every 18 seconds (Centers for Disease Control and Prevention, 2008b). This makes falling the most common cause of nonfatal injuries and hospital admissions for this population (Centers for Disease Control and Prevention, 2006). More than one-third of adults over the age of 65 (about 1.8 million people) experience at least one fall each year (Centers for Disease Control and Prevention, 2008b).

A press release from the National Safety Council (2008) helps put all these data into perspective:

> Falls among people 65 and older is now the leading cause of injury deaths. Furthermore, the mortality rate from falls for older Americans has increased 39% between 1999 and 2005. We must find a way to combat this growing public health concern before it is too late.

This trend is illustrated in figure 6.11.

The effects of this problem on older individuals was further emphasized by AARP president Jennie Chin Hansen, who stated the following at a U.S. Congressional briefing:

> As the nation's more than 79 million baby boomers head into their senior years, this is a problem that will only continue to escalate. . . . Each year, one in three Americans 65 and older falls and nearly 16,000 die from complications from a fall. That's more than the number of deaths that would have occurred if one 737 airliner had crashed every week of the year, killing all aboard (National Safety Council, 2008).

Given this analogy, the words of U.S. Congresswoman Lucille Roybal-Allard of California become even more meaningful:

> The CDC's alarming statistics showing that falls among seniors are a leading cause of senior disability and death should be a call to action to all of us. Senior falls are not inevitable, and therefore we need to focus our federal policies and programs on proven strategies to prevent falls and their disabling and often fatal consequences (Centers for Disease Control and Prevention, 2009).

When we look at these data, listen to the words of these experts, and recognize the change that the baby boomers will create in the average age of the U.S. population, the call to action is clear. We need prevention programs that will reduce the risk for falling.

Consequences of Falls

The frequency of falls and the resulting injuries are a serious problem that affects everyone. In 2004, more than 320,000 hospital admissions in

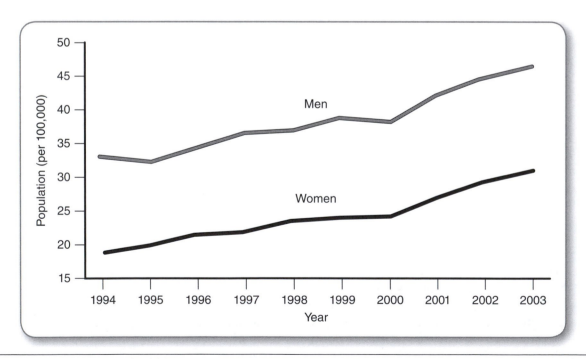

Figure 6.11 Age-adjusted fatal fall injury rates among men and women aged 65 years and older in the United States between 1994 and 2003.

the United States were due to hip fractures. This is a 3% increase over the figures reported in 2003 (Centers for Disease Control and Prevention, 2008b). Of these hip fractures, 9 out of 10 were caused by falls, especially falls that were to the side. In 2005, approximately 16,000 persons over the age of 65 died in the United States as a result of injuries from falling, making falls the leading cause of fatal as well as nonfatal injuries in older persons. It has been estimated that by 2040 the number of hip fractures per year in the United States will exceed 500,000.

But the number of injuries that occur due to falls is only part of the problem. We should also consider the consequences that these injuries have on the individual and on society. First let's consider the individual. People who fracture a hip due to a fall usually spend an average of 1 week in the hospital (Centers for Disease Control and Prevention, 2008b), and 25% of the independently living older persons who fall subsequently require a stay of at least 1 year in a nursing home. One of the most disturbing consequences in this litany of problems is that 1 out of every 5 older persons who fractures a hip dies within 1 year of the injury due to related complications.

Now let's take a look at the financial costs falls have on society. In 2000, the total direct costs of all fall injuries for Americans aged 65 and older exceeded $19 billion U.S. This amount is expected to increase to $43 billion U.S. by 2020 as the U.S. population becomes more gray.

Factors Associated With Falling

We can use a number of strategies to categorize the factors associated with falls. Here we will divide the factors into two categories: intrinsic factors and extrinsic factors. Intrinsic factors are those related to a person's physiology. Stephen Lord and colleagues (Lord et al., 2001) associate the following physiological factors with falling:

- *Vision.* Vision allows people to spot environmental hazards and gives information about the position and movement of the body in relation to the external environment. Declines in visual acuity, contrast, depth perception, and three-dimensional vision increase the risk of falling.

- *Vestibular (inner ear) sensation.* Even if you don't know the mechanisms behind the vestibular reflexes, you probably familiarized yourself with these reflexes as a child when you tried spinning around and around to make yourself dizzy. What you were doing was causing the fluids in your inner ear to flow over the little hair cells that tell the body where it is located within space. People have a 1 in 3 chance of experiencing reduced vestibular reflexes and a slower response to changes in body position. However, it appears that people can learn to use vision and proprioception (sense of body position and tactile sense) to compensate for these losses in order to reduce the likelihood of falling.

- *Peripheral sensation.* Reduced tactile sense at the ankle, vibration sense at the knee, and knee joint position sense are significant indicators of fall risk in both independently living individuals and individuals living in residential extended care. All of these senses are compromised significantly during the typical aging process.

- *Muscle strength.* Muscle strength and power decline exponentially after the age of 50. Reductions in lower-limb strength and power, especially of the hip flexors, dorsiflexors, and knee extensors, are predictive of falls. More recently, increasing weakness of the hip abductors and adductors has been shown to have a negative effect on dynamic balance.

- *Reaction time.* The reaction time of a 60-year-old is on average 25% slower than that of a 20-year-old. Additionally, people living in extended care have slower reaction times than those living in the community have, and fallers have slower reaction times than nonfallers have. These differences are seen both in simple reaction tasks and in complex reaction tasks requiring decision making.

- *Balance and mobility factors.* Numerous balance and mobility factors have been shown to be associated with fall probability. These include impaired stability when standing, impaired stability when leaning and reaching, inadequate responses to external perturbations, slow voluntary stepping, impaired gait and mobility, impaired ability when standing up, and impaired balance transfers.

- *Orthostatic hypotension.* Orthostatic hypotension is a sudden drop in blood pressure, usually greater than 20/10 mmHg, due to a change in posture from a sitting or lying position to an upright position. Symptoms include dizziness, faintness, or light-headedness. The incidence of orthostatic hypotension increases with age, and its prevalence in the elderly is reported to be 5% to 33%.

- *Cognition.* There is a proven relationship between reduced cognitive ability and increased probability of falling. For example, declines in general cognitive functioning, nonverbal and abstract reasoning, information processing speed, and immediate memory are all related to falls in older populations. Additionally, one of the most sensitive markers of fall probability is the inability to perform dual tasks, such as walking while trying to do math.

Extrinsic factors associated with falling include the following:

- *Medications, particularly sedative and psychotropic drugs.* Drugs are a major cause of postural hypotension. Drugs designed to control high blood pressure, such as diuretics, calcium antagonists, beta-blockers, ACE inhibitors, alpha-adrenergic blocking agents, and centrally acting antihypertensives, have more of an effect on older individuals than they have on younger people. Additionally, nitrates, antiparkinsonian drugs, antidepressants, and antipsychotics all have the potential to cause hypotension in older persons. Certainly exercise is a viable option for reducing the required doses of many of these drugs by promoting positive physiological changes.

- *Alcohol intake.* Drinking is responsible for a substantial proportion of unintentional falls resulting in hospital admission or death. Therefore, controlling alcohol consumption should be part of any program aimed at reducing falls. In fact, a history of drinking is associated with an increased risk of fatal injury from falls, motor vehicle crashes, and suicides in older persons.

- *Inappropriate footwear.* Wearing inappropriate footwear that lacks support, fits incorrectly, or does not adhere to the foot (such as flip-flops or slippers) can lead to falls and

related injuries. Improving knowledge and attitudes about proper choices in footwear should be a part of any program aimed at preventing falls.

- *Environmental factors.* Physical factors in the environment, such as stairs, poor lighting, loose rugs, extension cords, uneven sidewalks, or high curbs, can lead to falls and injuries. It is beyond the scope of this book to list and discuss environmental factors in any detail; however, an assessment of potential tripping hazards in the home or in the community is a critical factor in preventing falls.

Since this is a book about exercise, our conversation here focuses on the fall-associated factors that can be addressed through movement training. Additionally, exercises targeting strength and power are not discussed in this chapter, since they are addressed in the next chapter. That leaves us with balance and agility as the major training topics to be discussed in this chapter.

What Is Balance?

Balance is an important factor that affects the performance of standing as well as seated tasks and often limits daily functioning. Since balance activities usually require moving the body or other objects from one location to another, transitions from static to dynamic balance often become an important controlling element. Moreover, when balance must be incorporated into skilled movements such as navigating an uneven sidewalk, negotiating a curb, or moving around another person, the concept of agility enters the mix. To get a better appreciation for the importance of balance training, let's look at

- relationships between the center of gravity and the base of support,
- stable versus unstable equilibrium, and
- agility.

Relationships Between the Center of Gravity and Base of Support

The relationship between the center of gravity and base of support of any object determines the objects degree of balance, or equilibrium. For an object to be in a state of static equilibrium, or static balance, its center of gravity must be located

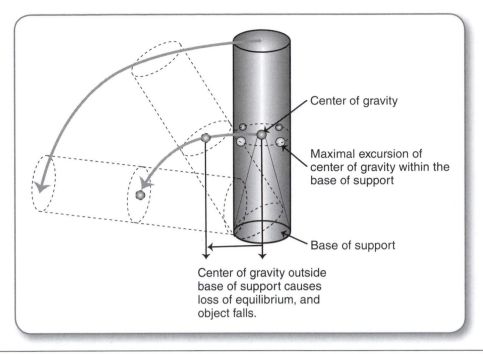

Center of gravity

Maximal excursion of center of gravity within the base of support

Base of support

Center of gravity outside base of support causes loss of equilibrium, and object falls.

Figure 6.12 The relationship between the center of gravity and the base of support affects the stability of a cylinder.

within its base of support. Once the center of gravity of an object moves outside the support base, the object falls (see figure 6.12).

In his classic text, *The Biomechanics of Sports Techniques,* James Hay (1973) lists three factors that control the stability of an object:

1. The position of the line of gravity relative to the boundaries of the base
2. The object's weight
3. The height of the center of gravity relative to the base

For humans like us (assuming this text is not sold to extraterrestrials), the center of gravity is located at approximately 55% of standing height for women and approximately 57% of standing height for men. This statement, of course, assumes that the person is standing up straight. Squatting moves the center of gravity closer to the feet (or base) and makes it easier to maintain balance. The ultimate position of stability, of course, is to lie on the ground, at which point you no longer have to worry about falling.

Stable and Unstable Equilibrium

Stable equilibrium is the state that occurs when an object tends to return to its original position

when its center of gravity is displaced. Examples of objects in a stable equilibrium are a pendulum and a rocking chair. People, on the other hand, spend the majority of their lives in some state of unstable equilibrium. This means that when our center of gravity moves away from our base, we tend to move farther away from our original position rather than return to it. In other words, we fall if we don't reestablish or widen our base (see figure 6.13).

Agility

Agility is the ability to control changes in direction and body position quickly and effectively. For our purposes, agility is the ability of clients to navigate around obstacles and regain their balance when faced with environmental challenges.

Strategies for Maintaining Balance

In a 2006 paper, Brian Maki and William McIlroy commented on the strategies used by older persons to maintain balance. One is a fixed-support strategy, in which a person uses the hip, knee, and ankle muscles to keep the center of gravity within the base of support (see figure 6.14, a-b). The second is a change-in-support strategy, which involves widening the base of support in order to keep the center of gravity within the base when the center of gravity is rapidly displaced

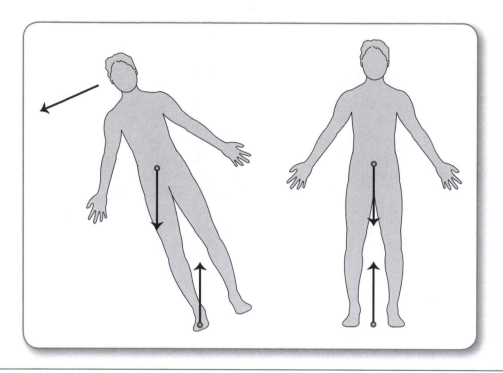

Figure 6.13 People fall once their center of gravity moves outside of their base unless they widen or move their base.

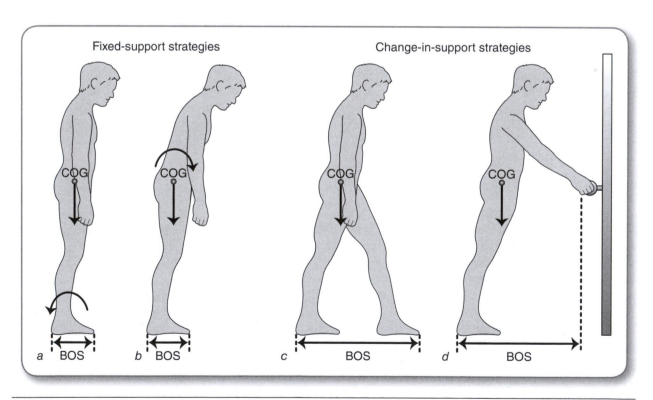

Figure 6.14 Recovery reactions used to maintain balance. Fixed-support reactions use forces developed by the muscles about the *(a)* ankle and *(b)* hip to maintain balance. Change-in-support reactions dramatically increase the base of support either by *(c)* stepping or *(d)* reaching, touching, and grasping. COG = center of gravity. BOS = base of support.

Based on Maki and McIlroy 2006.

(see figure 6.14, *c-d*). Since a shift in the center of gravity is usually the result of a rapid, unexpected change in body position, the response that allows a person to regain balance must also be rapid. Unfortunately, as people age their rapid stepping and reaching responses slow down, and they must adopt strategies that are different from those of younger individuals and that are often nonideal. These strategies are characterized by the following:

- Multiple sidesteps rather than crossing steps to regain lateral balance
- Limb collisions during lateral stepping and even walking
- Slow and poorly targeted reaching movements

Additionally, during recovery efforts older persons reduce their speed more, establish larger personal comfort zones, and make more mistakes when attempting to perform mental tasks. The research of Weerdesteyn, Nienhuis, and Duysens (2005) is helpful when it comes to devising an intervention strategy to prevent falls. These authors found that older persons have less success than younger persons have in avoiding obstacles placed in their paths during treadmill walking. This success declined even further when the time available for response was decreased. The authors also noted that older persons use greater variation in step length than younger persons use when negotiating obstacles.

TESTING BALANCE

There are a number of balance tests available in the literature. The three included in this section were chosen because they are simple to perform, are valid measures of balance, are reliable between testing sessions and raters, and are sensitive to change.

The Single-Leg Stance Balance Test

The single-leg stance balance test has been a clinical measure of balance since 1965. The test has been correlated with laboratory measures of postural sway and is a strong clinical tool for predicting falls. The test can be administered in an eyes-open or eyes-closed condition.

Equipment Needed

- A stopwatch
- A wall with a reference mark for the client to look at

Protocol

- Have the client stand, with feet together and arms down at the sides, about 3 feet (1 m) from a wall or other object that has a point that can be used as a visual reference.
- Demonstrate the technique before the individual attempts a trial.
- Instruct the client to raise one foot about 6 to 8 inches (15-20 cm) off the ground by bending that leg at the knee, keep both hands at his or her sides, and prevent legs from touching each other.. The stopwatch should be started as soon as the client has achieved this position.
- The client should stand on one leg as long as possible, keeping the standing leg straight, the arms at the sides, and the foot in one place while watching the reference mark (see figure 6.15).

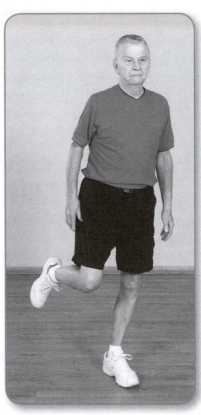

Figure 6.15   The single-leg stance balance test.

- Allow the client two practice trials before collecting data.
- Stop the test when the client's arms move away from the sides, the support foot moves across the floor, or the raised foot touches the floor.
- If desired, have the client repeat the test with the eyes closed.

Functional Reach Test

The functional reach test was developed by Duncan and colleagues in 1990. The test has since been shown to be an effective measure of frailty in older persons (Weiner, Duncan, Chandler, & Studenski, 1992). This test is simple to administer and perform and uses a minimal amount of equipment: a 36-inch (91.4 cm) measuring stick and Velcro strips. The variable being measured is the distance an individual can reach forward while maintaining a stable base of support. Test results correlate highly ($r = .83$) with classical pressure plate measurements of balance and have the sensitivity to detect age-related balance changes. While a number of other tests such as Romberg's test and the Tinetti balance test may be more effective measures of frailty and fall potential, the functional reach test provides an objective numerical score, is easily administered, and shows good reliability among tests and among testers. One problem with the test is that it requires two testers for effective administration.

Equipment Needed

- A measuring stick approximately 36 inches (91.4 cm) long
- Velcro or tape to hold the stick to a wall
- A helper

Protocol

- Have the person to be tested remove both shoes and socks and stand relaxed with the right shoulder perpendicular to the wall.
- Demonstrate proper form before starting the test.
- Affix the measuring stick to the wall, placing it parallel to the floor at the level of the client's right acromion.
- One tester should stand where it's easy to read the position of the client's knuckle as it moves along the measuring stick, and the other should lie on the floor to observe whether either of the client's heels loses contact with the floor.
- Instruct the client to fully extend the right arm horizontally (to approximately 90°), clench the right hand in a fist, and point the middle knuckle forward so that the initial reach (equivalent to the arm's length) can be measured (see figure 6.16).

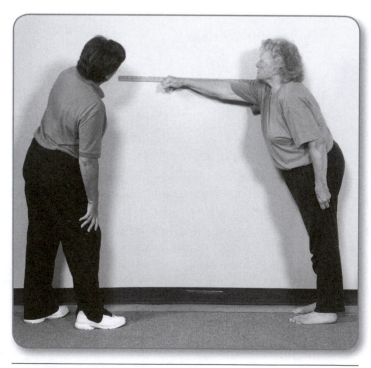

Figure 6.16   The functional reach test.

- Have the client lean as far forward as possible without losing balance.
- No specific strategy for completing the task is specified. The test is completed when one of the client's heels loses contact with the floor.
- Allow two practice trials before beginning the actual testing to familiarize the individual with the testing procedure. Evaluate the client's technique during the practice trials.
- The functional reach is the distance reached minus the initial reach.
- Two trials are performed.

8-Foot (2.4 m) Up-and-Go Test

The 8-foot (2.4 m) up-and-go test, also called the *get-up-and-go test,* is one of the most commonly used and reliable tests of muscular strength and mobility in the literature (Rikli & Jones, 1999). This version has been tested on more than 7,000 persons, and norms are available across age groups for comparison (Rikli & Jones, 1999). The variable being measured is the time it takes a person to get up from a chair with a seat height 17 inches (43 cm), walk 8 feet (2.4 m), return to the chair, and resume a seated position.

Equipment Needed

- A standard straight-back chair with a seat height of 17 inches (43 cm)
- A cone or similar position marker
- A stopwatch

Protocol

- Set up a chair against a wall and position a cone so that its base is exactly 8 feet (2.44 m) from the front edge of the chair seat.
- Ask the client to sit erect in the chair with the hands on the thighs, the back in contact with the chair back, and the feet flat on the floor.
- Demonstrate correct heel-to-toe walking with at least one foot in contact with the ground at all times (to ensure no running).
- Give the signal to go while simultaneously starting the stopwatch.
- At the starting signal the client rises from the chair (assistance with the arms is allowed), walks around the cone (see figure 6.17), and returns to the chair and sits in the original seated position.
- Allow the client one practice trial followed by two test trials.
- Use the average score to evaluate performance.

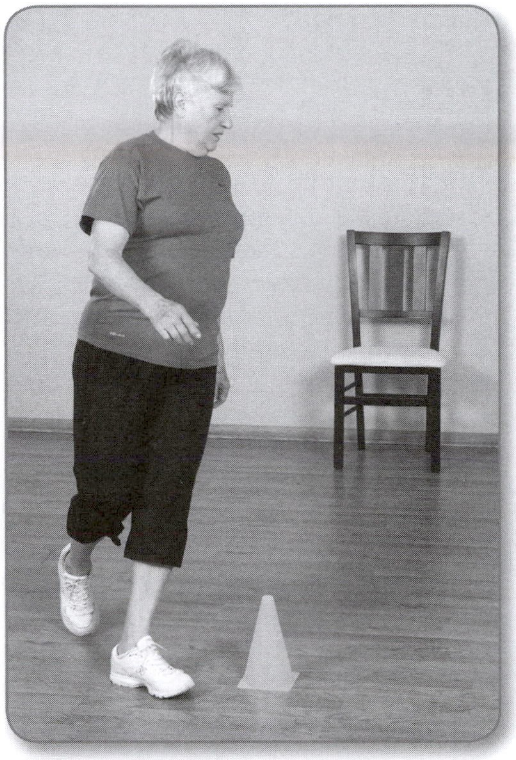

Figure 6.17 The 8-foot (2.4 m) up-and-go test.

Let's consider how to deal with the results of these diagnostic tests. Very often we perceive measurements like balance and agility differently than measures like strength and aerobic capacity. And while this may be true to some extent, these factors could become the major targets of our prescriptive exercise program if the above tests produce the lowest percentile ranks. If balance is the major goal, you should first determine if there is an underlying physical factor (usually lower body power or strength). If so, then balance can become the secondary target during the initial weeks of the training cycle. And during the second half of the cycle motor learning training drills can dominate "translating" your client's improvements into balance-related activities of daily living. You will see examples of these "translational" drills in Chapter 10. In addition, you will see how to structure these periodized training programs in Chapter 9.

BALANCE TRAINING

Although strength training and walking programs have some benefit for balance, it appears that the most effective programs for improving balance are multidimensional programs, especially those incorporating dynamic balance and agility training. By their very structures, these programs address the unstable equilibrium and agility concerns discussed in this chapter. Additionally, many of these programs can have a positive effect on reaction time, mobility, and proprioception if designed properly.

Tai Chi

The exercise method that has received the most positive scientific press as an intervention for preventing falls is tai chi (see figure 6.18). However, while tai chi has been shown to reduce falls, it has not been shown to be an effective training tool for increasing bone density, and therefore it should not be considered a panacea for the prevention of fall-related injuries. Having provided this disclaimer, let me say that there is a considerable body of research indicating that tai chi can improve static balance, improve proprioception, reduce the probability and incidence of falling, and diminish the fear of falling. Now that I have sung the praises of tai chi as a training technique for reducing falls, let's look at some other equally, if not more successful, exercise interventions.

Agility Training

Having made it this far in the book, you no doubt recognize that this is not a book about a single exercise modality and its miraculous ability to halt the aging process. Instead, it is a book about choosing the correct training tools to do the job. The emphasis is on the word *tools,* since effective training is usually the result of applying many different training modalities to a multifaceted

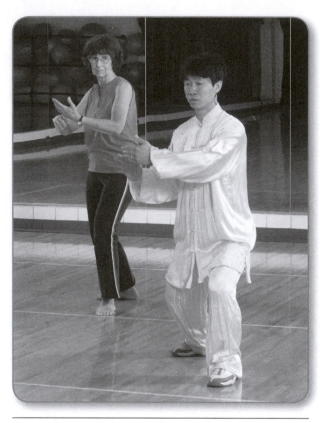

Figure 6.18 Tai chi is an effective method for improving static balance and proprioception.

problem (remember the diamond). Nowhere in the literature on exercise and aging is this multifaceted approach more evident than in fall prevention. There is a clear association between fall prevention and lower-body strength, power, and movement speed (see chapter 7). Additionally, strengthening the bones can reduce the probability of catastrophic injury if a fall does occur. Let's now examine another complementary training modality that can help in preventing falls: agility training. We are using the term *agility training* rather than *balance training* to reflect a statement made by Maki and McIlroy in their 2006 paper on the importance of rapid limb movement to balance recovery. These authors noted that "every time we move volitionally we perturb [throw off] our balance" (p. ii12). So every movement we make is actually a change in body position that we must control—in other words, every movement is an adventure in agility. The older we get, the greater the adventure.

Given the research findings, let's look at interventions that have used agility training as part of their programming. Two studies by Teresa Liu-Ambrose have shown the effectiveness of agility training in reducing fall risk. The first study looked at the separate effects of resistance, flexibility, and agility training on fall risk in women aged 75 to 85 years with low bone mass (Liu-Ambrose et al., 2004a). The authors observed significant decreases in fall probability with both the agility and resistance training programs. The agility training program was designed to improve

- eye–hand coordination,
- eye–foot coordination,
- dynamic balance,
- standing and leaning balance, and
- reaction time.

The researchers used ball games, relay races, dance movements, and obstacle courses to improve each of these parameters. For safety purposes, hip protectors were provided. In addition, the instructors supervised the drills and spotted the participants to reduce the potential for injury during training. In the second study, the researchers (Liu-Ambrose et al., 2004b) looked at balance confidence as a result of resistance or agility training. Using similar interventions they found that again resistance and balance training were effective interventions. The positive results of these studies indicated that resistance and agility training can have a positive impact on reducing falls and the associated likelihood of fractures.

Tatjana Bulat and colleagues (2007) examined the effects of an 8-week balance training program in community-living veterans of an average age of 78 years. Like the training program by Liu Ambrose, the Bulat program used specific exercises to address the elements central to fall prevention. Training was conducted in one session per week. Table 6.1 shows the training timetable, the progression in training, and the exercises used in the intervention. Notice the similarity between the elements trained in the Bulat study and the elements that were discussed earlier in this chap-

ter. The Bulat program improved all measures of balance, including the following:

- *Reaction time:* The time between the command to move and the patient's first movement.
- *Movement velocity:* The average speed of the movement of the center of gravity.
- *End-point excursion:* The end point, or the farthest point, in a person's lean toward a target.
- *Maximum excursion:* The maximum distance of a lean in any direction.
- *Directional control:* The measure of a person's ability to move toward a target while minimizing extraneous movements.

Agility training has also been shown to be an important component of mixed exercise interventions. Zhen-Bo Cao and colleagues (Cao et al., 2007) examined the success of a 12-week fall prevention program that included stretching exercises, balance ball exercises, step with body bar exercises, minihurdle walking, zigzag footwork, pool walking, ordinary walking, and sit-and-stand exercises. They found little effect on static balance, 10-meter walking speed, or sit-and-reach flexibility. But factors more reflective of the training stimuli showed significant improvements. Whole-body reaction time improved nearly 7%, while the 10-meter obstacle walk improved 5%.

We should look at one more topic to complete this discussion of balance and agility training: seated balance. Since the seated position provides both a large base (the gluteal muscles and feet) and a lower center of gravity, we sometimes forget that leaning and reaching from a seated position requires us to make adjustments in order to maintain balance. Sprigle and coworkers (Sprigle, Maurer, & Holowka, 2007) offer these recommendations for improving seated balance:

> While working with clients on seated stability and functional movement, clinicians should be encouraged to incorporate bilateral reach tasks because it has the strongest relationship to ADL performance. Researchers interested in studying postural control and stability during functional tasks should consider using uncompensated reach measures. (p. 40).

Table 6.1 Functional Balance Class Content

Week	Element trained	Sample exercises
1	Stance stability	Practice equal weight bearing. Resist self-initiated and external perturbations (perform minisquats, play tug of war with an elastic band). Progress to eyes-closed condition and using a compliant surface if tolerated.
2	Initiation of weight shift	Shift weight between anti and post and between left and right. Pass a ball (requires forced reaching and weight shifts). Look over the shoulder to promote weight shifting.
3	Advanced weight shifting	Perform week 2 exercises with a narrowed base of support, an instep stance position, or lights dimmed or eyes closed. Use a metronome or music to add an element of timing to tasks.
4	Introduction to stepping	Step repeatedly, alternating side taps or tap-ups to a 2-inch (5 cm) riser. Kick a stationary soccer ball.
5	Dynamic base of support	Practice resisted stepping (place an elastic band around waist and step away) and multidirectional stepping. Incorporate various surfaces if capable or alter visual input.
6	Vestibular stimulation	Perform gaze stabilization exercises in standing. Practice cone stacking side to side with associated head motion.
7	Multidirectional locomotion	Perform crossovers, braiding, and backward walking. Introduce direction-changing drills that require random, sudden changes in direction.
8	High-level coordination activities and multitasking	Introduce high-level gait training, speed changes, and ambulation with alternating claps. Dribble a soccer ball, play balloon volleyball, or negotiate an obstacle course.

Adapted by permission from Bulat et al. 2007.

Other Alternatives

Three other alternatives should be considered as part of an exercise intervention to improve balance. These alternatives are a bit high-tech but are successful. The first alternative is perturbation-based training. This type of training puts the individual into a condition that disturbs the relationship between the center of gravity and the base of support. One of the most common methods is the use of a perturbation platform that can be programmed to provide greater and greater levels of instability as the individual's balance improves. Numerous balance platforms are available and come with features that allow everything from simple amplitude control to the introduction of a virtual, dynamic environment that challenges all the senses.

The second high-tech alternative is the WBV training mentioned earlier in this book. Improve-ments in both laboratory and field test measure-ments have been reported with WBV training, making it an interesting alternative or additive training tool for the more traditional balance training methods.

Finally, some of the new video games offer promise for balance training and may act as wonderful additions to the training that you provide in the gym or wellness center. In our laboratory, we are currently examining how effective the Wii balance program is for improving static and dynamic balance, gait, and agility in persons aged 65 years and older.

SUMMARY

Exercise in conjunction with calcium and vitamin D supplementation may be the most effective and safest intervention for maintaining or even increasing bone density. When developing programs to increase bone density, high-intensity and high-speed movements and short but intense loading intervals are most effective. Remember that improvements in bone density and architecture are confined to the areas where the loading stresses are applied. For this reason, training to build bone requires us to think beyond the standard 8 to 10 flexion and extension methods and to begin exploring exercises that more effectively target areas such as the hip and femoral neck, which show minimal gains during standard training. Finally, varying loading patterns and training techniques provides unique overloads that encourage greater levels of adaptation across the training period. A periodized program using different levels and patterns of exercise across changing training cycles is the most effective way to accomplish these goals.

In addition to strengthening the bones, reducing fall probability is also important to preventing fall-related injury in clients. Tai chi, agility training, and multifactorial programs have all been shown to reduce fall probability and fear of falling. The most effective of these programs include the elements that we typically employ to regain or maintain balance in our daily lives. While programs designed to reduce falls certainly include strength and power training, maximum effectiveness cannot be expected unless agility and balance training are also included. Chapter 9 provides a template that allows you to seamlessly weave these practical training methods into a periodized program designed to maximize benefits and reduce the potential for overtraining and overuse injuries. Chapter 10, which describes drills that translate improvements in physical function into improvements in ADLs, presents a number of balance and agility drills.

Topical Bibliography

Structure of Bone

Ahlborg, H.G., Johnell, O., Turner, C.H., Rannevik, G., & Karlsson, M.K. (2003). Bone loss and bone size after menopause. *N Engl J Med* 349:327-334.

Borer, K.T. (2005). Physical activity in the prevention and amelioration of osteoporosis in women. *Sports Med* 35:779-830.

Brown, P., McNeil, R., Radwan, E., & Willingale J. (2007). The burden of osteoporosis in New Zealand: 2007-2020. www.iofbonehealth.org/download/osteofound/filemanager/policy_advocacy/pdf/white-papers/new-zealand-white-paper-2007.pdf

Burge, R.T. (2001). The cost of osteoporotic fractures in the UK: Projections for 2000-2020. *Journal of Medical Economics* 4:51.

Dennison, E., Cole, Z., & Cooper, C. (2005). Diagnosis and epidemiology of osteoporosis. *Curr Opin Rheumatol* 17:456.

European Foundation for Osteoporosis and Bone Disease and National Osteoporosis Foundation. (1997). Who are candidates for prevention and treatment for osteoporosis? *Osteoporos Int* 7:1.

Hagino, H., Katagiri, H., Okano, T., Yamamoto, K., & Teshima, R. (2005). Increasing incidence of hip fracture in Tottori Prefecture, Japan: Trend from 1986 to 2001. *Osteoporos Int* 16:1963.

National Osteoporosis Foundation. (2008). Osteoporosis: Quick facts. www.nof.org/professionals/Fast_Facts_Osteoporosis.pdf

Nguyen, T.V., & Eisman, J.A. (1999). Risk factors for low bone mass in elderly men. In E.S. Orwoll (Ed.), *Osteoporosis in men* (p. 335). San Diego: Academic Press.

Orimo, H., Hashimoto, T., Sakata, K., Yoshimura, N., Suzuki, T., & Hosoi, T. (2000). Trends in the incidence of hip fracture in Japan, 1987-1997: The third nationwide survey. *J Bone Miner Metab* 18:126.

Sambrook, P.N., Seeman, E., Phillips, S.R., & Ebeling, P.R. (2002). Preventing osteoporosis: Outcomes of the Australian Fracture Prevention Summit. *Med J Aust* 176(Suppl.): S1.

van Staa, T.P., Dennison, E.M., Leufkens, H.G., & Cooper, C. (2001). Epidemiology of fractures in England and Wales. *Bone* 29:517.

World Health Organization. (1994). *Assessment of fracture risk and its application to screening for postmenopausal osteoporosis.* Geneva: World Health Organization.

Exercise Training to Prevent Osteoporosis

Bautmans, I., Van Hees, E., Lemper, J., & Mets, T. (2005). The feasibility of whole body vibration in institutionalized elderly persons and its influence on muscle performance, balance and mobility: A randomised controlled trial. *BMC Geriatrics* 5:1-8.

Benton, M.J., & White, A. (2006). Osteoporosis: Recommendations for resistance exercise and supplementation with calcium and vitamin D to promote bone health. *J Com Health Nurs* 23:201-211.

Bulat, T., Hart-Hughes, S., Ahmed, S., Quigley, P., Palacios, P., Werner, D.C., & Foulis, P. (2007). Effect of a group-based exercise program on balance in elderly. *Clin Interv Aging* 2:655-660.

Burr, D.B., Robling, A.G., & Turner, C.H. (2002). Effects of biomechanical stress on bones in animals. *Bone* 30:781-786.

Cao, Z.B., Maeda, A., Shima, N., Kurata, H., & Nishizono, H. (2007). The effect of a 12-week combined exercise intervention program on physical performance and gait kinematics in community-dwelling elderly women. *J Physiol Anthropol* 26:325-332.

Fuchs, R.K., Williams, D.P., & Snow, C.M. (2001). Response of growing bones to a jumping protocol of reduced repetitions: A randomized controlled trial. *J Bone Min Res* 16:203.

Guney, E., Kisakol, G., Ozgen, G., Yilmaz, C., Yilmaz, R., & Kabalak, T. (2007). Effect of weight loss on bone metabolism: Comparison of vertical banded gastroplasty and medical intervention. *Obes Surg* 13:383-388.

Hannan, M.T., Tucker, K.L., Dawson-Hughes, B., Cupples, L.A., Felson, D.T., & Keil, D.P. (2000). Effect of dietary protein on bone loss in elderly men and women : The Framingham Osteoporosis Study. *J Bone Min Res* 15:2504-2512.

Hart, J., Liskova, M., & Landa, J. (1971). Reaction of bone to mechanical stimuli I: Continuous and intermittent loading of tibia in rabbit. *Folia Morphol (Praha)* 19:290-300.

Ilich, J.Z., Brownbill, R.A., & Tamborini, L. (2003). Bone and nutrition in elderly women: Protein, energy, and calcium as main determi-

nants of bone mineral density. *Eur J Clin Nutr* 57:554-565.

Katzeff, H.L., Yang, M.U., Presta, E., Leibel, R.L., Hirsch, J., & Van Italli, T.B. (1990). Calorie restriction and iopanoic acid effects on thyroid hormone metabolism. *Am J Clin Nutr* 52:263.

Lanyon, L.E., & Rubin, C.T. (1984). Static vs dynamic loads as an influence on bone remodelling. *J Biomech* 17:897-905.

Lau, E.M.C., Woo, J., Leung, P.C., Swaminathan, R., & Leung, D. (1992). The effects of calcium supplementation and exercise on bone density in elderly Chinese women. *Osteoporosis Int* 2:168-173.

Legrand, E., Chappard, D., Pascaretti, C., Duquenne, M., Krebbs, S., Rohmer, V., Lix Basle, M., & Audrani, M. (2000). Trabecular bone microarchitecture, bone mineral density, and vertebral fractures in male osteoporosis. *J Bone Min Res* 15:13-19.

Liu-Ambrose, T., Khan, K.M., Eng, J.J., Janssen, P.A., Lord, S.R., & McKay, H.A. (2004). Resistance and agility training reduce fall risk in women aged 75 to 85 with low bone mass: A 6- month randomized, controlled trial. *JAGS* 52:657-665.

Liu-Ambrose, T., Khan, K.M., Eng, J.J., Lord, S.R., & McKay, H.A. (2004). Balance confidence improves with resistance or agility training. Increase is not correlated with objective changes in fall risk and physical abilities. *Gerontology* 50:373-382.

Martin-St. James, M., & Carroll, S. (2006). High-intensity resistance training and postmenopausal bone loss: A meta-analysis. *Osteoporosis Int* 17:1225-1240.

Martyn-St. James, M., & Carroll, S. (2006). Progressive high-intensity resistance training and bone mineral density changes among premenopausal women: Evidence of discordant site-specific skeletal effects. *Sports Med* 36:683-704.

NIH Consensus Development Panel on Osteoporosis Prevention, Diagnosis, and Therapy. (2001). Osteoporosis prevention, diagnosis, and therapy. *JAMA* 285:785-795.

Rizzoli, R., Ammann, P., Chevalley, T., & Bonjour, J.P. (2001). Protein intake and bone disorders in the elderly. *Joint Bone Spine* 68:383-392.

Robling, A.G., Hinant, F.M., Burr, D.B., & Turner, C.H. (2002a). Improved bone structure and strength after long-term mechanical loading is greatest if loading is separated into short bouts. *J Bone Min Res* 17:1545-1554.

Robling, A.G., Hinant, F.M., Burr, D.B., & Turner, C.H. (2002b). Shorter, more frequent mechanical loading sessions enhance bone mass. *Med Sci Sport Exerc* 34:196-202.

Rubin, C., Turner, A.S., Mallinckrodt, C., Jerome, C., McLeod, K., & Bain, S. (2002). Mechanical strain, induced noninvasively in the high-frequency domain, is anabolic to cancellous bone, but not cortical bone. *Bone* 30:445-452.

Suominen, H. (2006). Muscle training for bone strength. *Aging Clin Exp Res* 18:85-93.

Surgeon General. (2004). *The 2004 Surgeon General's report on bone health and osteoporosis: What it means to you.* Washington, DC: Department of Health and Human Services.

Turner, C.H., & Robling, A.G. (2002). Designing exercise regimens to increase bone strength. *Exercise and Sports Science Review* 31:45-50.

van der Maulen, M.C., Beaupre, G.S., & Carter, D.R. (1993). Mechanobiologic influences in long bone cross-sectional growth. *Bone* 14:635-642.

Verschueren, S.M., Roelants, M., Delecluse, C., Swinnen, S., Vanderschueren, D., & Boonen, S. (2004). Effects of 6-month whole body vibration training on hip density, muscle strength, and postural control in postmenopausal women: A randomized controlled pilot study. *J Bone Min Res* 19:352-359.

Weerdesteyn, V., Nienhuis, B., & Duysens, J. (2005). Advancing age progressively affects obstacle avoidance skills in the elderly. *Hum Mov Sci* 24:865-880.

Better Balance and Agility

Brauer, S.G., Woollacott, M., & Shumway-Cook, A. (2002). The influence of a concurrent cognitive task on the compensatory stepping response to a perturbation in balance-impaired and healthy elders. *Gait Posture* 15(1): 83-93.

Centers for Disease Control and Prevention. (2006). Injury prevention and control: Data and statistics (WISQARS). www.cdc.gov/ncipc/wisqars.

Centers for Disease Control and Prevention. (2008). Hip fractures among older adults. www.cdc.gov/ncipc/factsheets/adulthipfx.htm

Centers for Disease Control and Prevention. (2008). *Preventing falls among older adults.* Washington, DC: Department of Health and Human Services.

Centers for Disease Control and Prevention. (2009). Falls among older adults: An overview. www.cdc.gov/homeandrecreationalsafety/falls/adultfalls.html

Cummings, S.R., Kelsey, J.L., Nevitt, M.C., & O'Dowd, K.J. (1985). Epidemiology of osteoporosis and osteoporotic fractures. *Epidemiol Rev* 7:178-208.

Cummings, S.R., Rubin, S.M., & Black, D. (1990). The future of hip fractures in the United States. Numbers, costs, and potential effects of postmenopausal estrogen. *Clin Ortho Rel Res* 252:163-166.

Dunne, R.G., Bergman, A.B., Rogers, L.W., Inglin, B., & Rivara, F.P. (1993). Elderly persons' attitudes towards footwear—a factor in preventing falls. *Public Health Rep* 108(2):245-248.

Englander, F., Hodson, T.J., & Terregrossa, R.A. (1996). Economic dimensions of slip and fall injuries. *J Forensic Sci* 41:733-746.

Gerdhem, P., Ringsberg, K.A., & Akesson, K. (2006). The relation between previous fractures and physical performance in elderly women. *Arch Phys Med Rehabil* 87:914-917.

Gérin-Lajoie, M., Richards, C.L., & McFadyen, B.J. (2006). The circumvention of obstacles during walking in different environmental contexts: A comparison between older and younger adults. *Gait Posture* 24:364-369.

Grabiner, M.D., & Jahnigen, D.W. (1992). Modeling recovery from stumbles: Preliminary data on variable selection and classification efficacy. *J Am Geriatr Soc* 40(9):910-913.

Hausdorff, J.M., Yogev, G., Springer, S., Simon, E.S., & Giladi, N. (2005). Walking is more like catching than tapping: Gait in the elderly as a complex cognitive task. *Exp Brain Res* 164:541-548.

Hay, J.G. (1973). *The biomechanics of sports techniques.* Englewood Cliffs, NJ: Prentice Hall.

Hayes, W.C., Myers, E.R., Morris, J.N., Gerhart, T.N., Yett, H.S., & Lipsitz, L.A. (1993). Impact near the hip dominates fracture risk in elderly nursing home residents who fall. *Calcif Tissue Int* 52:192-198.

HealthandAge.com. (2008). Live well, live longer. www.healthandage.com.

Heitmann, D.K., Gossman, M.R., Shaddeau, S.A., & Jackson, J.R. (1989). Balance performance and step width in noninstitutionalized, elderly, female fallers and nonfallers. *Phys Ther* 69:923-931.

Ivers, R.Q., Cumming, R.G., Mitchell, P., & Attebo, K. (1988). Visual impairment and falls in older adults: The Blue Mountains Eye Study. *J Am Geriatr Soc* 46:58-64.

Komatsu, T., Kim, K.J., Kaminai, T., Okuizumi, H., Kamioka, H., Okada, S., Park, H., Hasegawa, A., Mutoh, Y., Mutoh, Y., & Yamamoto, I. (2006). Clinical factors as predictors of the risk of falls and subsequent bone fractures due to osteoporosis in postmenopausal women. *J Bone Miner Metab* 24:419-424.

Kool, B., Ameratunga, S., Robinson, E., Crengle, S., & Jackson, R. (2008). The contribution of alcohol to falls at home among working-aged adults. *Alcohol* 42(5): 383-388.

Leibson, C.L., Toteson, A.N.A., Gabriel, S.E., Ransom, J.E., & Melton III, J.L. (2002). Mortality, disability, and nursing home use for persons with and without hip fracture: A population-based study. *J Am Geriatr Soc* 50:1644-1650.

Lord, S.R., & Dayhew, J. (2001). Visual risk factors for falls. *J Am Geriatr Soc* 49:508-515.

Lord, S.R., Sherrington, C., & Menz, H.B. (2001). *Falls in older people: Risk factors and strategies for prevention.* Cambridge, UK: Cambridge University Press.

Magaziner, J., Hawkes, W., Hebel, J.R., Zimerman, S.I., Fox, K.M., Dolan, M., Felsenthal, G., & Kenzora, J. (2000). Recovery from hip fracture in eight areas of function. *J Gerontol Med Sci* 55A: M498-M507

McGinnis, P.M. (2007). *Biomechanics of sports and exercise* (2nd ed.). Champaign, IL: Human Kinetics.

Menant, J.C., Steele, J.R., Menz, H.B., Munro, B.J., & Lord, S.R. (2008). Effects of footwear features on balance and stepping in older people. *Gerontology* 54(1):18-23.

Menz, H.B., Morris, M.E., & Lord, S.R. (2006). Footwear characteristics and risk of indoor and outdoor falls in older people. *Gerontology* 52(3):174-180.

Mulch, G., & Petermann, W. (1979). Influence of age on results of vestibular function tests. Review of literature and presentation of caloric test results. *Ann Otol Rhinol Laryngol Suppl* 88(Suppl. 56): 1-17.

National Safety Council. (2008). Falls leading cause of injury death for people 65 and older; medical costs of $19 billion per year to more than double by 2020. www.nsc.org/Pages/NSCHoldsCalltoActiononCapitolHill.aspx.

Nevitt, M., Cummings, S.R., Kidd, S., & Black, D. (1989). Risk factors for recurrent non-syncopal falls. *JAMA* 261:2663-2668.

Peel, N.M., Bartlett, H.P., & McClure, R.J. (2007). Healthy aging as an intervention to minimize injury from falls among older people. *Ann NY Acad Sci* 1114:162-169.

Robbins, A.S., Rubenstein, L.V., Josephson, K.R., Schulman, B.L., Osterweil, D., & Fine, G. (1989). Predictors of falls among elderly people—results of two population-based studies. *Arch Intern Med* 149:1628-1633.

Rogers, M.W., & Mille, M.L. (2003). Lateral stability and falls in older people. *Exerc Sport Sci Rev* 31:182-187.

Shumway-Cook, A., Guralnik, J.M., Phillips, C.L., Coppin, A.K., Ciol, M.A., Bandinelli, S., & Ferrucci, L. (2008). Age-associated declines in complex walking task performance: The Walking InCHIANTI Toolkit. *J Am Geriatr Soc* 55:58-65.

Sorock, G.S., Chen, L.H., Gonzalgo, S.R., & Baker, S.P. (2008). Alcohol-drinking history and fatal injury in older adults. *Alcohol* 40(3): 193-199.

Springer, S., Giladi, N., Peretz, C., Yogev, G., Simon, E.S., & Hausdorff, J.M. (2006). Dual-tasking effects on gait variability: The role of aging, falls, and executive function. *Mov Disord* 21:950-957.

Stevens, J.A., Corso, P.S., Finkelstein, E.A., & Miller, T.R. (2006). The costs of fatal and non-fatal falls among older adults. *Injury Prevention* 12:290-295.

van den Bogert, A.J., Pavol, M.J., & Grabiner, M.D. (2002). Response time is more important than walking speed for the ability of older adults to avoid a fall after a trip. *J Biomech* 35:199-205.

van Schoor, N., Smit, J.H., Pluijm, S., Jonker, C., & Lips, P. (2002). Different cognitive functions in relation to falls among older persons. Immediate memory as an independent risk factor for falls. *J Clin Epidemiol* 55(9): 855-862.

Verhaeverbeke, I., & Mets, T. (1997). Drug-induced orthostatic hypotension in the elderly: Avoiding its onset. *Drug Safety* 17(2):105-118.

Whipple, R.K., Wolfson, M.D., & Amerman, P.M. (1987). The relationship of knee and ankle weakness to falls in nursing home residents: An isokinetic study. *Journal of the American Geriatrics Society* 35:13-20.

Testing Balance

Bohannon, R.W. (2006). Single limb stance times: A descriptive meta-analysis of data from individuals at least 60 years of age. *Topics in Geriatric Rehabilitation. Transportation and Mobility* 22:70-77.

Bohannon, R.W., Larkin, P.A., & Cook, A.C. (1984). Decrease in timed balance test scores with aging. *Phys Ther* 64:1067-1075.

Cho, C.Y., & Kamen, G. (1998). Detecting balance deficits in frequent fallers using clinical and quantitative evaluation tools. *J Am Geriatr Soc* 46:426-430.

Duncan, P.W., Weiner, D.K., Chandler, J., & Studenski, S. (1990). Functional reach: A new clinical measure of balance. *J Gerontol A Biol Sci Med Sci* 45:M192-M197.

Ekdahl, C., Jarnlo, G.B., & Andersson, S.I. (1989). Standing balance in healthy subjects. Evaluation of a quantitative test battery on a force platform. *Scand J Rehabil Med* 21:187-195.

Mann, G.C., Whitney, S.L., Redfern, M.S., Borello-France, D.F., & Furman, J.M. (1996). Functional reach and single leg stance in patients with peripheral vestibular disorders. *J Vestib Res* 6:343-353.

Rikli, R.E., & Jones, C.J. (1999). Development and validation of a functional fitness test for community-residing older adults. *Journal of Aging and Physical Activity* 7:129-161.

Sherrington, C., & Lord, S.R. (2005). Reliability of simple portable tests of physical performance in older people after hip fracture. *Clin Rehabil* 19:496-504.

Sprigle, S., Maurer, C., & Holowka, M. (2007). Development of valid and reliable measures of postural stability. *J Spinal Cord Med* 30:40-49.

Thomas, J.I., & Lane, J.V. (2005). A pilot study to explore the predictive validity of 4 measures of falls risk in frail elderly patients. *Arch Phys Med Rehabil* 86:1636-1640.

Vellas, B.J., Wayne, S., Romero, L., Baumgartner, R.N., Rubenstein, L.Z., & Garry, P.J. (1997). One-leg balance is an important predictor of injurious falls in older persons. *J Amer Geriatr Soc* 45:735-738.

Weiner, D.K., Duncan, P.W., Chandler, J., & Studenski, S.A. (1992). Functional reach: A marker of physical frailty. *Journal of the American Geriatrics Society* 40:203-207.

Balance Training

Lee, M.S., Pittler, M.H., Shin, B.C., & Ernst, E. (2008). Tai chi for osteoporosis: A systematic review. *Osteoporos Int* 19:139-146.

Li, Y., Devault, C.N., & Van Oteghen, S. (2007). Effects of extended tai chi intervention on balance and selected motor functions of the elderly. *Am J Chin Med* 35:383-391.

Maki, B.E., & McIlroy, W.E. (2006). Control of rapid limb movements for balance recovery: Age-related changes and implications for fall prevention. *Age Ageing* 35:ii12-ii18.

Richerson, S., & Rosendale, K. (2007). Does tai chi improve plantar sensory ability? A pilot study. *Diabetes Technol Ther* 9:276-286.

Rose, D. (2009). *Fallproof! A comprehensive balance and mobility training program.* Champaign, IL: Human Kinetics.

Voukelatos, A., Cumming, R.G., Lord, S.R., & Rissel, C. (2007). A randomized, controlled trial of tai chi for the prevention of falls: The Central Sydney Tai Chi Trial. *J Am Geriatr Soc* 55:1185-1191.

Zijlstra, G.A., van Haastregt, J.C., van Rossum, E., van Eijk, J.T., Yardley, L., & Kempen, G.I. (2007). Interventions to reduce fear of falling in community-living older people: A systematic review. *J Am Geriatr Soc* 55:603-615.

References

Benton, M.J., & White, A. (2006). Osteoporosis: Recommendations for resistance exercise and supplementation with calcium and vitamin D to promote bone health. *J Com Health Nurs* 23:201-211.

Bulat, T., Hart-Hughes, S., Ahmed, S., Quigley, P., Palacios, P., Werner, D.C., & Foulis, P. (2007). Effect of a group-based exercise program on balance in elderly. *Clin Interv Aging* 2:655-660.

Cao, Z.B., Maeda, A., Shima, N., Kurata, H., & Nishizono, H. (2007). The effect of a 12-week combined exercise intervention program on physical performance and gait kinematics in community-dwelling elderly women. *J Physiol Anthropol* 26:325-332.

Centers for Disease Control and Prevention. (2006). Injury prevention and control: Data and statistics (WISQARS). www.cdc.gov/ncipc/wisqars.

Centers for Disease Control and Prevention. (2008a). Hip fractures among older adults. www.cdc.gov/ncipc/factsheets/adulthipfx.htm

Centers for Disease Control and Prevention. (2008b). *Preventing falls among older adults.* Washington, DC: Department of Health and Human Services.

Centers for Disease Control and Prevention. (2009). Falls among older adults: An overview. www.cdc.gov/homeandrecreationalsafety/falls/adultfalls.html

Hay, J.G. (1973). *The biomechanics of sports techniques.* Englewood Cliffs, NJ: Prentice Hall.

Ilich, J.Z., Brownbill, R.A., & Tamborini, L. (2003). Bone and nutrition in elderly women: Protein, energy, and calcium as main determinants of bone mineral density. *Eur J Clin Nutr* 57:554-565.

Liu-Ambrose, T., Khan, K.M., Eng, J.J., Janssen, P.A., Lord, S.R., & McKay, H.A. (2004a). Resistance and agility training reduce fall risk in women aged 75 to 85 with low bone mass: A 6- month randomized, controlled trial. *JAGS* 52:657-665.

Liu-Ambrose, T., Khan, K.M., Eng, J.J., Lord, S.R., & McKay, H.A. (2004b). Balance confidence improves with resistance or agility training. Increase is not correlated with objec-tive changes in fall risk and physical abilities. *Gerontology* 50:373-382.

Lord, S.R., Sherrington, C., & Menz, H.B. (2001). *Falls in older people: Risk factors and strategies for prevention.* Cambridge, UK: Cambridge University Press.

Maki, B.E., & McIlroy, W.E. (2006). Control of rapid limb movements for balance recovery: Age-related changes and implications for fall prevention. *Age Ageing* 35:ii12-ii18.

National Osteoporosis Foundation. (2008). Osteoporosis: Quick facts. www.nof.org/professionals/Fast_Facts_Osteoporosis.pdf

National Safety Council. (2008). Falls leading cause of injury death for people 65 and older; medical costs of $19 billion per year to more than double by 2020. www.nsc.org/Pages/NSCHoldsCalltoActiononCapitolHill.aspx.

NIH Consensus Development Panel on Osteoporosis Prevention, Diagnosis, and Therapy. (2001). Osteoporosis prevention, diagnosis, and therapy. *JAMA* 285:785-795.

Rikli, R.E., & Jones, C.J. (1999). Development and validation of a functional fitness test for community-residing older adults. *Journal of Aging and Physical Activity* 7:129-161.

Sprigle, S., Maurer, C., & Holowka, M. (2007). Development of valid and reliable measures of postural stability. *J Spinal Cord Med* 30:40-49.

Suominen, H. (2006). Muscle training for bone strength. *Aging Clin Exp Res* 18:85-93.

Surgeon General. (2004). *The 2004 Surgeon General's report on bone health and osteoporosis: What it means to you.* Washington, DC: Department of Health and Human Services.

van der Maulen, M.C., Beaupre, G.S., & Carter, D.R. (1993). Mechanobiologic influences in long bone cross-sectional growth. *Bone* 14:635-642.

Weerdesteyn, V., Nienhuis, B., & Duysens, J. (2005). Advancing age progressively affects obstacle avoidance skills in the elderly. *Hum Mov Sci* 24:865-880.

Weiner, D.K., Duncan, P.W., Chandler, J., & Studenski, S.A. (1992). Functional reach: A marker of physical frailty. *Journal of the American Geriatrics Society* 40:203-207.

Muscular Strength, Power, and Endurance Training

Sarcopenia, the loss of muscle tissue due to aging, becomes a progressively greater problem as people move from their 50s to their 60s, 70s, 80s, and beyond. Researchers and clinicians have defined sarcopenia as a muscle mass that is more than 2 standard deviations below the mean muscle mass of healthy young adults. This means that a person with sarcopenia has muscles that are significantly smaller than the muscles of about 98% of healthy 20-year-olds. How many older people are affected by sarcopenia? A lot! It has been estimated that from age 60 to age 80 the prevalence of sarcopenia in the general population progresses from 15% to 32% for men and from 23% to 36% for women. After the age of 80 these values increase to about 51% for women and 55% for men. The long and short of this story is that sarcopenia appears to be an inevitable consequence of aging, although the levels of muscle loss appear to vary considerably among older individuals. So what makes one person lose more muscle mass than another person loses? To answer this question, let's examine the possible reasons for age-related muscle loss and its potential effects on successful aging. Afterward, we'll look at the most effective training interventions for dealing with the structural and functional declines linked to sarcopenia.

SARCOPENIA: WHAT MAKES IT HAPPEN?

Roubenoff (2000) produced a model showing how aging, reduced physical activity, and other intrinsic factors can lead to sarcopenia, sarcopenic-related reductions in physical reserves, and increased levels of frailty (see figure 7.1). In this chapter, we will discuss the neuromuscular and biochemical factors associated with declines in muscle performance as well as the specific training strategies that can address losses in muscle mass and strength. In addition, we will examine other factors that reduce mobility, decrease independence, and make clients more susceptible to injuries that may lead to temporary or even permanent disability.

Neuromuscular Causes of Sarcopenia: The Nerve and the Muscle Fiber

The neuromuscular changes that appear to have a direct effect on the age-associated loss in muscle mass include the following:

1. *Shrinking cross-sectional areas of all muscle fibers (muscle cells).* This is especially true for the type II fast-twitch fibers.

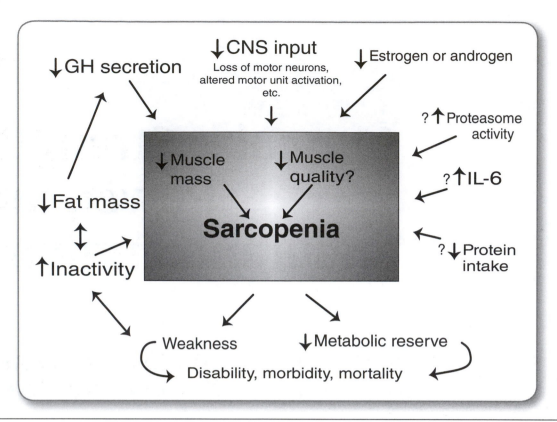

Figure 7.1 Factors contributing to sarcopenia.

Reprinted by permission from Macmillan Publishers Ltd: *European Journal of Clinical Nutrition*, from R. Roubenoff, 2000, "Sarcopenia and its implications for the elderly," 54(3): S40-S47, copyright 2000.

2. *Fewer motor nerves and an increase in the size of the remaining motor units.* As shown in figure 7.2, when motor nerves die off due to the aging process (especially the faster ones), the muscle fibers they support also die. A few fibers, however, are rescued by neighboring motor nerves. This rescue process increases the size of the rescuing motor units and changes the ratio of fast-twitch fibers to slow-twitch fibers.

3. *Structural changes in the neuromuscular junction.* The neuromuscular junction is where the nerve sends a chemical signal (acetylcholine) to the muscle in order to tell the muscle what to do (see figure 7.3a). One change that occurs with aging is an unraveling of the folds on the muscle cell membrane that contain the receptors that pick up the chemical message (the acetylcholine) sent by the nerve (see figure 7.3b). This unraveling flattens the cell membrane, increasing the distance between the receptors and reducing the quality of the chemical transmission. A second age-related change is myelin sheath infiltration.

Myelin is the fatty insulation that wraps around the nerves and acts like the insulation wrapped around an electrical wire. When myelin moves into the space between the muscle and the nerve (called the *synaptic cleft)*, it partially blocks the acetylcholine message sent from the nerve, once again reducing transmission between nerve and muscle (see figure 7.3b). Each of these age-related changes reduces both the speed and the quality of the messages sent from the nerves to the muscles and ultimately affects how well the muscles contract.

4. *Reduced calcium flow inside the muscle, which leads to slower, less powerful contractions.* The muscles contain small sacs called sarcoplasmic reticula. Sarco means "flesh" or "muscle," plasmic means "fluid," and reticula are collections of tubes. So the sarcoplasmic reticula are merely a bunch of tubes in the muscle that collect and release calcium, telling the muscle when to contract and relax. The speed at which calcium is released from and pumped back into the sar-

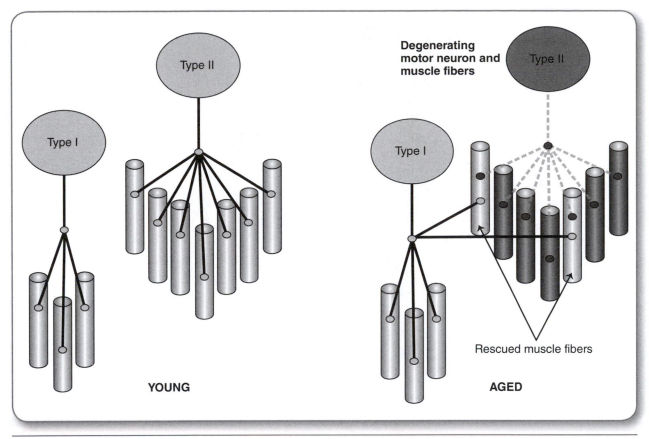

Figure 7.2   Illustration of healthy (light grey) and degenerating (dark grey) motor units showing the denervation and reinnervation processes that occur with aging.

coplasmic reticula dictates how forcefully and quickly the muscles contract.

5. *Less satellite cell activity.* Satellite cells are immature cells that surround the muscle fibers (thus the name satellite). They can produce new muscle cells (fibers). They can also fuse two existing muscle cells and form new muscle nuclei that control the building of new proteins (protein synthesis) within the muscle fiber. The loss of satellite cell activity decreases the muscle's potential for both repair and hypertrophy.

Biochemical Causes of Sarcopenia

Falling levels of muscle-building (anabolic) hormones, such as growth hormone (GH), insulin-like growth factor (IGF), and testosterone, have been associated with decreases in muscle mass in older persons. These declines are so common during the aging process that they have been termed *andropause* (drop in testosterone) and

somatopause (drop in GH and IGF) to reflect the more common term *menopause*.

In addition to the reduced levels and activities of anabolic hormones, aging is accompanied by declines in the capacity to produce energy and build (synthesize) protein. Muscle protein, especially, is affected by aging. In fact, the age-related changes in muscle fiber type are directly related to the age-associated inability to synthesize the heavy chains of myosin, a major contractile protein of skeletal muscle. The nature of these heavy chains affects the activity of the enzyme myosin ATPase, which dictates the fiber type of a muscle.

EFFECTS OF RESISTANCE TRAINING ON THE CAUSES OF SARCOPENIA

Resistance training has been shown to positively affect neurological, hormonal, and mechanical factors associated with muscle maintenance and

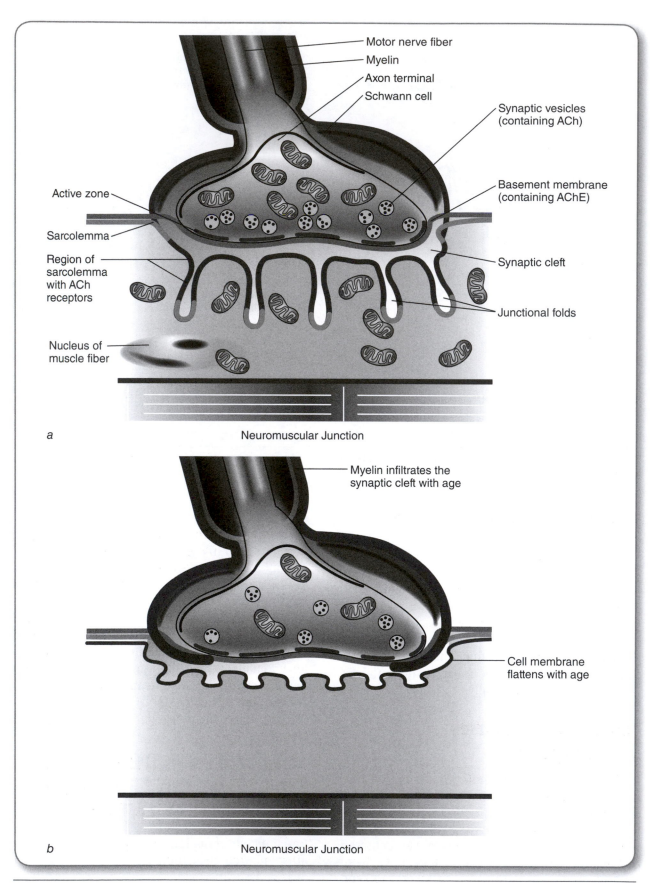

Figure 7.3 (a) The neuromuscular junction and (b) its age-related changes.

growth. It should come as no surprise that you could fill up a small warehouse with articles touting the benefits of resistance exercise in reducing sarcopenia and its impacts on independence, falls, and mobility.

Resistance Training and Neuromuscular Causes of Sarcopenia

The neuromuscular structures retain the capacity to respond to training well into the later years. Resistance training can counteract the loss in muscle tissue and the decrease in neural control that occur with aging. This being the case, let's examine the effects of resistance training on the neuromuscular causes of sarcopenia:

1. Resistance training increases the cross-sectional areas of the muscle fibers of older persons, especially the areas of type II fibers, which are the fibers most dramatically affected by the aging process.

2. Resistance training increases the firing rate of the motor nerves in older people as well as improves the ability of the nerves to call up (recruit) motor units to meet increasing needs. These changes increase the force-producing capacities of the muscles, especially during the early stages of training.

3. High-intensity training, such as resistance and complex agility training, can actually increase the number of branches or the complexity of the neuromuscular junction and so decrease the effects of age-induced unraveling at the neuromuscular junction.

4. Resistance training increases calcium flow through the muscles and so allows older muscles to perform like muscles that are many years younger.

5. Resistance training counteracts the normal age-related decline in satellite cell numbers, allowing the muscle to repair itself more effectively and to reach higher levels of hypertrophy.

APPLICATION POINT Resistance training can have a positive effect on all aspects of the neuromuscular decline that accompanies aging.

Resistance Training and Biochemical Factors

Several studies have shown that resistance training can increase levels of testosterone and GH; however, these increases are consistently lower in older people than they are in younger persons. Additionally, most researchers have reported that IGF and the binding factor that allows it to function are increased by resistance training.

All the energy systems, especially the anaerobic ones, are affected positively by training. These improvements are evidenced by the increase in blood glucose utilization that is seen in middle-aged and elderly subjects following high-intensity weight training. They are also demonstrated by increases in anaerobic and aerobic enzymes that occur after resistance training by older persons. As we will see, however, the degree of change observed in the body's energy systems is related directly to the type of resistance training employed. Finally, myosin ATPase activity, and therefore muscle fiber type, has been shown to be changed by resistance training (see figure 7.4).

APPLICATION POINT You can use the resistance training techniques presented in this book to counteract the biochemical changes that occur with aging and thus bend your clients' aging curves.

RESISTANCE TRAINING TO REDUCE THE EFFECTS OF SARCOPENIA

So far in this chapter we have defined sarcopenia, examined its potential causes, and shown that resistance training can positively affect each of these causes. Now let's look at how reducing sarcopenia can affect quality of life and help older clients to steal back some of the years that Father Time has insidiously stolen away. As you have no doubt realized by now, the aging process affects a multitude of physical factors, and so an effective exercise prescription must target the factors that have the greatest effects on each client. We can use resistance training to target different needs by changing the nature of the training program. As you can see from table 7.1, there are numerous factors that resistance training can address, and

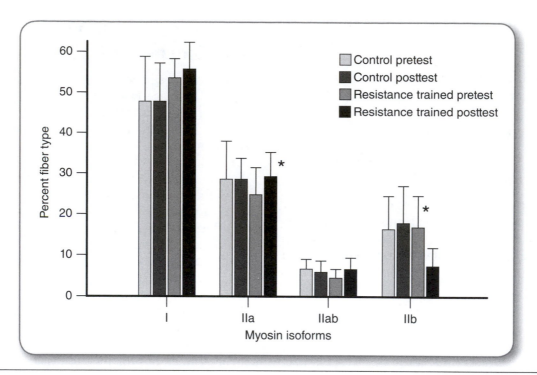

Figure 7.4   Changes in fiber type in resistance-trained and nonexercising controls.
* Indicates an increase in type IIa fibers and a reduction in type IIb fibers due to resistance training.

there are specific training protocols that can be used to address each factor. Let's look at some of these factors in turn.

Muscular Strength

The term *strength* can be defined as the maximal force a muscle can produce under a specific type of contraction. In the gym and in the laboratory, strength is often described as the most weight a person can move using a particular movement or motor pattern. For example, at the gym it's almost impossible to eavesdrop on a group of young men discussing lifting without hearing the question, "How much can you bench?" In the laboratory, a subject's 1RM is commonly used to assess the success of a resistance training program. Both of these measures are expressions of what is known as *dynamic constant resistance,* or *isoinertial, strength.* Isoinertial strength is measured when the muscle is shortening or lengthening. When you get up from a chair you are shortening your

Table 7.1   Standard Recommendations for Targeting Specific Goals During Resistance Training

	Sets	Repetitions	Intensity	Rest period (s)
Muscular strength	1-4	5-8	Heavy	60-180
				90-210
Muscular endurance	1-3	15-20	Low	30-60
	2-5	10-15	Low	15-45
Power	1-5	1-5	Moderate to heavy	120-210
Hypertrophy	1-4	8-12	Moderate	60-120
Maximal strength	1-3	1-3	Very heavy	180-300
	3-5	1	Maximum	180-420

quadriceps (thigh) muscles. The strength you produce when a muscle is shortening is called *concentric strength*. When you sit down in a chair, that same quadriceps muscle is lengthening and the strength you produce is called *eccentric strength*. Special assessment machines called *isokinetic dynamometers* can be used to determine strength at specified and constant testing speeds. This is called *isokinetic strength*. Finally, strength can be measured against an immovable object, meaning that there is no visible movement of the joint being used. This is called *isometric strength*. The most common isometric measurement is grip strength. Each of these methods has been used to evaluate strength in older individuals.

Strength and Independence

Several studies have shown that leg strength is associated with the ability to rise from a chair, with a person's gait speed, and with fall incidence. In other studies, leg strength has been found to be a major predictor of frailty and mortality and to be strongly associated with the ability to perform daily activities. Given the association between muscular strength and independence and between muscular strength and fall prevention, it is not surprising that there is an enormous volume of literature demonstrating the positive effects of resistance training on muscular strength.

Resistance Training for Muscle Strength and Hypertrophy

Since the breakthrough studies published by Maria Fiatarone (Fiatarone et al., 1990) and Walter Frontera (Frontera, Meredith, O'Reilly, Knuttgen, & Evans, 1988) more than a decade ago, there have been innumerable studies demonstrating the positive effects of resistance training on strength and muscle size in older persons. However, the variables associated with developing a resistance training protocol have received far less attention. These variables include training load, number of repetitions, number of sets, training sessions per week, muscle groups targeted, and motor patterns.

Training Load

Interestingly, and perhaps reflective of the desire to deal with sarcopenia, most studies to date have employed resistance levels of 8RM to 12RM (70%-80% of maximum strength), which are commonly used for hypertrophy training, rather than loads of 1RM to 8RM (75%-100% of maximum strength),

which are commonly associated with strength in the training literature. Although strength training professionals agree that higher loads produce greater strength gains, it seems prudent to use the 8RM to 12RM loads when working with older clients, since these loads are proven effective and safe for older persons. Until clinical research and application have proven the safety and efficacy of using these heavier loads, especially in your less fit or more physically frail clients, it is my suggestion that the standard guidelines—using heavier loads for strength development—be abandoned in favor of these more hypertrophy-based loading protocols. One caveat to this recommendation occurs when a client begins any training program. As we will see in chapter 9, before starting any training program or after a long time of detraining, a client should go through a period of tissue adaptation to strengthen and hypertrophy muscle and connective tissue before working with the training load necessary to increase strength. This recommendation is supported by two separate studies conducted in untrained older persons that showed that lower loads (40%-50% of maximum strength) can produce improvements similar to those produced at higher intensities, at least during the early stages of a training program.

Number of Repetitions

As you probably deduced while reading the previous section on training loads, there is a clear association between the number of repetitions performed and the load used. In fact, standard progressive resistance protocols often use the completion of all repetitions in a set as an indication to increase the training load. As noted, the number of repetitions commonly used to maximize strength and hypertrophy in older persons is between 8 and 12; however, lower repetitions with greater loads may prove more effective at increasing strength, so you may consider using greater loads and lower repetitions with your well-trained older clients.

Number of Sets

There has been a good deal of discussion concerning the number of sets necessary to maximize strength development. In their review of the topic in 1998, Carpinelli and Otto concluded that "there is little scientific evidence, and no theoretical physiological basis, to suggest that a greater volume of exercise elicits greater increases in strength or hypertrophy" (p. 73). However, a 2004 review noted that 7 of 8 studies published between 2000 and 2004 showed that multiset and periodized multiset programs were better than single-set programs at increasing strength and muscle size (Galvao & Taaffe, 2004). Moreover, two meta-analyses (Rhea, Alvar, & Burkett, 2002; Rhea, Alvar, Burkett, & Ball, 2003) that made adjustments for differences among study methods reported that multiset training was superior to single-set training for the development of muscle strength in both trained and untrained individuals.

Although there are no controlled studies comparing multiset to single-set training for strength development in older persons, there are a number of helpful hints that we can use to make an educated decision about the number of sets to prescribe. First, most of the studies examining the effects of resistance training on older persons have used multiple sets; however, there are a few studies that have used single sets and produced comparable results. Second, the review papers on the topic indicate that the differences between single-set and multiset responses are greater in trained versus untrained individuals. Third, the amount of damage resulting from a single bout of resistance training has been shown to be similar in older and younger individuals, and the recovery is similar regardless of age.

APPLICATION POINT   Single sets may be effective during both the tissue adaptation and early stages of strength training, but it may be necessary to use multiple sets to produce strength improvements in older clients who reach higher training levels.

Training Sessions Per Week

Most studies that have produced positive strength increases in older persons have followed the classic pattern of training on 3 days per week; however, some studies have used 2 training days per week and have seen comparable results, especially for long-term training. Additionally, in a study comparing training frequencies, training 1 day per week compared favorably to training 2 and 3 days per week (Taaffe, Duret, Wheeler, & Marcus, 1999). When motor performance is the goal, the results are more consistent. One study showed that training once per week resulted in greater increases in ADL performance (Hunter et al., 2001), while another showed that training 1, 2, or 3 times per week had a similar effect on ADL performance (Taaffe et al., 1999), indicating

that a single day may provide sufficient stimulus for improvement.

As was the case with training sets and training intensity, most of these results were produced by subjects who were in the early stages of training, and they may not be applicable to older clients who have a higher training status. In chapter 9, we will examine how to manipulate these variables to maximize performance.

Muscle Groups Targeted

Since the muscles work in specific sequences to perform daily tasks, there are three important factors to consider when the goal of strength training is to enhance ADL performance:

1. The muscle groups to be targeted (based on a client's inability to perform specific ADLs)
2. The method of overload (free weights, plate-loaded machines, pneumatic machines, and so on)
3. The movement pattern, or the kinetic chain of movement (based on a client's specific ADL decrements)

Although humans use all of the muscles in many different sequences when performing daily activities, certain muscles are more active than others are during specific activities. For example, the lower-body muscles, such as the quadriceps, hamstrings, gastrocnemius, and soleus, are very active during stair ascents and descents, walking, and rising from a chair. On the other hand, the upper-body and core (waistline) muscles play a dominant role during food preparation, grooming, and dressing.

Declining lower-body strength has been associated with a higher probability of falling. Because of their lower muscle mass, older persons require more gluteus, quadriceps, and calf muscle activity than younger persons require to step over an obstacle. This increases the risk of falling, especially during repetitive activities such as climbing stairs or negotiating curbs or uneven sidewalks. One muscle group that has been conspicuously ignored in resistance training is that of the ankle dorsiflexors, and yet the majority of studies including this group in their analyses see reduced dorsiflexor strength as a major predictor of falling.

Given the dominance of specific muscle groups in certain tasks, such as the quadriceps in climbing the stairs, we can tailor a training program to each client's individual needs by assessing the client's (1) results on the strength tests presented in this chapter, (2) reported decrements in specific ADLs, and (3) history of falls.

Motor Patterns: The Kinetic Chain

As noted earlier, the performance of daily activities involves a number of different motor patterns in which different muscles work in a specific sequence to accomplish a task. A simple example is taking a gallon of milk from a countertop and placing it on a refrigerator shelf. Although this may seem like a purely upper-body movement, it actually starts with a push-off and rotation of the feet achieved by the upper- and lower-leg musculature. The force is then transferred to the upper body through the core muscles, and only then are the upper-body muscles used to complete the task as the arm is first flexed and then extended (see figure 7.5).

Several recent studies comparing training that simulates everyday tasks to classic weight training have demonstrated how important it is to train the motor patterns that the client uses in daily life. Although resistance training programs can have a positive effect on ADL performance, more and more studies are showing that ADL-specific training programs can improve ADL performance better than standard resistance training programs can. These studies should not be considered as condemnations of resistance training. Instead, they should be thought of as another opportunity to enhance functionality. Let me give you an example. Suppose you were training a football team in the weight room, and you made the team the strongest football team on earth, but you never took your team to the practice field to learn the game. How many games would you win? Most likely you would win none. On the other hand, if you had your team practice on the field but never brought your team to the weight room, you would lack the strength to compete with stronger opponents. It's the same when it comes to ADL performance and fall prevention: You need both strength and practice. Therefore, in chapter 9 we will see a method that incorporates both resistance training and ADL simulation into a comprehensive program.

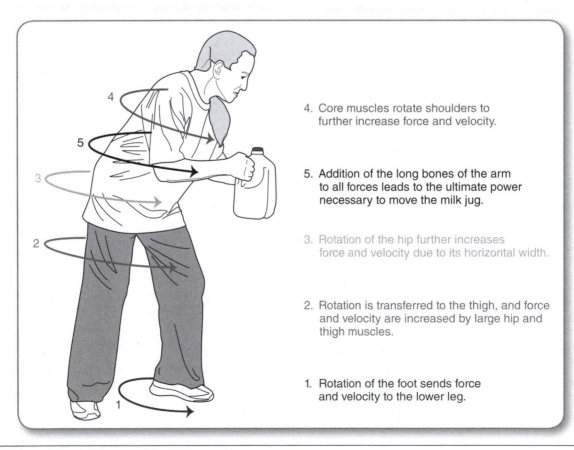

4. Core muscles rotate shoulders to further increase force and velocity.

5. Addition of the long bones of the arm to all forces leads to the ultimate power necessary to move the milk jug.

3. Rotation of the hip further increases force and velocity due to its horizontal width.

2. Rotation is transferred to the thigh, and force and velocity are increased by large hip and thigh muscles.

1. Rotation of the foot sends force and velocity to the lower leg.

Figure 7.5   The kinetic chain for moving a milk jug.

Muscular Endurance

Let's begin this discussion by examining the terms involved so we're all on the same page (no pun intended). I have chosen to use the term *muscular endurance* rather than *endurance* to distinguish between two different—although related—factors, *muscular endurance* and *cardiovascular endurance*. The term *muscular endurance* has been defined as the ability to perform multiple repetitions against a set of submaximal loads, the ability to maintain force production at a high power output, and (more simply) the ability to maintain a specific power output. *Cardiovascular endurance*, in contrast, can be defined as the capacity of the cardiovascular and respiratory systems to maintain sufficient oxygen for prolonged activity. This section is about muscular endurance; cardiovascular endurance is addressed in the following chapter. The decline of muscular endurance with age is well established, and this decline seems to be greater in individuals with chronic respiratory problems. Although the loss of muscular endurance might be related to age-associated declines in strength, there are other factors that might be of equal, if not greater, importance. These include

- reduced quality and quantity of messages relayed from the central nervous system,
- decreased electrical signals along the muscle cell membrane,
- less calcium flow within the muscle, and
- declining anaerobic and aerobic capacities.

Muscular Endurance and Activities of Daily Living

Unfortunately, there are a limited number of studies examining the relationship between muscular endurance and ADL performance. However, the information we do have confirms that muscular endurance is an important factor in performing ADLs. For example, during routine tasks the ankle dorsiflexors of older persons experience much greater fatigue than that experienced by the dorsiflexors of younger persons. Obviously, activities such as walking, shopping, and climbing stairs are repetitive and are therefore negatively affected by lower muscular endurance. Additionally, fatigue may increase the risk of injury during ADL performance.

Muscular Endurance, Dynamic Balance, and Falls

Substantial evidence demonstrates a relationship between lower-limb muscular endurance and falling. For example, fallers have significantly lower knee extension endurance than nonfallers have, and lower-body fatigue increases the risk of falling when stepping over objects. Muscle fatigue has even been linked to a reduced ability to feel the position of a limb (a phenomenon called *proprioception*) during stepping. Therefore, you can improve clients' abilities to maintain balance by increasing their lower-body neuromuscular endurance.

Resistance Training for Muscular Endurance

Muscle fatigue in the elderly may in part be caused by a decline in strength, since when performing any given task older persons use a higher percentage of their maximum strength than younger persons use. Therefore, strength training should improve muscular endurance. However, the relationship between strength and muscular endurance is not absolute, and using resistance training to target muscular endurance requires a lower load and a larger number of repetitions. Campos and colleagues (2002) confirmed the existence of a strength–endurance continuum by showing that a high-repetition training program (20RM-28RM for two sets with 1 minute of rest between sets) produced greater improvements in muscular endurance than a low-repetition program (3RM-5RM for four sets with 3 minutes of rest between sets) and an intermediate program (9RM-11RM for three sets with 2 minutes of rest between sets) produced. These results strengthen the argument that high-repetition, low-intensity resistance training should be used to improve muscular endurance.

APPLICATION POINT High-repetition, low-load training can effectively target muscular endurance, and the importance of improving muscular endurance to increase independence and reduce fall probability is an important topic in training older persons.

Power

Let's start this section with a definition. Defining power is a bit difficult since there are many kinds of power. You may have heard terms such as *speed strength, explosive power,* and many others thrown around the weight room. When it comes to exercise and training, however, two terms are usually used: *metabolic power* and *mechanical power.* Metabolic power is the rate at which your body can use fuel to produce energy. There are two levels of metabolic power commonly associated with exercise: anaerobic power and aerobic power. In this chapter we are discussing work that *predominantly* uses anaerobic power. We will discuss aerobic power in the next chapter, which is on aerobic training. The term *anaerobic power* is often used synonymously with the term *power.* This is a mistake that often leads to misconceptions in both the description and the application of training.

Anaerobic power is a measure of how fast the two anaerobic systems, the creatine phosphate system and the anaerobic glycolysis system, replenish ATP. The maximum rates at which these two systems can replenish ATP are approximately 75% and 50% of the rate at which ATP is broken down; this makes them the most *powerful* metabolic systems in the body. But it is mechanical power that has the strongest correlation with ADL performance and fall probability. To understand mechanical power, we'll need to revisit physics and biology 101.

What Is Power?

Perhaps you remember from high school physics that

power = force × velocity, where

force = mass × acceleration.

When you accelerate the mass of your body against gravity, such as when climbing a flight of stairs or rising from a chair, your muscles are exerting force. But what about velocity? Velocity is a vector. Remember vectors? Vectors have both magnitude and direction. In other words, velocity not only tells us how fast we're moving but also tells us in what direction we're moving. Speed, on the other hand, only tells us how fast we're going. Physicists call speed a *scalar.* To understand vectors and scalars, let's look at an example demonstrating why these two terms aren't synonymous. If you are lifting a weight at 1 meter per second (m/s), the speed and velocity of that weight are both 1 m/s. But if you are attempting to lift a weight at 1 m/s while someone else pushes it down at 1 m/s, the speed at which the weight is traveling is still 1 m/s, but the velocity is –1 m/s since the weight is moving in a direction opposite the intended direction. Weight trainers know of this concept as a *negative* or *forced negative.*

Now let's look at the interactions between force and velocity and how they affect power. If you are lifting the maximum load you can lift (1RM) against gravity, the force you need to lift that weight is very large and the velocity at which you are moving the weight is very slow. If the load is increased so that you can't move it, your velocity becomes 0 m/s (you are performing an isometric exercise). On the other hand, if the weight is reduced to a minimum, you become able to move it at maximum velocity. This is the force–velocity relationship in skeletal muscle that is represented by the famous *force–velocity curve* (see figure 7.6). Somewhere along the force–velocity curve there is an optimal load where the product of force times velocity yields the highest power (indicated in figure 7.6). Figure 7.7 shows how changes in the force necessary to overcome a load and the velocity at which that load can be moved affect power. We will discuss why these concepts are important in the training section of this chapter.

Definitions of Some Resistance Training Variables

velocity	A vector (has quantity and direction) that indicates the direction and rate at which a distance is covered.
speed	A scalar (has only quantity) that indicates the rate at which a distance is covered regardless of direction.
power	Force times velocity. Since work is equal to the force applied over a distance and velocity is the rate at which a distance is covered, power can also be considered the rate of doing work.

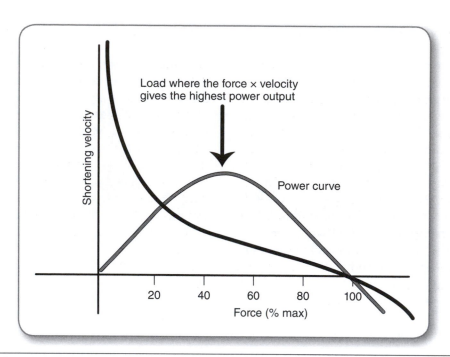

Figure 7.6 The force–velocity curve.

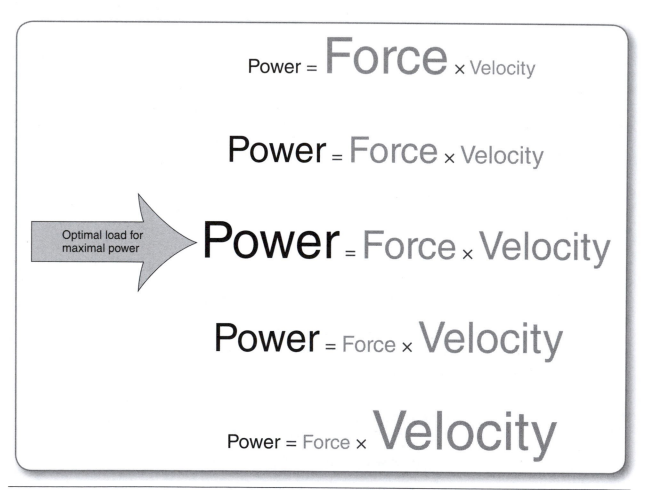

Figure 7.7 Variations in force and velocity change the resulting power outputs.

Declines in Power With Aging: Potential Mechanisms

From age 65 to age 89, explosive lower-limb extensor power declines 3.5% annually, while strength drops only 1% to 2% per year. Additionally, the average decline in anaerobic power from age 20 to age 70 is 8.3% per decade.

The fact that power declines more rapidly than strength does should not be surprising. Remember that a muscle's cross-sectional area drops exponentially with aging. Also recall that the greatest losses occur in the type II, or fast-twitch, fibers. These changes provide a double whammy when it comes to power, since they affect both the force and the velocity of the muscle. In addition to changes in muscle fiber type and cross-sectional area, there are also changes in some of the supporting cast members, including

- slower electrical signals moving down the motor nerves,
- decreased myelin insulation around the motor nerve,
- reduced nerve-to-muscle (neuromuscular) transmission, and
- decreased calcium flow within the muscle.

Unfortunately, all of the physiological cards of aging are being dealt against the hand held by power.

Power and Activities of Daily Living

Power is one of the major performance variables associated with independence. In fact, leg extensor power correlates significantly with a number of ADLs, including rising from a chair, walking (specifically, walking speed), and climbing stairs. There is general agreement that testing for leg extensor power should be included among the diagnostic tests of any program designed to reduce physical frailty. Skelton, Greig, Davies, and Young (1994) showed that knee extensor power per unit of body weight (termed *relative power*) affects chair rise time and step height. Since then other researchers have reported that leg power is a strong predictor of self-reported functional status in older women and in older people with limited mobility. It is believed that the higher levels of disability observed in elderly women compared with elderly men are due to a lower ratio between power and body weight and a smaller capacity to produce power. These findings have helped to establish the link between power and independence in older persons.

Power and Falls

A substantial volume of research shows the importance of leg power in fall prevention. In 1984, Aniansson, Ljungberg, Rundgren, and Wetterqvist used muscle biopsy techniques to show that patients experiencing hip fractures have significant losses in muscle cross-sectional area, especially in the faster, more powerful, type II muscle fibers. Later, Whipple, Wolfson, and Amerman (1987) showed the strong association between falling and knee and ankle isokinetic power in institutionalized elders. Skelton, Kennedy, and Rutherford (2002) found that women who fall have 24% less explosive power in their weaker limb than women who did not fall have. They also noted that in older women who live independently, poor lower-limb explosive power combined with power differences (asymmetry) between limbs may be a better predictor of future falls than the more traditional measurements of strength. This finding should alert us to the need to work for balanced power production between limbs. In 2006, Sayers and colleagues found that older persons showing slower walking times for the 400-meter walk test and lower power when performing the leg press at 70% of 1RM and 40% of 1RM had a higher incidence of falls. In addition, participants in this study produced slower velocities when performing the leg press at 40% of 1RM. A final point may be helpful for rehabilitation after injuries such as falls: Individuals with higher power outputs show faster recovery rates.

Resistance Training for Power

The use of high-speed resistance training to increase power in older persons has been gaining acceptance over the past two decades and is now an accepted training method for older persons. The beginnings of this concept can be traced back to presentations in the early 1990s that reported the positive effects of high-speed training on both power and functional performance (Flipse et al., 1993; Signorile, Sochet, et al., 1995; Signorile, Suidmak, et al., 1995). Since then, several researchers have demonstrated the effectiveness of this training technique in increasing both power and movement speed.

However, before applying high-speed training techniques to yourself or to a client, you should consider the following:

- The equipment, techniques, and training environment to be used
- The optimal loads to maximize power, ADL performance, or specific muscle performance
- The development of a strength base before beginning high-speed training
- The correct patterns of training (periodization) to maximize results and reduce the potential for overtraining or overuse injuries

Equipment, Techniques, and Training Environment

High-speed training has been used successfully in research studies using free weights, stack-loaded machines, pneumatic machines, tubes and bands, and even sandbags. However, when free weights and stack-loaded machines are employed, two factors must be considered: inertia and momentum. Inertia is resistance to change in motion, while momentum is mass in motion, or mass times velocity. When a person working with free weights or stack-loaded machines accelerates a weight to a high velocity, the weight continues to move at a high velocity until gravity slows it to a stop. Unfortunately, gravity usually slows the weight to a stop only well after the end ROM of the lift has been reached. What this means is that the potential for injury at the end ROM of an exercise is increased because the weight continues to move after the limb stops. This is especially true during the eccentric portion of lifts, when gravity is actually accelerating the weight. This problem has been noticed by researchers, and the majority of studies using these types of equipment restrict high-speed work to the concentric portion of the lifts. One way to address safety is to use devices that minimize momentum, such as pneumatic devices, bands, and rubber tubing. If you do use free weights or stack-loaded machines with clients, you should take care to explain to uninitiated clients that they should begin slowing the weight well before reaching the end ROM of the lift. In fact, it would be prudent to have clients practice the deceleration portion of the contraction before applying any training loads. The resulting learning effect will reduce the potential for injury. Other

options for high-speed work are to use medicine balls and light plyometrics, but again you should know proper technique before starting and you should increase training intensity gradually. Finally, the swimming pool provides an excellent environment for high-speed training. Resistance (drag) increases exponentially with movement speed, while the water provides a more forgiving environment. In fact, the pool may provide one of the most effective training environments, especially for frail individuals or people with a history and associated fear of falling.

> **APPLICATION POINT** Since velocity is the major factor affecting power in older persons, the use of high-speed training techniques is important if you intend to increase power and its related benefits in your clients.

Optimal Loading for Power and Performance

Optimal loading is not a simple topic to address. In older persons, power can be increased by using loads ranging from 20% to 80% of a person's maximum strength. Additionally, not every muscle group has the same response to high-speed training. Factors such as joint structure, bone length, and fiber type can affect the capacity of a muscle to respond to high-speed training. Different joints have different capacities to produce force and speed and so require you to use different loads during training to maximize power gains (see figure 7.8).

Another factor to remember is that people have the capacity to train for power anywhere along the force–velocity curve. I call this capacity to target specific goals by selecting different points of load and velocity *surfing the force–velocity curve*. For example, decrements in balance and gait speed are best addressed with loads at about 40% of 1RM, while reduced ability to rise from a bed or chair or to climb stairs is better addressed with resistances at 60% to 70% of 1RM (see figure 7.9).

Building a Strength Base

Beginning high-speed training without developing a strength base is not prudent for a number of reasons:

1. High-speed work requires the capacity to decelerate a limb as the movement approaches end ROM. Therefore, eccentric

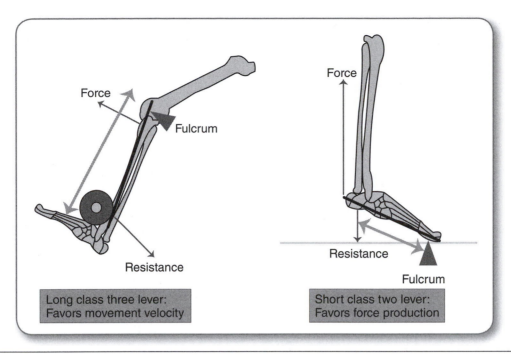

Figure 7.8   Lever systems and their effects on force and power.

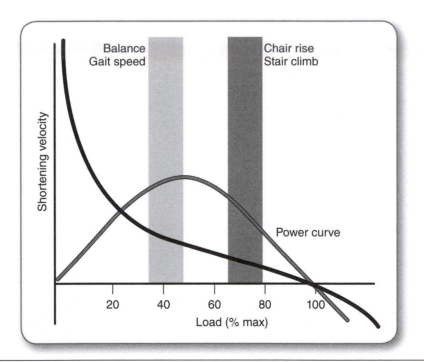

Figure 7.9   The best locations along the force–velocity curve for training selected ADLs.

strength should be developed before high-speed training is attempted.

2. Muscles and connective tissues need to be toughened up before being asked to deal with the momentum and inertial forces associated with high-speed training. There-fore, an initial strength and hypertrophy cycle should be completed.

3. Although velocity is the major controlling factor in the loss of power production in older persons, strength is still important. Therefore, strength should be developed.

Periodization to Reduce Overtraining and Maximize Benefits

It is clear from both research and practical application that cycles using targeted training coupled with scheduled recovery are the most effective strategy for improving neuromuscular performance. In Chapter 9 of this book I will provide templates for strength, power, and endurance cycles. In addition, Chapter 9 and the DVD will offer you case studies showing how to apply periodization theory to address specific diagnostic profiles.

TESTING NEUROMUSCULAR PERFORMANCE

The 30-second chair stand test, modified ramp power test, 30-second arm curl test, and gallon jug shelf test measure upper-body and lower-body strength and power. These tests not only measure power during simulated daily activities but also have strong correlations with laboratory tests that have significantly higher equipment costs and time requirements. Because loss of speed is inherent to the aging process (due to the loss of the faster-contracting motor units) and because speed tests have strong associations with independence and fall probability, a walking speed test is also included in this chapter.

30-Second Chair Stand

This test measures the number of stands that a person can perform during 30 seconds. Chair stand tests have been used for many years to evaluate lower-body functional performance; the most common chair stand method is to measure the time necessary to complete 5 or 10 stands. However, the effectiveness of this method was often tainted by the fact that the tests showed a significant basement effect because many subjects could not complete the required number of stands. Therefore, Jones and coworkers (1999) developed the 30-second chair stand test presented here. The test was developed as a functional measure of leg strength, and norms have been established across a large sample of older persons.

Although some researchers have questioned the factors contributing to performance during sit-to-stand tests, a number of researchers have reported significant correlations between these tests and leg extensor strength.

Equipment Needed

- A standard straight-back chair with a seat height of 17 inches (43 cm)
- A stopwatch

Protocol

- Demonstrate proper form.
- Have the client begin this test seated in a standard straight-back chair with a seat height of 17 inches (43 cm). The client's back should be straight, feet should be flat on the floor, and arms should be crossed at the wrists and held against the chest.
- Provide a practice trial of 1 to 3 repetitions to familiarize the client with the test. Use the practice trial to evaluate the client's form.
- Give the signal to go while simultaneously starting the stopwatch.

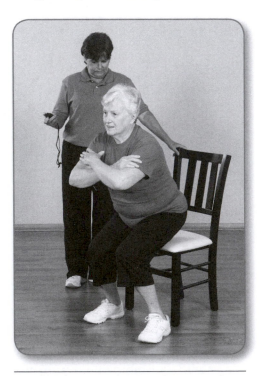

Figure 7.10   The 30-second chair stand test.

- The client rises to a full standing position and then sits down, touching the seat of the chair, and repeats as many times as possible within 30 seconds (see figure 7.10).
- Count the number of times the client stands. For a stand to be counted, the client must have completed the movement fully.
- Provide encouragement while ensuring that the client maintains good form.

This test can also be used to measure power since it involves moving body mass against gravity as rapidly as possible. In our laboratory, we have developed an equation to compute power using the number of stands completed during the first 20 seconds of this test (Smith et al., 2010). The equations are as follows:

Average power in watts = –504.845 + 10.793 × body weight in kilograms + 21.603 × number of stands in 20 seconds.

Peak power in watts = –715.218 + 13.915 × body weight in kilograms + 33.425 × number of stands in 20 seconds.

Obviously, to use these equations, you must also know the person's body weight.

Modified Ramp Power Test

Stair-climbing has been shown to be a valid and reliable field test of power. However, since stair-climbing tests require bounding up a set of stairs, they possess a higher potential for falling and related injuries than ramp tests possess. Additionally, skill, coordination, leg length, and approach distance have a greater effect on stair-climbing tests than they have on ramp tests. This is especially true for women due to their smaller stature and shorter stride lengths. Therefore, several researchers have concluded that ramp tests produce significantly greater power than stair tests produce.

The ramp test presented here is a modification of earlier tests developed using younger individuals. In our laboratory, we have used this test successfully with people of all ages (from 18 to 102 years) and all levels of functionality, including people using walking aids. This modified version of the ramp test uses the standard access ramp found in most facilities (with a rise-to-run ratio of 1:12) rather than the 30.5° or 35° ramps used previously for younger people. The lower incline makes the test accessible to a greater segment of older persons and increases the contribution of velocity to the production of power. This increase in the contribution of velocity is important since it makes the patterns of muscle utilization and the force–velocity relationships more specific to walking. The variable measured during the modified ramp power test is the time required to complete the task. You can use a digital timer or a stopwatch to record the time. Figure 7.11 shows a diagram of the test setup and a picture of a person performing the task. The following is the formula used to compute power from this test:

$$Power = \frac{mass \times distance \times g}{time}$$

where

power = mechanical power in watts,
mass = body mass in kilograms,
distance = vertical distance between the starting and finish lines in meters,
time = time necessary to complete the task in seconds, and
g = acceleration due to gravity, which is 9.8 m/s^2.

Equipment Needed

- A standard access ramp
- A ruler or tape to measure the vertical distance from the position of the starting line to the position of the finish line
- Cones or similar markers to mark the approach, start, and finish lines
- A stopwatch or other timing device with sensors (such as the photocells used by many of the commercially available athletic speed assessment systems)

Protocol

- Mark a starting line at the beginning of the ramp and a finish line about 4 meters up the ramp (the finish line in figure 7.11a is 3.79 m from the starting line). The absolute distance along the ramp is not important since the test uses the vertical distance from the starting line and finish line as the value to be entered into the equation.
- First, demonstrate proper technique.
- Have the client begin the test from a standing position 4 meters from the ramp.
- Tell the client to move up the ramp as quickly as possible (see figure 7.11b).

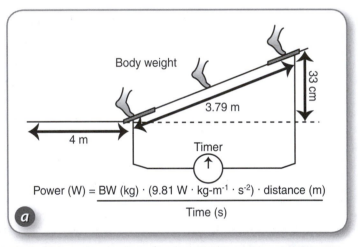

Figure 7.11 The modified ramp power test. (a) Test setup. Note the 4-meter approach and the rise-to-run ratio of 1:12, a lower incline than is used in a standard ramp test. (b) The execution of the test.

$$\text{Power (W)} = \frac{\text{BW (kg)} \cdot (9.81\ \text{W} \cdot \text{kg-m}^{-1} \cdot \text{s}^{-2}) \cdot \text{distance (m)}}{\text{Time (s)}}$$

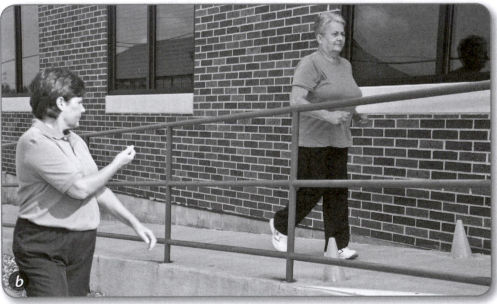

- Begin the test when the individual passes the starting line and end the test when the individual passes the finish line.
- Provide encouragement while ensuring that the individual maintains good form.
- Have the client complete one practice trial followed by two recorded trials.

30-Second Arm Curl Test

The arm curl test is an evaluation of upper-body strength. Due to the low resistance used and the simplicity of the movement, it can be used in any clinical setting with minimal training and personnel. Strength is quantified by counting the total number of arm curls the subject can perform within 30 seconds. As with many of the other tests from Rikli and Jones (1999), norms are available for age 60 and older.

Equipment Needed

- A standard straight-back chair with a seat height of 17 inches (43 cm)
- A 5-pound hand weight for women and a 7.5-pound hand weight for men
- A stopwatch

Protocol

- Demonstrate proper form.
- Have the individual sit in a chair. The client's back should be straight and feet should be flat on the floor. The dumbbell should be held in the dominant hand in a handshake (hammer) position. The elbow should be completely extended and the arm should be perpendicular to the floor (see figure 7.12a).
- Kneel on the client's dominant side. Place one hand behind the triceps to stabilize the upper arm and prevent backward drift of the elbow and place a finger in the antecubital space to prevent forward drift of the arm and to feel the forearm in order to ensure that a full curl has been performed.

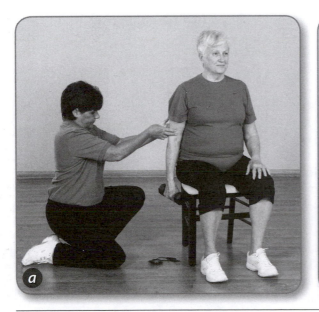 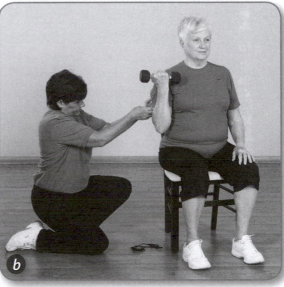

Figure 7.12   The 30-second arm curl test. (a) The starting position showing the tester preventing the arm swinging by placing her hands behind the upper arm and in the bicep fold. (b) The client has completed one contraction with the hand rotated inward (supinated).

- Have the client complete a practice trial of 1 to 2 repetitions to become familiar with the test.
- Use the practice trial to evaluate the client's form.
- Give the signal to go while simultaneously starting the stopwatch.
- The client performs the curl by flexing at the elbow while supinating (outwardly rotating) the hand and then returns the weight to the starting position (see figure 7.12*b*).
- The client performs as many curls as possible within the 30-second time period.
- Provide encouragement while ensuring that the client maintains good form.

It might be argued that strength is easy to evaluate with maximal lifting (1RM) tests and that these tests have been shown to have a minimal risk for injury in older persons. However, when considering safety and liability, these tests should be limited to controlled laboratory environments.

Gallon Jug Shelf Test

This test provides an assessment of a common IADL. The maneuver simulates activities such as retrieving food from a low shelf in a refrigerator or retrieving an object from a shelf in a closet (Signorile et al., 2007). Before asking the client to perform any lifts, you should provide exact instructions on lifting technique. These include keeping the back as straight as possible, keeping the head up, not leaning forward, using the legs as the primary source of power for the lift, and aborting the task at any sign of stress or discomfort. The objects to be lifted are five 1-gallon (3.8 L) jugs filled with water. This provides a weight of approximately 8.3 pounds (3.8 kg) per jug. This test measures the time needed to transfer the five jugs from a low shelf to a high shelf.

Equipment Needed

- A bookcase with adjustable shelves that are wide enough to hold all five 1-gallon (3.8 L) jugs
- Five 1-gallon (3.8 L) jugs filled with water
- A stopwatch

Protocol

- Adjust the heights of the shelving so that the top of the lower shelf is at the base of the client's patella (knee) and the top of the upper shelf is aligned with the client's acromion process (shoulder). Begin the test with the five jugs lined up on the bottom shelf.
- Demonstrate proper lifting form.
- Provide a practice trial of one repetition (which means moving all five jugs) to familiarize the client with the test. Use the practice trial to evaluate the client's form.
- Have the individual begin by standing up straight in front of the bookcase.

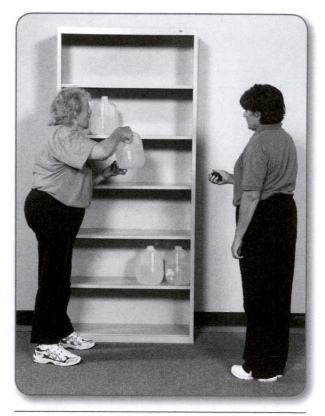

Figure 7.13 The gallon jug shelf test.

- Give the signal to go while simultaneously starting the stopwatch.
- The individual bends at the knees and hips, keeping the back as straight as possible, and grasps the first jug.
- The person then stands, holding the jug as close to the body as possible, and places the jug on the top shelf (figure 7.13).
- This process is repeated until all five jugs are placed on the top shelf.
- Record the time it takes to lift all five jugs to the top shelf.
- Allow the client to complete two trials. Provide a 2-minute rest between trials.

15-Foot Walk Test

Slower speeds are inherent to the aging process due to the loss of the faster-contracting motor units. Additionally, walking speed and other timed assessments have strong associations with independence and fall probability. Thus it is prudent for us to include a test for speed in our testing battery. Due to its status in the hierarchy of testing, a gait speed test will work well as the assessment for speed.

Two major considerations in choosing a walking speed test are the length of the test and the walking speed (usual versus maximal walking speed). To address these considerations, we should take into account what we want to measure. Shorter distances are more appropriate for anaerobic, power-based evaluations, while longer distances are better for aerobic, endurance-based evaluations. A review of the literature reveals that distances between 3 and 4 meters are often used for short-distance testing. Additionally, the 15-foot walking speed is highly predictive of performance over longer distances (Rolland et al., 2004).

There are several factors to consider when choosing between usual and maximal walking speed. First, usual walking speed may predict functional dependence for subjects aged 75 years and older, while maximal walking speed appears to be more sensitive in predicting functional dependence for people aged 65 to 74 years. Second, variations in lateral balance have little effect on preferred walking speed but do affect balance at higher speeds.

One other factor to consider when using a walking speed test is the individual's ability to accelerate to maximal walking speed. Many researchers have reported that an initial acceleration phase is necessary before maximal steady-state walking speed can be achieved. Distances employed for the acceleration phase have varied considerably. In a study to determine the distance necessary to reach steady-state maximal walking speed, Lindemann and colleagues (2007) indicated that the first 2.5 meters of a gait speed test should be excluded from the analysis. In their study examining leg extension power and walking speed in community-dwelling subjects 80 years old and older, Rantanen and Avela (1997) used an approach distance of 3 to 4 meters. The test described for this chapter uses a 15-foot walk with a 15-foot approach to evaluate gait velocity. As was the case for the ramp test, either photocells or a stopwatch can be used for the test.

Equipment Needed

- Four cones or similar markers
- A stopwatch or other timing device
- Four orange pylons

Protocol

- Set four orange pylons (with photocells if desired) in a straight line on a flat surface at 0, 15, 30, and 40 feet along the walking path (see figure 7.14).
- Demonstrate correct heel-to-toe walking with at least one foot in contact with the ground at all times (to ensure no running).

- Emphasize that the client should walk as quickly as possible from the first pylon through the last pylon in order to increase the probability that maximal speed will be maintained in the testing area, which is between the second and third pylons.
- Give the signal to go and start the stopwatch when the client reaches the second pylon at 15 feet. Then stop the watch as the client reaches the third pylon at 30 feet.
- Repeat this test two times.

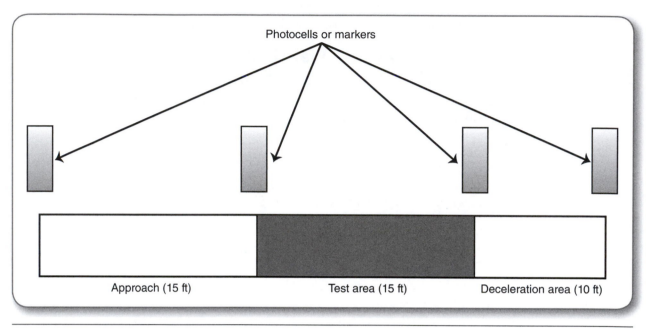

Figure 7.14 The 15-foot walking speed test.

RESISTANCE TRAINING EXERCISES

Let's start our discussion on resistance training with the usual disclaimer. Be sure that your client checks with the doctor before beginning any training program. Existing neurological problems, existing or previous muscular or skeletal injuries, low bone density, hormonal irregularities, and a host of other medical concerns may increase the risk of injury during resistance training. Also, there is a misconception that resistance training is an anaerobic exercise and therefore does not involve the cardiovascular system. This is simply wrong, wrong, wrong. Resistance exercise, like any exercise, requires an increase in metabolic rate that must be supported by the cardiovascular system.

Remember that as people age their connective tissues stiffen and weaken and their muscle mass and bone mass decline. Any training program should be preceded by a period of gradual strengthening and toughening of the tissues. The length of this tissue adaptation period is shorter for younger and well-conditioned persons and longer for older and poorly conditioned persons.

As you read through this section of resistance training exercises, you should realize the following:

- Resistance can be provided by machines, barbells, dumbbells, bands and tubes, kettlebells, body weight, or fluid drag (water resistance). Each of these approaches has its own advantages and shortcomings.
- All exercises should be performed through the entire ROM. Contrary to popular belief, strength training can actually increase the ROM of a joint when performed correctly.
- Proper technique should be mastered before training begins.
- The proper breathing method is to exhale during the exertion (concentric or positive) phase and inhale during the return (eccentric or negative) phase.

The resistance training exercises presented here are organized by body segment and exercise environment, including the gym, home, and pool. Both single-joint and multijoint exercises are included. The instructions in the following exercises speak directly to the client, so you can read the instructions to the client if desired.

Lower-Body Exercises   156

Hip and Thigh   156
  Leg Press   156
  Leg Extension   157
  Squat   158
  Lunge   159
Hamstrings   160
  Leg Curl   160
Hip Flexors   162
  Hip Flexion Exercise   162
Hip Extensors   163
  Hip Extension Exercise   163
Hip Adductors   164
  Hip Adduction   164
Hip Abductors   165
  Hip Abduction   165
Lower Leg   166
  Heel Raise   166

Dorsiflexors   168
  Toe Raise   168
Upper-Body Exercises   170
Chest and Anterior Shoulders   170
  Seated Chest Press   170
  Flat Bench Press   170
  Fly   172
Upper Chest and Deltoids   172
  Inclined Bench Press   172
Upper and Middle Back   173
  Row   173
Latissimus Dorsi   175
  Lat Pull-Down   175
Shoulders   177
  Overhead Press   177
  Lateral Raise   178
  Shrug   179

Rotator Cuff   180
  Internal Rotation   180
  External Rotation   182
Arm Muscles   184
  Biceps Curl   184
  Triceps Push-Down   186
  Triceps Extension   187
  Triceps Kickback   189
  Wrist Curl   190
Core Musculature   191
  Crunch   191
  Side Plank   192
  Bridge   193
  Hip Rotator Exercise   193
  Quadruped   194
  Superman   195

LOWER-BODY EXERCISES
HIP AND THIGH

▰ Leg Press ▰

Environment   This exercise can be performed in the gym.

Application   The quadriceps and hip muscles make up the largest muscle groups of the body. They are vital in the maintenance of balance, mobility, and independence. Leg presses are one of the safest and easiest exercises to learn for these muscles. There are a number of different leg press machines, the most common of which are the horizontal and diagonal machines (see figure 7.15).

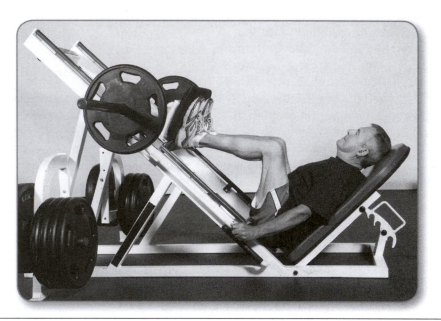

Figure 7.15   The diagonal leg press machine.

Position   Before beginning the exercise, adjust the machine so that the knees and hips form a 90° angle when the feet are in place on the foot plate or pedals. The hips and gluteal muscles should stay in contact with the seat padding during the entire exercise, and there should be a slight arch in the lower back.

Execution   Extend the knees forcefully, but do not lock them.

Variations

- Move the feet farther apart to increase the utilization of the adductor (inner thigh) muscles, or bring the feet closer together to increase the activity of the quadriceps.
- Anecdotal information suggests that using a higher foot position increases the activity of the hamstring and gluteal muscles.

Safety   Remember to exhale when pressing and inhale when lowering the weight. Holding the breath can cause a dangerous increase in blood pressure. Additionally, control the weight and avoid bouncing, since doing so may cause undue stress or injury.

▬ Leg Extension ▬

Environment   This exercise can be performed in the gym, home, or pool.

Application   The leg extension isolates the quadriceps muscles, especially the vastus medialis, which is the teardrop-shaped muscle on the inner side of the thigh. This is especially true toward the last 30° of extension.

Position   For the machine exercise in the gym, sit with the seat adjusted so your knees are in line with the machine's axis of rotation when the footpad is at your ankle. Ideally, your head should rest against the back pad for a more stable body position.

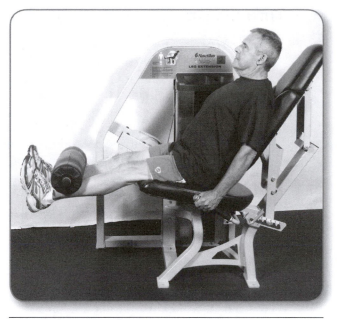

Figure 7.16   A leg extension performed on a stack-loaded leg extension machine.

Execution   Perform the exercise by kicking out until the legs are nearly fully extended (see figure 7.16). Slowly bring the legs back to the starting position.

Variations

- Externally rotating the legs during leg extensions places a greater emphasis on the vastus lateralis (outer thigh) muscle, whereas internally rotating the legs targets the vastus medialis. Some researchers even argue that internal rotation targets both vasti muscles.

- At home, this exercise can be done using rubber tubing or ankle weights and a chair (see figure 7.17). To use rubber tubing, place one foot through the handle loop, wrap the tubing around the leg of the chair so that there is no slack in the tubing, and step on the tubing with your other foot to hold it in place while you extend the leg. Switch legs and perform the exercise on the other side.

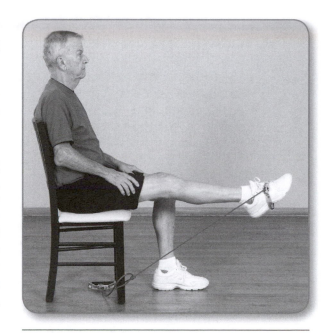

Figure 7.17   The leg extension performed at home with rubber tubing and a chair.

- In the pool, the exercise can be performed in waist-deep to shoulder-deep water. Stand with your back to the wall with one knee bent and extended forward. Kick the leg out and then bring the leg back to the original position. Pretend to be a Rockette at Christmas!

Safety   When performing the machine or chair exercises, try to prevent the gluteal muscles from rising up off the seat. For all forms of the leg extension, do not lock the knees at the end of the extension.

Squat

Environment   This exercise can be performed in the gym, home, or pool.

Application   The squat has been called the *king of all exercises.* Because the load is applied at the shoulders (when using a bar) or through the shoulder girdle (when using dumbbells or bands), this is not an exercise for beginners. The squat trains all the trunk (stabilizing) muscles and the lower-body muscles to varying extents. Using a bar requires sufficient strength and flexibility to be developed before the squat is attempted. Clients must understand the technique completely before adding any load. It is best to start by sitting on a chair and using no load to develop proper form. Once the squatting technique has been mastered, the exercise can be progressed to include the bar.

Position   Start with the feet slightly wider than shoulder-width apart. If you are using a bar, rest it across the trapezius muscles, holding it securely with the hands. Remember to keep the head up and chest out throughout the lift. When using a bar, you *must* perform the exercise either in a squat rack or with the help of knowledgeable spotters. When using a squat rack, set the bar at a height that allows you to place it on the trapezius muscles when the knees are slightly bent. Get under the bar and lift it off the rack, then step backward to clear the rack.

Execution   Start the movement by leading with your buttocks (in effect sitting back without bending your knees). As you continue to lower yourself into the sitting position and begin to bend the knees, try to keep the head up (you will still feel a slight forward bending at the waist). Continue the sitting motion until the thighs are parallel to the ground (see figure 7.18). Then pause and drive upward with the legs while exhaling forcefully. Concentrate on pushing against the ground with the heels while driving the hips forward.

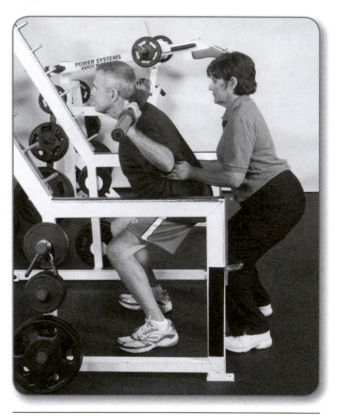

Figure 7.18   The barbell squat performed in a squat rack.

Variations

- There are four major variations of the free weight squat:

  1. The first variation is bar position. The bar can be held at either a high (top of the posterior deltoids) or low (upper trapezius) position. It can also be rested on the clavicles for a front squat.

  2. The second variation is squatting depth, which usually includes three levels: the full squat (below 90°), the parallel squat (to 90°), or the half squat (to approximately 135°).

  3. The third variation is stance width, which can vary from slightly narrower than shoulder-width apart to the ultrawide sumo position.

4. The fourth variation is the location of the center of gravity. A pendulum bar or dumbbells can be used to lower the center of gravity from the shoulders to below the waist. The squat can also be performed in a Smith machine (though I do not recommend this) or can be performed without weights, either while standing freely on the floor or sliding up a wall (the wall squat).

- The squat can be performed with tubing, bands, or water for resistance. The same motion is used for dumbbell, tubing, band, and pool squatting. In the pool you can increase resistance by opening the hands or wearing webbed gloves or paddles and facing the palms in the direction of the movement.

Safety   The first and most obvious safety tip for squatting is to never overestimate your abilities. The bar squat is one of those exercises in which the body is the only thing standing between the weight and the earth. Second, never squat without a safety rack or experienced spotters. Third, maintain the back in a neutral or slightly extended position by keeping the head up throughout the lift. Fourth, the squat may be the only exercise in which holding the breath during the concentric portion of the lift is a good idea. Intraabdominal pressure protects the back during the squat and holding the breath increases intraabdominal pressure. Finally, the squat places considerable compressive force on the skeleton, especially the vertebrae, so this exercise should not be performed by people with osteopenia or osteoporosis unless they have been cleared by their physician and are working out in an extremely controlled environment.

Lunge

Environment   This exercise can be performed in the gym, home, or pool.

Application   The lunge is the fourth exercise in this series of exercises targeting the lower body. It is more challenging than the squat is since the legs alternately perform two different biomechanical movements and the lunging action requires greater balance than the more symmetrical squat requires.

Position   Begin the exercise by standing upright with the arms at the sides holding onto dumbbells or with the bar positioned high on the trapezius muscles.

Execution   Step forward a comfortable distance with one foot. Keep the feet shoulder-width apart to maintain balance. Bend the forward leg until the thigh is parallel with the ground and the rear knee is nearly touching the ground. Do not allow the lead knee to go past the toes. Hesitate at the bottom and return to the starting position (see figure 7.19).

Variations

- The lunge can be done as a stationary or walking exercise. Additionally, the

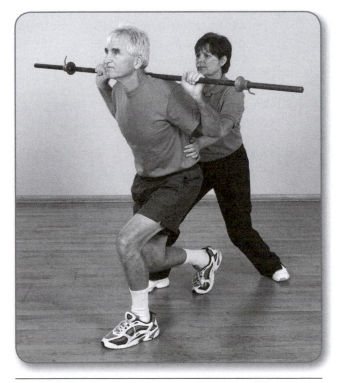
Figure 7.19   Performing a lunge with a barbell.

lunge can be performed with the front or rear leg on a step to increase the load on those legs, respectively.

- Another variation is to exaggerate the height of the front step by using the hip and knee flexors. This variation not only engages the hip and knee flexors but also requires greater balance because it prolongs the single-leg stance used during the lunge.

- The lunge can be performed while holding the weights overhead. This engages the shoulder muscles and makes it more difficult to maintain balance because it moves the center of gravity farther from the base (the feet). Obviously, these variations are for the advanced lifter, and spotters should be available to help if necessary.

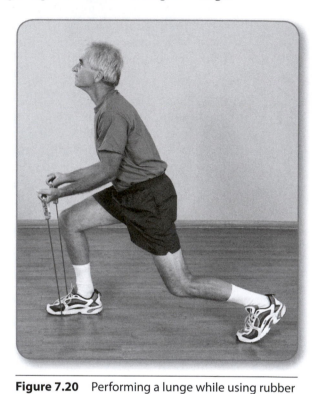

- The lunge can also be performed with dumbbells or rubber tubing (see figure 7.20) or while in the pool. If the lunge is performed with a band or tubing, it is by necessity a stationary exercise. Hold the middle of the band or tubing under the front foot and hold the arms at a right angle. Keeping the front foot flat on the ground so the band or tube remains in place, bend both knees lowering the body in a nearly vertical plane. Maintain tension throughout the exercise by holding onto the ends of the band or tubing and keeping your arms bent at a right angle.

Figure 7.20 Performing a lunge while using rubber tubing for resistance.

- When performing the lunge in the pool, move to waist-deep water and increase the resistance by forcefully pushing upward with your open hands or using handheld drag devices while attempting to stand.

Safety   Never allow the front knee to move forward past the toes. Ensure that the rear knee does not drift inward. Remember to keep the legs shoulder-width apart during the walking lunge.

HAMSTRINGS

Leg Curl

Environment   This exercise can be performed in the gym, home, or pool.

Application   The hamstrings are important for gait and balance and for initiating many ADLs. Additionally, developing balanced strength between the quadriceps and hamstrings is highly desirable for the structural health of the knee.

Position   To prepare for the lying leg curl, lie prone on the pad. Then align the knees with the pivot point of the machine and adjust the footpad so that it is at the level of the Achilles tendons. Ideally, your face should be close to the pad to reduce stress on the neck.

Execution Begin the exercise by bringing the pad toward the buttocks (see figure 7.21). Hold the movement for an instant and then slowly lower the weight. Do not raise your body off the pad to complete the exercise—instead, reduce the weight.

Variations

- In addition to offering the lying leg curl machine, many gyms offer a seated (see figure 7.22) or a standing leg curl machine. The procedures for using these machines are the same as those for all stack-loaded machines. Adjust the weight according to your ability. Position yourself in the machine, being certain that the knee joint or joints is in line with the pivot point of the machine and the footpad is on the Achilles tendon or tendons. Curl the leg or legs toward the buttocks. Ideally, your head should rest against the back pad for a more stable body position.

- The standing leg curl can also be performed at home by using a chair for support and tubing for resistance. Stand erect with one end of the tubing around one ankle and the other end attached to the chair leg. Without moving the upper leg, bend the knee so that the lower leg pulls on the tubing. Then lower the leg to the starting position. Repeat on the other side.

- To perform the standing leg curl in the pool, stand in waist-deep to shoulder-deep water. Face the pool wall and hold onto the overflow. Use a flotation device such as a noodle to add resistance. Extra resistance can also be applied by using drag devices such as ankle fins or aquatic drag shoes.

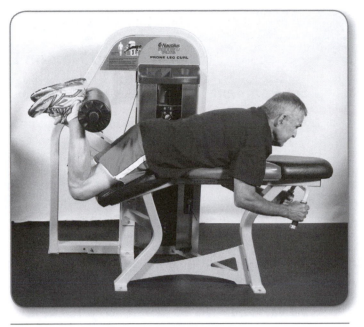

Figure 7.21 Performing the leg curl on a lying leg curl machine.

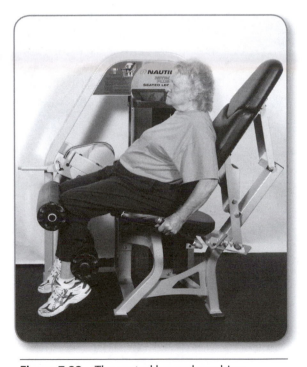

Figure 7.22 The seated leg curl machine.

Safety Use a weight you can handle. Too many times we allow our egos to control our good sense. Adding too much weight to the leg curl can cause the back to arch or, in the case of the lying leg curl, the hips to lift. This places both the low back and hamstrings at risk for acute injury. Another safety measure is to be sure the settings on the machine are set to accommodate your personal ROM. Incorrect settings can lead to serious injury, especially at the end of a set when the muscles are fatigued.

HIP FLEXORS

Hip Flexion Exercise

Environment   This exercise can be performed in the gym, home, or pool.

Application   The hip flexors are often ignored during the planning of training programs. However, these muscles are important to gait performance and fall prevention, especially when a person is clearing obstacles such as uneven sidewalk slabs, curbstones, thresholds, and rug bars.

Position   Hip flexion is one of the positions accommodated by the four-way hip machine. Begin the exercise with the padded arm in the bottom position. Place the thigh of one leg against the pad and hold onto the stability bar for balance.

Execution   Keeping the back straight, bring the knee up until the thigh is parallel to the ground. Then return to the starting position.

Variations

- The straight-leg hip flexion exercise is a variation that can be performed in the gym, home, or pool. The low pulley position available on most multistation machines can be used for this exercise. Stand facing away from the machine and hold the handles of the machine for stability. Keeping the knee straight, kick out from the hip.

- The straight-leg hip flexion exercise can also be performed by using elastic tubing to provide resistance. Attach the tubing to a chair leg and hold onto the chair for support (see figure 7.23).

- The movement can also be performed in the pool. Stand parallel to the wall in waist-deep to shoulder-deep water and support yourself by holding onto the side of the pool or the overflow. If desired, use drag devices to increase the resistance during the exercise.

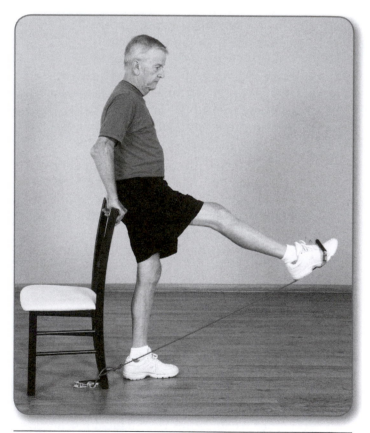

Figure 7.23   The hip flexion exercise can also be performed by using rubber tubing and holding onto a chair or other stationary object for support.

Safety   Again, using too much weight can cause low back or hip injury. You should be able to complete the hip flexion exercise without the chest leaning forward or the hips rotating in an attempt to compensate for inadequate muscle strength.

HIP EXTENSORS

Hip Extension Exercise

Environment   This exercise can be performed in the gym, home, or pool.

Application   Hip extension strength has been shown to be an important factor in maintaining proper gait. When a person's hip extensor muscles are weak and cannot function optimally, that person often assumes a posterior lean rather than an anterior lean during foot strike. The posterior lean increases the potential for falls and injury.

Position   Hip extension is the second of the positions on the four-way hip machine. Begin with the padded machine arm under the thigh of the bent leg. Hold the bent leg parallel to the floor and balance on the other leg, holding onto the stability bar for support.

Execution   Keeping the back straight, bring the raised knee back as far as is comfortable. Then return the knee to the starting position.

Variations

- A straight-leg hip extension can also be used in the gym, at home, or in the pool. In the gym, use the low pulley position on a multistation machine. To begin, stand facing the machine and hold onto the handles of the machine for stability. Keeping the knee straight, kick back from the hip.

- At home, use elastic tubing to provide resistance. Attach the tubing to a chair leg and hold onto the chair for support (see figure 7.24).

- In the pool, stand parallel to the wall in waist-deep to shoulder-deep water. Maintain balance by holding onto the coping or overflow. If desired, use drag devices to increase the resistance during the exercise.

Safety   Again, beware of using too much weight. Too much weight causes undue stress on the low back due to hyperextension. As with the hip flexion exercise, avoid hip rotation.

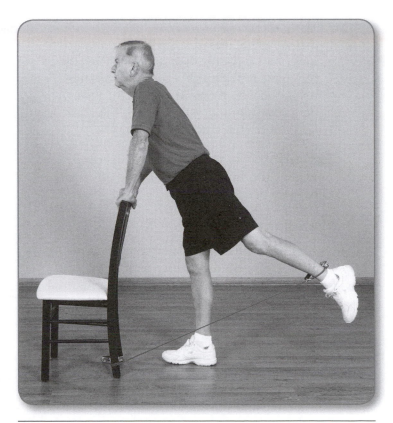

Figure 7.24   The straight-leg hip extension exercise can be performed at home by using rubber tubing and holding onto a chair or other stationary object for support.

HIP ADDUCTORS

Hip Adduction

Environment   This exercise can be performed in the gym, home, or pool.

Application   Strength and contractile speed of the hip adductors and abductors have been shown to be associated with both dynamic balance and recovery from falls. Since many of the falls resulting in hip fractures occur to the side or the rear, the training of these muscles can't be ignored. Poor balance during the 8-foot (2.4 m) up-and-go test and a history of falling are two factors indicating the need for adductor and abductor training. If balance, agility, or gait is an issue, the training of these muscles is a must.

Position   Hip adduction machines provide one of the safest and most effective tools for training the hip adductors. Begin in a seated position with the legs separated and the pads of the machine in contact with the inner aspects of the legs near the lower thigh and knee. Adjust the depth of the seat so that the hip joints are aligned with the pivot points on the machine (see figure 7.25). Ideally, your head should rest against the back pad for a more stable body position.

Execution   Bring the thighs together to adduct the hips. Return the legs to their original position.

Variations

- Straight-leg adductions can be performed in the gym, the home, or the pool. In the gym, use the low pulley position of a multistation machine. Stand with the leg to be exercised next to the machine and hold onto the machine handles for stability. Adduct the straight leg at the hip by pulling the leg across the body.
- At home, use an elastic band for resistance and a chair for support. A short band can be looped around the support leg and the exercising leg to create resistance (see figure 7.26), while a somewhat longer band can be attached to the chair leg or stood upon.

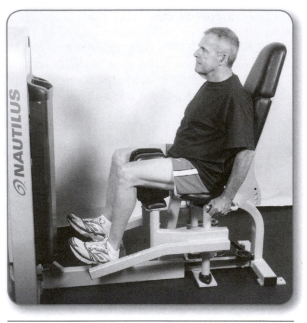

Figure 7.25   Hip adduction using a stack-loaded machine.

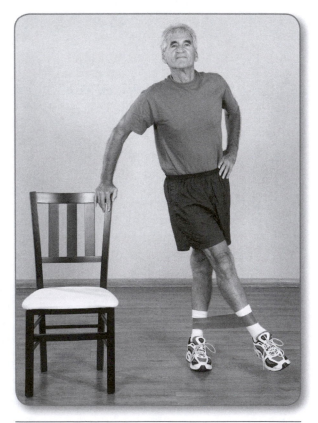

Figure 7.26   Hip adduction using a rubber band for resistance and a chair for support.

- In the pool, stand in waist-deep to shoulder-deep water and use the coping or overflow for support.

Safety   An initial concern with using the seated adduction machine is establishing the correct ROM to prevent strain or acute injury of the adductor muscles. When performing the standing exercises, it is especially important to choose a load that allows you to perform the hip adduction without shifting the position of the hips or forcing a lateral bend at the waist. Both of these conditions can damage the adductors and low back.

HIP ABDUCTORS

Hip Abduction

Environment   This exercise can be performed in the gym, home, or pool.

Application   As noted earlier, abduction strength affects both gait and balance. Like adductor training, abductor training is often ignored, especially by men. However, training these muscles affects not only independence but also safety.

Position   Hip abductor machines resemble hip adductor machines; however, their function is to train the opposite movement. The exercise is again performed in a seated position, but this time the pads of the machine are in contact with the outer thighs and knees. Position yourself in the machine and adjust the depth of the seat to align the hip joints with the pivot points on the machine (see figure 7.27). Ideally, your head should rest against the back pad for a more stable body position.

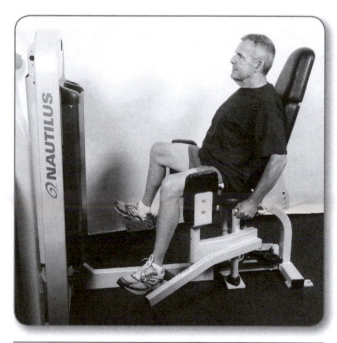

Figure 7.27   Performing hip abduction on a stack-loaded machine.

Execution   Bring together (abduct) the legs. Then return the legs to the starting position.

(HIP ABDUCTION continued on following page)

Variations

- The straight-leg hip abduction can be performed in the gym, at home, or in the pool. The straight-leg hip abduction is the final of the four exercises performed while using the low pulley position of a multistation machine. Begin by standing sideways to the pulley with the leg to be exercised away from the machine. Wrap the strap around the far ankle and hold onto the handles of the machine for stability. Move the leg away from the machine—that is, abduct the leg at the hip.

- At home, use rubber tubing for resistance and a chair for stability (see figure 7.28).

- In the pool, stand perpendicular to the pool wall. Keep about an arm's length away from the pool wall and hold onto the overflow for support. Then move the far leg away from the support leg as far as feels comfortable.

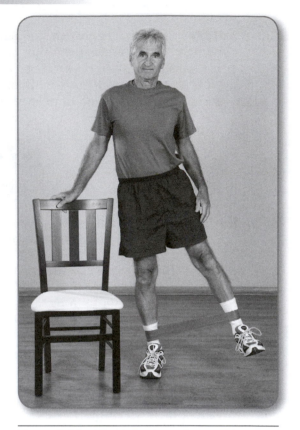

Figure 7.28 Hip abduction using a rubber band for resistance.

LOWER LEG

Heel Raise

Environment   This exercise can be performed in the gym, home, or pool.

Application   The heel raise targets the calf muscles (gastrocnemius and soleus). These muscles are very active throughout the stance phase of the gait cycle, and their strength has been associated with walking speed and fall probability.

Position   To use the standing heel raise machine, stand on the step and adjust the shoulder pads to create a slight bend in the knees. Adjust the feet so that only the balls of the feet are in contact with the step. The heels should be off the step. Straighten the legs to load the muscles.

Execution   Perform the exercise by standing on tiptoe, lifting the body as high as possible and keeping the legs straight (see figure 7.29). Then slowly return to the starting position.

Variations

- Alternative versions of the heel raise can be performed in all three training environments. The seated heel raise is very effective at training the soleus muscle since it reduces the contribution of the gastrocnemius muscle to the exercise. To begin, sit on

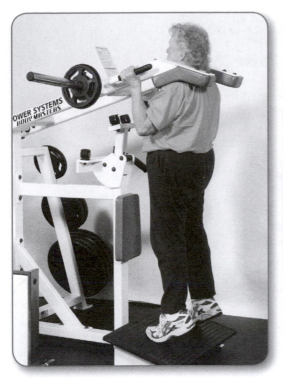

Figure 7.29   Performing the heel raise on the standing heel raise machine.

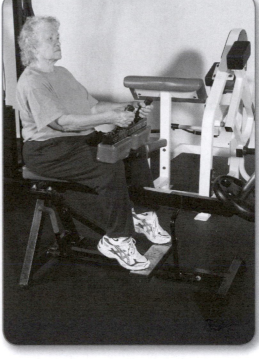

Figure 7.30   The seated heel raise machine.

the seated heel raise machine and place the balls of your feet on the foot plate. The heels should be hanging off the plate. Then adjust the pad so that it presses against the thighs. Push down on the foot plate to raise the heels. This action should raise the thigh pad. Hold at the top of the movement and then lower the heels to the starting position (figure 7.30).

- The standing heel raise can be performed at home by using a pair of handheld weights for resistance (see figure 7.31). To achieve maximal ROM, perform the exercise on a block or a step. Bands or rubber tubing can also be used for resistance.

- In the pool, the heel raise can be performed by standing facing the pool wall and holding onto the overflow for support.

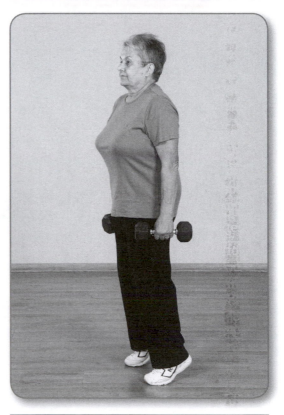

Figure 7.31   The standing heel raise using handheld weights.

DORSIFLEXORS

Toe Raise

Environment   This exercise can be performed in the gym, home, or pool.

Application   The muscles on the front of the lower leg are the dorsiflexors. The major muscle group here is the tibialis anterior. The strength and power of this muscle group consistently have been correlated with the probability of falling and with effective mobility. These muscles are responsible for lifting the ball and toes of the foot—a critical function for clearing potential fall hazards such as cracks in the sidewalk and rug bars. Although there are clear indications that these muscles are vital to maintaining independence and to fall prevention, only a very few commercially available machines target them (see figure 7.32). However, there is a piece of portable equipment called the *dynamic axial resistance device, or DARD,* that has been available for years and that adds resistance to dorsiflexion exercises (see figure 7.33*a*). A simple gym exercise targeting the dorsiflexors is a loaded toe raise (see figure 7.33*b*).

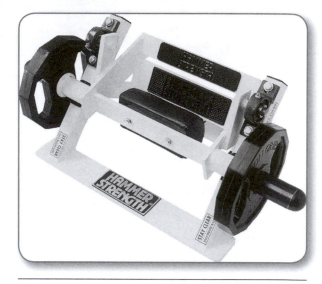

Figure 7.32   A Hammer dorsiflexion machine.

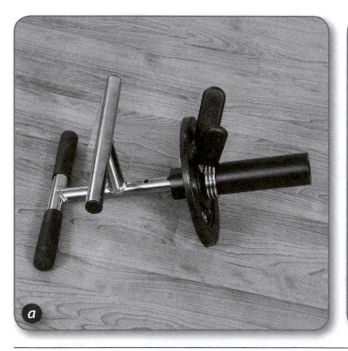

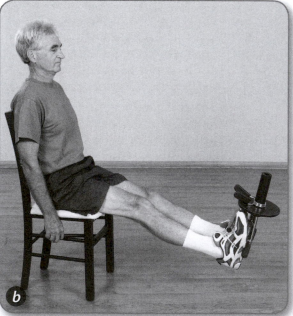

Figure 7.33   The *(a)* portable DARD adds resistance to *(b)* dorsiflexor exercises.

Position   The loaded toe raise requires a towel and a weight that you can move through the entire ROM of the exercise. Wrap the weight in the towel to form a sling for the weight. Using the towel to stabilize the weight, place the weight on the toes and forefoot while the foot is flat on the ground.

Execution   Use the toes and forefoot to lift the weight. Then return the weight to the starting position (see figure 7.34).

Variations

- Toe raises can also be performed at home with no loading. The exercise can be performed on the floor, but greater ROM can be obtained by performing the exercise on a step or platform. To begin, stand on the heels at the edge of the step with the toes pointed downward, while holding tightly onto the rail for balance. Point the toes up toward the ceiling and then return the feet to the starting position.

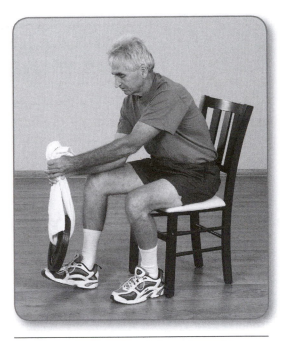

Figure 7.34   Using a weight and towel to target the dorsiflexors.

- Elastic bands or tubes can be used to add resistance to the dorsiflexion exercise, but using them requires a stable inanimate object or a friend. Either have a friend wrap a band or elastic tube around your toes while holding onto the other end or wrap the tube around an inanimate object and place the handles around your feet while you're sitting on the floor. Start the exercise with the ankles held at 90°, making sure that the tube or band is under tension. To perform the exercise, pull the toes toward the body and then return the feet to the starting position.

Safety   When using weights for the loaded toe raise, be sure that the weight is stable and that you have a good grip on the towel. Losing control of the weight can cause injury. Since the DARD is a pure isolation device with no end point in the ROM, be careful not to load the device beyond your capacity or be sure you have spotters available. For band exercises, be careful that the band does not slip off the feet. This can be detrimental to the health of the person assisting with the exercise.

UPPER-BODY EXERCISES
CHEST AND ANTERIOR SHOULDERS

Seated Chest Press

Environment   This exercise can be performed in the gym.

Application   The muscles of the chest and anterior (front) shoulders are needed to perform a plethora of movements associated with ADLs and IADLs. Additionally, upper-body strength is important for using handrails, armrests, and walking devices and proves useful in a last-ditch effort to prevent injury during a fall.

Position   To begin the exercise, sit in the seat of the chest press machine and check the level of the handles. Adjust the handles so that they are at chest level.

Execution   Keeping the back against the seat pad and the head in a neutral position, perform the exercise by pushing out on the handles until the arms are nearly straight. Hold and return to the starting position.

Variations   There are two basic types of chest press machines. One is a straight press in which the handles move directly forward from the starting position, and the other is a biaxial machine that combines the pressing action with a gradual movement toward the midline of the body.

At home, the chest press can be performed by using tubing or bands in a standing or seated position (see figure 7.35). Place the tube or band behind your back or the back of the chair. Hold one end in each hand at either side of the chest and make sure the tubing or band is under tension. To perform the exercise, push straight out from the chest toward the center line of the body, stop near full extension, and then return to the starting position.

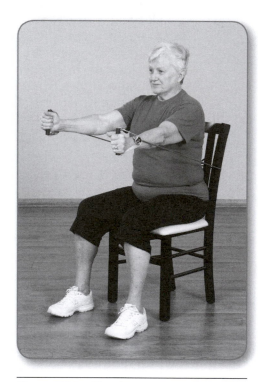

Figure 7.35   The chest press performed using rubber tubing.

Safety   The chest press is one of the safest exercises targeting the chest muscles. However, remember to set the ROM before performing the exercise to prevent undue stress on the vulnerable shoulder joint. Also, be sure not to lock the elbows into full extension at the end of the concentric movement.

Flat Bench Press

Environment   This exercise can be performed in the gym.

Application   It's impossible to go to a gym or heath club during prime time without seeing mobs of postpubescent males clustered around the flat benches and without hearing the number one question asked in most weight rooms: "What do you bench?"

If the squat is the king of all exercises, then the bench press is the king of all upper-body exercises.

Position   Start in the prone position on a flat bench and look straight up at the bar. Grasp the bar, placing the hands slightly wider than shoulder-width apart (see figure 7.36). Lift the bar from the uprights (some newer benches have swing supports that help with this action).

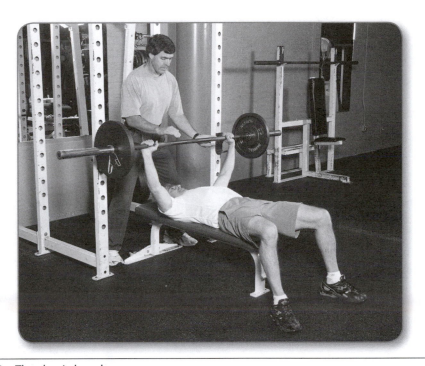

Figure 7.36   The classic bench press.

Execution   Start the exercise by slowly lowering the bar toward the chest. At the bottom of the lift, when the bar is nearly touching the chest, stop the weight and forcefully drive the bar upward to the starting position. When the set is complete, rack the weight.

Variations   You can vary your grips depending on the muscles you wish to target. A narrow grip targets the outer fibers of the chest and triceps, while a wide grip targets the fibers closer to the sternum.

Safety   While it is perhaps the most effective exercise for increasing upper-body strength and power, the bench press is not without risk and should not be performed without experienced spotters who can help with the weight should you lose control or fail to complete a repetition. The bench press is an exercise that can trap the body under the bar if you fail or flaw during a lift. Here are some don'ts for the bench press: Don't place your feet on the bench. Instead, keep them on the floor. Don't arch your back to complete the lift. Instead, seek help from your spotter and consider using less weight for subsequent sets. Don't try to test your maximum bench press. It serves no purpose and can lead to serious injury and even death. Don't emulate the lifters who lower the weight quickly and bounce it off their chests. While it might allow you to lift a few more pounds, it provides no additional benefit and may prove hazardous to your health. The bench press is a wonderful training tool, but it must be respected. To paraphrase Uncle Ben in *Spider-Man:* Great overload requires great responsibility.

◼◼ Fly ◼◼

Environment   This exercise can be performed in the gym, home, or pool.

Application   The fly machine isolates the chest and anterior deltoids to a greater degree than the chest or bench press does because it takes the triceps out of the exercise. Additionally, the fly allows greater ROM than the pressing exercises allow.

Position   To align yourself correctly in the machine, place the hands on the handles and adjust the seat height so that the forearms are on the pads and the elbows are bent at 90°.

Execution   Begin the exercise by simultaneously bringing the pads together. Hold the pads together briefly and then return them to the starting position.

Variations

- The dumbbell fly can be performed on the flat bench or on a stability ball (see figure 7.37). Lie supine on the bench. Hold a dumbbell in each hand. Begin the exercise with the arms out, slightly bent, and parallel to the floor. Bring the arms together simultaneously, as if hugging a big bear. Hold the contracted position for a moment before slowly returning to the starting point.

- Flys can also be performed in the pool. Stand in shoulder-deep water or squat in water of a lesser depth. Hold the arms out to the side with the hands just below the surface of the water. Using your hands, paddles, or webbed gloves and your forearms, push the water forward and toward the midline of the body as if you are squeezing the water between your arms. As you return the arms to the starting position, turn your hands for extra resistance. This will provide a small overload on the back musculature.

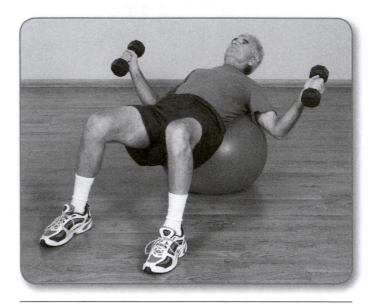

Figure 7.37   The chest fly performed on a stability ball.

UPPER CHEST AND DELTOIDS

◼◼ Inclined Bench Press ◼◼

Environment   This exercise can be performed in the gym or home.

Application   The inclined bench press targets the upper portion of the chest muscles and to a greater extent the anterior deltoids. The anterior deltoids are the front shoulder muscles.

Position   Use a bench that is on a 45° angle. If you are using a barbell, place the bar on the support brackets just above your clavicles. If you are using dumbbells, hold the dumbbells just above the fronts of the shoulders (see figure 7.38).

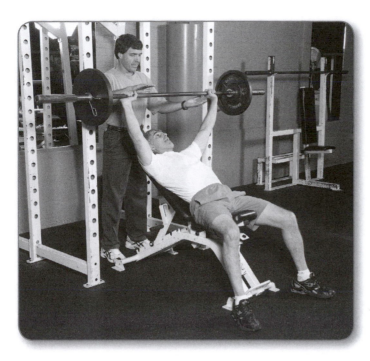

Figure 7.38 Performing the inclined bench press with a barbell.

Execution   The action of the inclined bench press is the same as that used for the flat bench press. Straighten the arms to a nearly fully extended position and then return to the starting position.

Variation   Using dumbbells to perform the inclined bench press increases ROM at the cost of resistance.

Safety   All the precautions taken when performing the flat bench press apply to the inclined bench press, with one additional precaution. The position of the bar in the inclined bench press makes the weight more difficult to control and puts the rotator cuffs at greater risk for injury.

UPPER AND MIDDLE BACK

Row

Environment   This exercise can be performed in the gym, home, or pool.

Application   Translocation, or moving an object from one surface to another, and many other ADLs depend on the functional performance of the muscles of the upper and middle back. Consider the number of everyday activities that require a person to bring an object toward the body—the list is extensive. The following exercises target these muscles.

Position   To perform the seated row, sit down with the back slightly arched, the chest out, and the head aligned with the spine. Extend the legs forward and place the feet on the foot plate while maintaining a slight bend of the knees. Extend the arms in front of the body and grab the machine handles. If you are using a seated row machine, adjust the seat so that the chest pad is centered on the sternum and you are pulling on solid lever arms. If you are using the cable row machine, grasp the single handle attached to the cable (see figure 7.39).

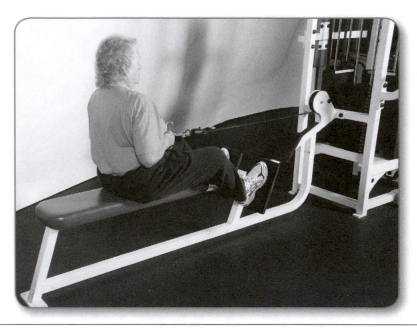

Figure 7.39 The seated row using a cable weight-stack machine.

Execution Pull the elbows back toward the body, keeping the elbows tight at the sides. Pause slightly when the bar reaches the upper abdomen or the handle is pulled to the body. Slowly return to the starting position. To get the most out of the exercise, imagine bringing the shoulder blades together as if trying to squeeze a ball between them.

Variations

- The bent-over row is one of the oldest exercises using free weights. Begin with the left foot on the floor and the right knee on a bench. Lean forward and support the upper body with the right arm so that the back is as parallel to the ground as possible. Hold the weight in the left hand with the left arm hanging straight down. Bring the weight up toward the chest by contracting the back muscles and bending the elbow. Then return the weight to the starting position (see figure 7.40). Switch sides and repeat.

- The reverse fly also targets the muscles of the upper back. Lie prone on a bench with the legs extended backward and the toes on the floor for stability. Grasp a dumbbell in each hand. Keeping the arms straight, bring the shoulder blades together and raise the arms until they are at the level of the bench. Then return to the starting position.

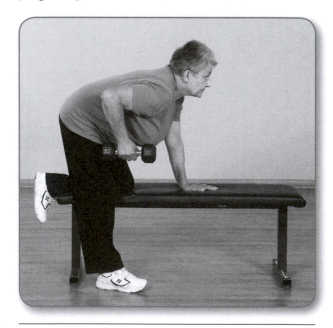

Figure 7.40 The bent-over row with a dumbbell.

- There are three exercises that use bands or tubing to target the upper shoulder muscles.
    1. The first is the standing row. Hold one end of a band in each hand; the hands should be shoulder-width apart. Keeping both arms partially extended, lift the

hands out to the sides, concentrating on bringing the shoulder blades together. Once you have reached end ROM, slowly return the hands to the starting position.

2. The second exercise is the seated row (see figure 7.41). Sit with the legs fully extended and loop the middle of the exercise tube around the insteps of the feet. Grasp a handle in each hand and fully extend the arms. Then perform the exercise exactly as you would when performing the seated cable row.

3. The third exercise is a kneeling reverse fly. Begin the exercise on all fours. Hold one handle of the tube in one hand and place the tube itself under the other hand so that the tube is taut. Keeping the arm relatively straight, pull the arm directly out to the side so that the hand reaches a position just below shoulder level. Complete the exercise by returning to the starting position.

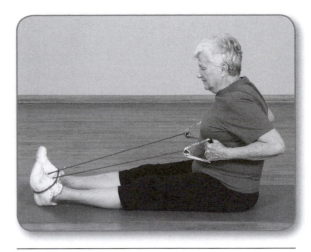

Figure 7.41   The seated row with rubber tubing for resistance.

• When performing the rowing exercise in the pool, the movement portion is the same as it is for the other rowing exercises. Stand in shoulder-deep water while holding buoyant dumbbells or other drag devices in each hand. Bring both arms back simultaneously or in an alternating pattern. This exercise is designed to target the shoulders, so minimize the involvement of the low back muscles by keeping the trunk as stable as possible.

LATISSIMUS DORSI

Lat Pull-Down

Environment   This exercise can be performed in the gym, home, or pool.

Application   The latissimus dorsi, or lats, are the winglike muscles running down the back from the armpits to the waist area. Functionally these muscles are used for activities such as climbing a ladder, using an overhead object to pull the body up, or pushing up out of a chair or bed. The most common machine used to perform the lat pull-down is the pulley and cable system (see figure 7.42).

Position   To start the exercise, place the legs under the thigh pad. Grasp the bar with the palms facing forward at a width about 1.5 times wider than shoulder-width apart.

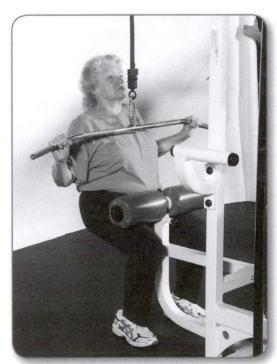

Figure 7.42   Lat pull-down machine.

Execution Lean back slightly and pull the bar down in front of the body to the collarbone, passing it close to the face and chin. While pulling down, attempt to squeeze the shoulder blades together. Keep the chest up and out throughout the lift. After a pause, slowly return the bar to the starting position.

Variations

- The lat pull-down can be performed on solid-arm machines rather than cable and pulley machines. Solid-arm machines actually dictate the movement pattern, so the concerns about bar positions are not applicable to solid arm machines.

- You're probably familiar with the pull-up from your old high school gym class. In addition to being a wonderful exercise for the lats, it is also one of the most difficult exercises to perform. But there is hope. The assisted pull-up machine (see figure 7.43) allows you to either kneel or sit on a platform while performing the pull-up. By adding weight to counterbalance your body weight, you can make yourself light and make the pull-up easier to perform. Executing the pull-up is just as you remember! Hang from the overhead bar or handles with the palms of the hands facing forward. Pull the body up until the chin clears the bar, and then return to the starting position.

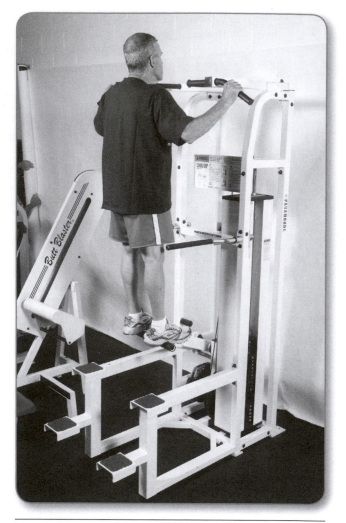

Figure 7.43 Assisted pull-up machine.

- When at home, you can use bands or tubing to simulate the lat pull-down and pull-up machines (see figure 7.44). Begin the exercise by holding the band overhead with the hands just wider than shoulder-width apart. Lower the band to chest level, pulling outward until the arms are straight and the band makes contact with the chest. Once the movement is completed, slowly return the band to the overhead position. A second option for using bands at home is to loop the band over a door or some other stable object. This allows you to perform the pull-down exercise in a manner that is even closer to the machine exercises.

- When in the pool, you can perform a straight-arm lateral push-down. Stand in shoulder-deep water while holding a buoyant dumbbell or other drag device in each hand. Extend the arms outward to shoulder level. Keeping the arms straight, bring the hands down to the sides, keeping the palms facing down. Then bring the hands back to the starting position, with the palms up.

Safety The lat pull-down incorporates the muscles of the rotator cuff. Two controversies surround the cable pull-down: grip width and the point at which the concentric portion of the exercise should end. While most texts agree that using a grip width that is slightly wider than shoulder width is most effective for targeting the lats, some practitioners argue that it is more effective to pull the bar behind the neck rather than to the clavicle. Data from our lab have shown that there is no need to pull the bar behind the neck—the most effective variation is to pull to the clavicle. In fact, pulling the bar behind the neck increases the possibility of impingement or cervical injury.

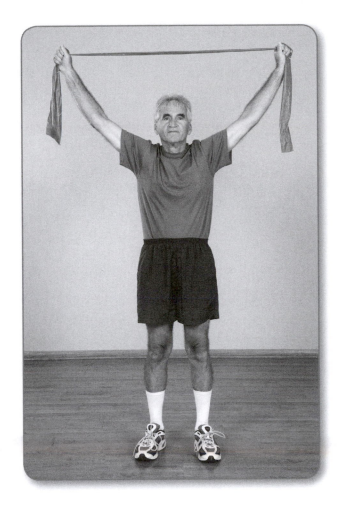

Figure 7.44 Using rubber bands to target the lats.

SHOULDERS

Overhead Press

Environment   This exercise can be performed in the gym, home, or pool.

Application   The shoulder muscles are important for everyday activities such as reaching, lifting, and carrying. In addition, the shoulder muscles (deltoids) are important for maintaining posture and for stabilizing the upper body during the performance of many ADLs. Exercises in which weight is lifted directly overhead are commonly used to overload the shoulder muscles. These exercises can be performed with machines or free weights. While using free weights increases the use of the accessory muscles to control the movement, machine exercises are safer for beginning lifters.

Position   Whether you are using a barbell or dumbbells to perform the overhead press, sit on a bench, keeping the upper body stable and the feet firmly on the ground. A spotter can help you remove the bar from the bench stanchions so that you can start the lift at shoulder level.

Execution   Push the barbell or dumbbells directly overhead until the arms are near full extension. Hold the position for a moment and then return to the starting position (see figure 7.45). This exercise should be spotted.

Variations

- When using dumbbells, start with the weights at shoulder level. When using a machine, set the seat so that the handles are at shoulder level.
- The overhead press can also be performed at home by using an elastic band or tubing.

Safety When using free weights such as barbells or dumbbells, be sure to have a spotter available to help you.

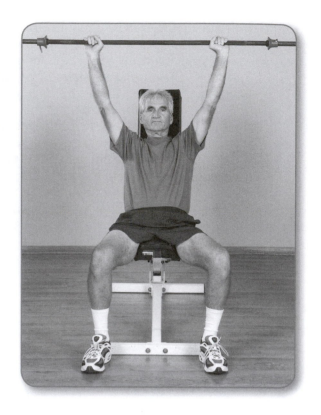

Figure 7.45 The overhead press performed with a barbell.

Lateral Raise

Environment This exercise can be performed in the gym, home, or pool.

Application The lateral raise concentrates on the medial, or middle, deltoids. However, the other portions of the shoulder muscles are also utilized (see figure 7.46).

Position When using a lateral raise machine, adjust the seat height so that the chest pad is in contact with the chest and the arm pads are in contact with the upper arms. Be sure to keep the upper body stable while performing this exercise.

Execution Keeping the arms bent at the elbows, raise the arms directly to the side. Stop at the level of the shoulders, and then return the pads to the starting position.

Variations

- Lateral raises target the middle deltoids. They can be performed seated or standing. To perform a dumbbell version of the lateral raise, hold a dumbbell in each hand. Start with the hands at the sides with the palms facing the body. Lift the dumbbells to the

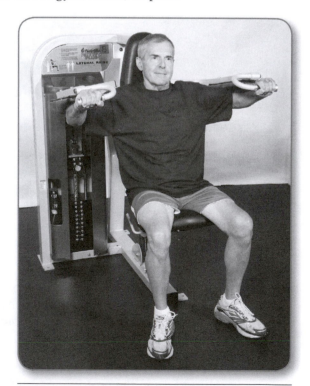

Figure 7.46 Performing the lateral raise on a machine.

side, stopping at shoulder level. Return to the starting position.

- Front raises target the anterior deltoids and can also be performed seated or standing. To perform a front raise, hold a dumbbell in each hand. Start with the hands at the sides with the palms facing backward. Lift the arms to the front, stopping at shoulder level. Return to the starting position.

- When at home, you can use bands or tubing to perform the lateral or front raise (see figure 7.47).

- When in the pool, you can perform the lateral or front raise by using resistive gloves or paddles. Raise the arms to shoulder level, keeping the elbows slightly bent. Lift out to the side for lateral raises or to the front for front raises. Pause at the top position and then slowly lower the arms.

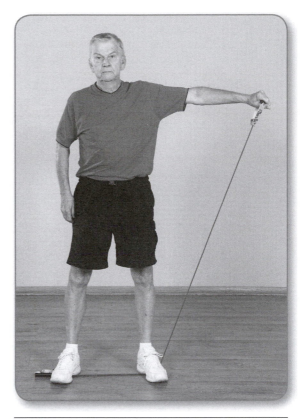

Figure 7.47   The lateral raise performed by using elastic tubing.

Shrug

Environment   This exercise can be performed in the gym or home.

Application   Shrugs target the posterior shoulder muscles and the upper trapezius muscles (the large muscle group at the base of the neck). The exercise can be performed with dumbbells, a barbell, or specially designed machines.

Position   Whether you are using dumbbells, a barbell, or a machine, the performance is very much the same. Hold the bar, dumbbells, or handles in the hands and let the arms hang at the sides of the body.

Execution   Without bending the arms, bring the shoulders up toward the ears and slightly back in a sort of "I don't know" gesture (see figure 7.48). Once you have reached the top position of the exercise, hesitate, and then return to the starting position.

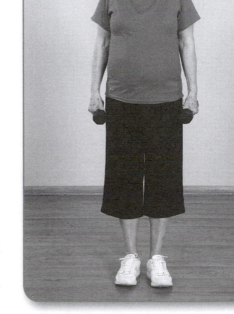

Figure 7.48   The shoulder shrug.

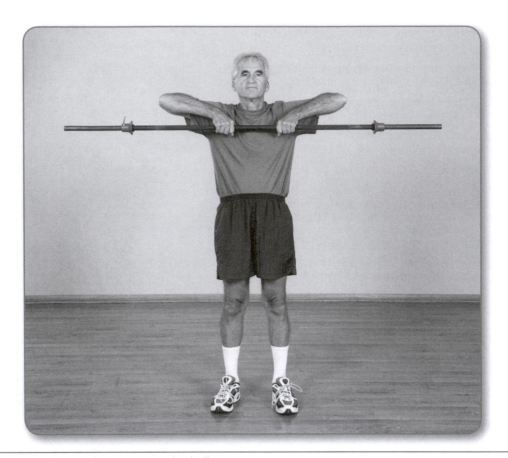

Figure 7.49 The upright row using a barbell.

Variation The upright row also targets the rear deltoid and upper trapezius. The exercise is typically performed while standing. Begin with the barbell or dumbbells held at thigh level, hands shoulder-width apart, with the arms passively extended by the weight. Lift the weight by contracting the trapezius and rear deltoid muscles while bending the arms at the elbows to bring the weight to the level of the collarbone (see figure 7.49). Hold and return the weight to the starting position. This exercise incorporates more of the deltoid muscles than the shrug incorporates.

ROTATOR CUFF

Internal Rotation

Environment This exercise can be performed in the gym, home, or pool.

Application One of the most common injuries seen in older persons is damage to the rotator cuff. Rather than undergoing a complicated surgical repair and prolonged rehabilitation, why not perform a bit of preventative maintenance by training the musculature that helps maintain the integrity of this joint?

Position To perform the internal rotation with the cable system, grasp the handle of the cable in one hand and flex the elbow to 90°. Keeping the elbow locked close to the body, rotate the arm so that the forearm points directly out to the side.

Execution   Bring the handle of the cable to the front midline of the body (see figure 7.50). Be sure to keep the elbow in place.

Variations

- This movement can be performed by using rubber tubing for resistance. Attach one end of the tubing to a stable object and grasp the other end in one hand. Then perform the internal rotation as described for the cable system.

- To perform the internal rotation in the pool, use the hand or a drag device for resistance. In all cases, try varying the planes of motion so you can strengthen the rotator cuff through various ROMs.

- You can also perform this exercise with a hand weight. When using a hand weight, lie on the side of the exercising arm (see figure 7.51). Using a hand weight while standing is ineffective since gravity offers little resistance in the plane of the movement.

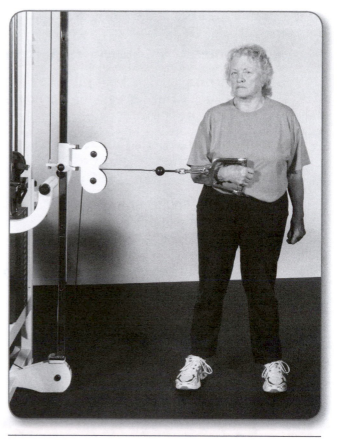

Figure 7.50   The internal rotation performed with a cable system.

Safety   Remember that the incredible freedom of movement about the shoulder puts the rotator cuff at greater risk for injury. Limit the resistance and carefully control the pattern of the movement.

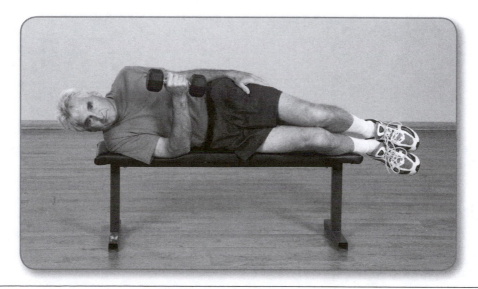

Figure 7.51   Lying internal rotation using a hand weight for resistance. Ideally, the head will be supported with a head rest or pillow.

External Rotation

Environment   This exercise can be performed in the gym, home, or pool.

Application   As noted, the rotator cuff is susceptible to injury, especially in older persons. External rotations are the second major type of exercises used to strengthen this muscle group.

Position   To perform the external rotation with the cable system, begin with a cable in one hand. Flex the elbow to 90° and keep it locked close into the body. As opposed to the internal rotation exercise, rotate the arm so that the forearm is across the body.

Execution   Rotate the arm so that the hand points directly to the side. Be sure to keep the elbow in place (see figure 7.52).

Variations

- As was the case with the internal rotation, the external rotation can be performed with a tube or band or can be performed in the pool. However, in the pool the application of resistance is limited by the inability to turn the hands in the direction to optimize resistance.

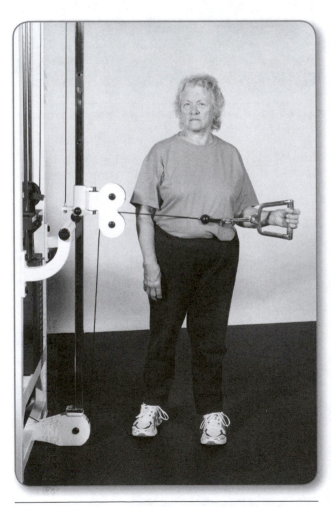

Figure 7.52   The external rotation performed with a cable system.

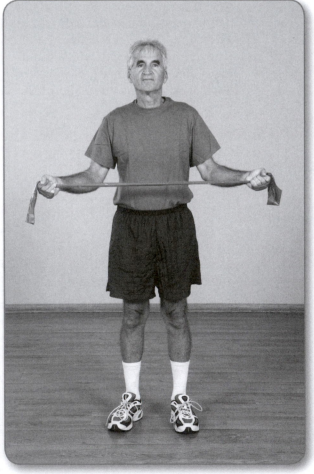

Figure 7.53   External rotation performed by using a band.

- Since the movement is away from the center line of the body, you can perform an external rotation by holding a band or tube between the hands and rotating the hands outward (see figure 7.53).
- If you are using a hand weight to perform the external rotation, be sure to lie on the side opposite the exercising arm (see figure 7.54).

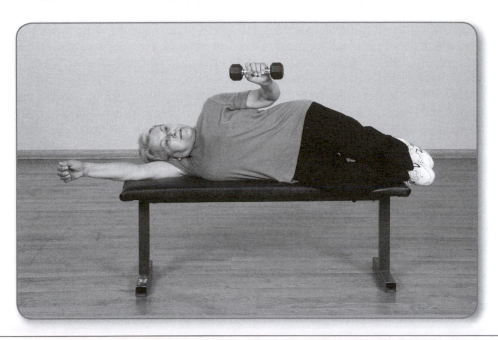

Figure 7.54   Lying external rotation performed by using a hand weight. Ideally, the head will be supported with a head rest or pillow.

ARM MUSCLES

Biceps Curl

Environment   This exercise can be performed in the gym, home, or pool.

Application   As children, we learn that the biceps is almost synonymous with the word *muscle. Make a muscle* always means "Show me your biceps!" Since this book is about performing as if we are young again, the biceps should certainly have a warm place in all of our hearts. But are these muscles important to daily activities? The simple answer is to think about the number of times we bend our arms throughout the day. Additionally, any time we hold an object at chest level, we are using an isometric contraction of the biceps. If the biceps are the most recognizable muscles in the body, then the biceps curl is the most recognizable exercise. In its simplest form the exercise is performed in the standing position with either a dumbbell or a barbell for resistance; however, the dumbbell biceps curl can also be performed in a seated position.

Position   To perform a barbell biceps curl, hold the bar so that the arms are straight and the palms of the hands are facing away from the body. Stand with a slight bend in the knees. Maintain good upper-body alignment and keep a straight back.

Execution   Maintaining the hand position, keep the elbows close to the sides of the body while bending at the elbows to bring the bar to the chest (see figure 7.55). Pause at the top and then return to the starting position.

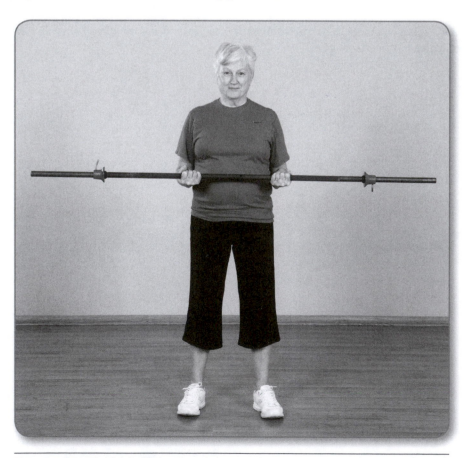

Figure 7.55   The barbell biceps curl.

Variations

- If you are using dumbbells, hold them at your sides with your palms facing toward your body. Curl the weights upward while rotating the palms from an inward-facing to a forward-facing position.

- To isolate the biceps muscle even more, try the concentration curl. Sit on the edge of a bench with a dumbbell in one hand and the corresponding elbow resting against the inside of the thigh. Curl the weight, keeping the palm facing up to maximize biceps activation.

- A variation of the concentration curl is the so-called *preacher* or *deacon curl*. Sit on the preacher curl bench. Place the backs of the arms against the pad, straighten the arms, and grasp the bar. The preacher curl bench is often incorporated into a stack machine.

- You can use bands and tubes to perform the biceps curl by holding one end in one hand and stabilizing the other end with your other hand (see figure 7.56), your foot (see figure 7.57), or an inanimate object.

- To perform the biceps curl in the pool, stand in shoulder-deep water both arms extended down at the sides, palms facing forward. Keeping the body stable, curl the arms upward, using the water for resistance. By turning the hands downward on the return movement you can also work the triceps. To increase resistance, use webbed gloves, paddles, or other drag devices.

Safety As with many of the exercises in this chapter, excess loading is often the factor that causes injury. All you need to do is look around the gym to see how using too much weight can affect the standing biceps curl. To compensate for a lack of biceps strength, lifters often arch their backs and shift toward their dominant side to complete the lift. This action puts the back at risk for acute injury. Additionally, performing heavy lifts without sufficient recovery can cause overuse injury to both the muscle and the connective tissue, especially during isolation exercises such as the concentration and preacher curls.

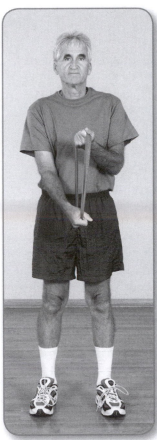

Figure 7.56 Biceps curls performed with a band for resistance.

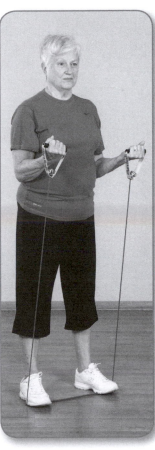

Figure 7.57 Biceps curls performed with rubber tubing for resistance.

Triceps Push-Down

Environment   This exercise can be performed in the gym.

Application   Any movement requiring arm extension involves the triceps muscles. Passing the salt, putting a book back on a shelf, and pulling down the shades all use the triceps muscles. There are a large number of exercises that target this muscle group. One of them is the machine push-down. The machine push-down is performed in a seated position and simulates the triceps action used when rising from a chair or the bed.

Position   Adjust the seat of the push-down machine so that when the hands are on the handles, the arms are maximally flexed without forcing a rise in the shoulders. Then sit in the seat and grasp the handles.

Execution   To perform the exercise simply push down on the handles. Hesitate at the bottom, and then return to the starting position.

Variations   The triceps push-down can be performed on a cable pulley station (see figure 7.58). Stand facing the cable pulley station with a short bar attached to the cable. Grab the bar with an overhand grip, with the palms facing down and the elbows flexed so that the forearms meet with the biceps. Slightly bend the knees and maintain a natural arch of the lower back, keeping the chest up. Keep the elbows near your sides so they can act like a hinge. Start the exercise by extending the arms downward to a nearly full extension. Stop at the bottom of the exercise, and then slowly allow the bar to return to the starting position. The rope or V-bar attachment can also be used to perform the cable push-down.

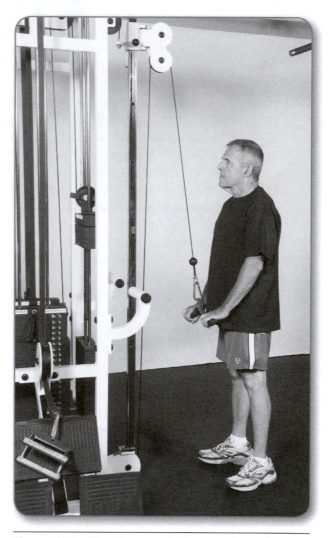

Figure 7.58   The triceps push-down performed on a cable pulley station.

Safety   Although this may sound redundant, the major problems experienced during the triceps push-down are the result of using too much weight. When performing the seated push-down, people often allow their body to rise off the seat so they can use their body weight to aid in the exercise. This means that the load is well beyond the contractile strength of the triceps and is most likely beyond the structural strength of the muscle and connective tissue. In the cable push-down excess weight usually leads to elevated shoulders and flared elbows, which puts undue stress on the rotator cuff. Additionally, many lifters use forward flexion of the trunk to increase force generation, placing further stress on the shoulder joint.

▰ Triceps Extension ▰

Environment   This exercise can be performed in the gym, home, or pool.

Application   The triceps extension isolates the triceps muscles by placing the arms in a position where other muscle groups can provide little additional force during the exercise.

Position   To set yourself up in a triceps extension machine, adjust the seat height so that the upper arms are slightly lower than parallel to the ground and the elbows are aligned with the pivot point of the machine arm. The hands should be comfortable when holding the handles (see figure 7.59).

Execution   Starting with the elbows flexed, push outward on the handles until the arms are nearly straight. Stop, hold, and then return to the starting position.

Variations

- The overhead triceps extension can be performed with a dumbbell (see figure 7.60), a rubber tube (see figure 7.61), or a band for resistance. To reduce the potential for injury, work one side at a time. Grasp the resistance in one hand and point the elbow toward the sky so that the hand and the resistance are going down your back. Reach up to the sky by straightening the elbow, stop, and then return to the starting position.

- Another variation on the triceps extension is the dip. The most common of the dip exercises is the parallel dip (see figure 7.62*a*). Stand between the dip bars and climb the stairs so that you can place a hand on each bar with the elbows straight. Pull the heels up to the buttocks or step off the step so that the legs are hanging. Lower your body by bending at the elbows. Once the elbows reach a right angle, push back up. Since this exercise requires you to lift your own body weight, you may not be able to complete it due to your age or training status. Thankfully, there is an assisted dip machine that uses the same technology (and is often the same machine) as the assisted pull-up machine. This machine uses weights to counterbalance your body weight so that you can complete the exercise (see figure 7.62*b*).

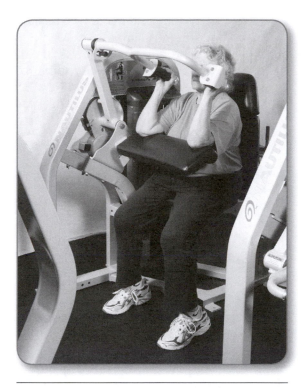

Figure 7.59   A triceps extension machine.

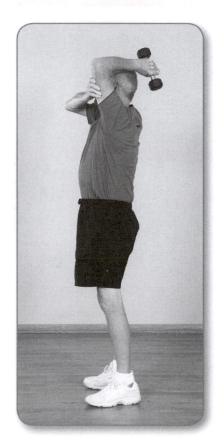

Figure 7.60   The triceps extension performed by using a dumbbell.

- Another variation of the dip, the bench dip, can be performed on a bench or chair (be careful about stability!). The bench dip provides greater concentration on the triceps than the parallel dip provides and requires less strength since it does not require you to lift your entire body weight. Sit in the middle of a bench with both legs extended on one side and the heels of the hands on the bench next to each hip. Then walk the feet forward and pull the buttocks away from the bench so that you are supported on your feet and hands. Now bend the elbows, lowering your body toward the floor. Stop before the shoulders start to elevate, and then push yourself back to the starting position so that the arms are in nearly complete extension. Remember to keep your core stable.

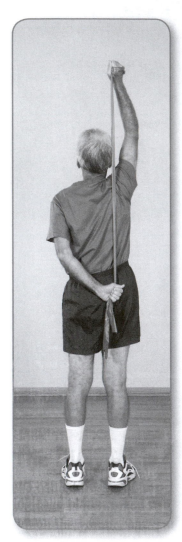

Figure 7.61 The triceps extension performed by using rubber tubing.

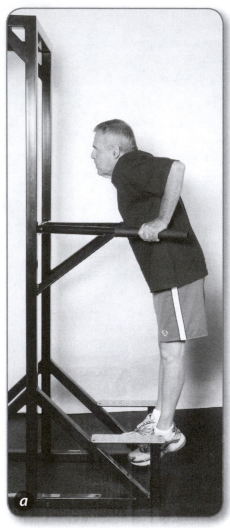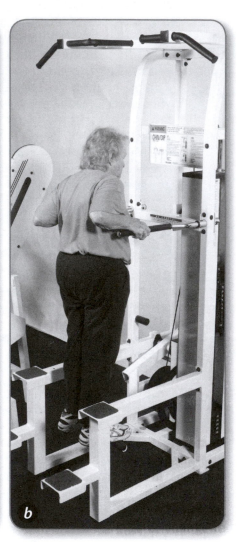

Figure 7.62 The triceps extension performed by the dip exercise: *(a)* the parallel dip and *(b)* using the assisted dip machine.

Triceps Kickback

Environment   This exercise can be performed in the gym, home, or pool.

Application   The triceps kickback is normally performed with a dumbbell. This exercise is performed within a limited ROM when compared with the other triceps exercises described in this chapter.

Position   Begin the exercise bent at the waist and supporting yourself by resting one arm on a bench or on your thigh. Hold the dumbbell in the other hand. Be sure to hold the arm parallel to the trunk throughout the exercise.

Execution   Begin the exercise with the working arm bent to 90°. Extend it back to near full extension and then return to the starting position, keeping the elbow in position throughout the movement (see figure 7.63).

Variations

- You can also use rubber tubing or bands to perform the kickback. Grab the end or handle of the rubber band or tubing. Bend slightly at the waist and step on the tube or band so that there is tension when the upper arm is parallel to the body and the elbow is bent to 90°. Now straighten the arm back to a position just short of full extension. Hold, and then return to the starting position. Do not allow any drift in the upper arm (see figure 7.64).

- The movement pattern and body position for the triceps kickback are the same in the pool as on land. The level of the water must wash over your back as you bend over. When performing the kickback, keep the elbows in a stable position and be sure that the palms of the hands are facing backward into the direction of the movement in order to provide resistance.

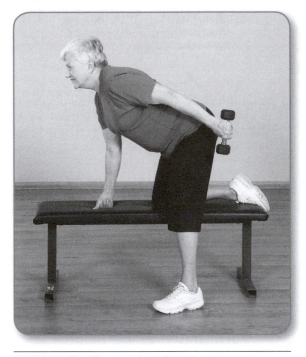

Figure 7.63   The triceps kickback using a dumbbell.

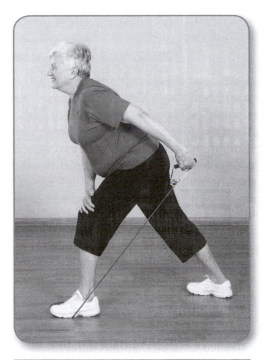

Figure 7.64   The triceps kickback performed by using rubber tubing for resistance.

▰ **Wrist Curl** ▰

Environment   This exercise can be performed in the gym or home.

Application   Although forearm exercises are often ignored in exercise programs for older clients, grip strength is an important single marker of independence in older persons. Given that the hands are the anatomical tools that link the body to the instruments used in most IADLs, it seems imprudent to ignore the muscles that control their performance. The wrist curl works the muscles that flex the wrist.

Position   Place the forearm on the edge of a bench or over the knee and grasp a dumbbell in your hand. Next allow the wrist to extend downward.

Execution   Curl the dumbbell up until the wrist is fully flexed (see figure 7.65). Hold the top position for a second, and then slowly lower the weight using only the wrist (not the arm).

Variations

- You can use a band or tubing to perform the wrist curl by securing one end of the device to the bench or stepping on the device to provide sufficient tension.

- The companion exercise to wrist flexion is wrist extension. When performing the wrist extension, the body position is the same as it is for wrist flexion except that the palm of the hand is now facing downward. This way the angle at the wrist must increase (extend) when the weight is lifted (see figure 7.66).

- One of the most recognizable training tools for working the forearm is the grip strength exerciser. This tool can range in structure from a simple compliant ball to a spring-type device. The exercise is simple to perform: Squeeze in and slowly release.

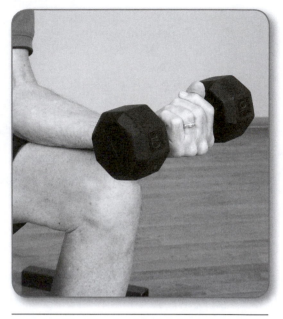

Figure 7.65   The dumbbell wrist curl.

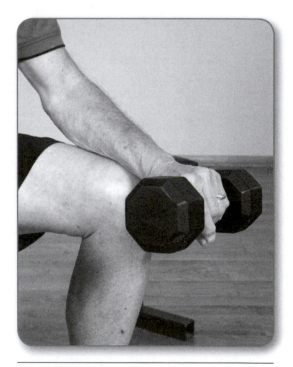

Figure 7.66   The dumbbell wrist extension.

CORE MUSCULATURE

Crunch

Environment   This exercise can be performed in the gym or home.

Application   Crunches are designed to target the rectus abdominis, the major muscle responsible for trunk flexion (sitting up). There is considerable information connecting strong abdominal muscles to improved back health.

Position   When performing the crunch on the floor, lie on your back with the knees bent and the feet flat. Place the arms across the chest.

Execution   Roll up, bringing the shoulder blades off the ground. Pause and then return to the starting position (see figure 7.67).

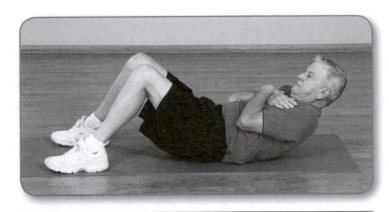

Figure 7.67   The crunch.

Variations

- When performing this exercise on a ball, the same technique applies; however, you must find a balance point (usually with the ball cradled in the lower back) before beginning. Then sit up, driving the buttocks into the ball while keeping the body as stable as possible.

- A further modification is the reverse crunch. Lie on your back on the floor. Place the arms across the chest, crossing them at the wrists. Keeping the knees bent, roll the knees toward the shoulders until the thighs form a right angle with the hips. Hold for a second then slowly lower the legs to the starting position. For greater stability, perform the exercise with your arms flat on the ground and adducted slightly, palms down.

- The side crunch is the last exercise in the crunch series (see figure 7.68). This exercise is most easily performed on a ball or bench. When on a ball, establish a good relationship between your center of gravity and base of support so that the ball can't slide or roll out from under you. Since the legs are extended, it may help to split them forward and backward to increase the

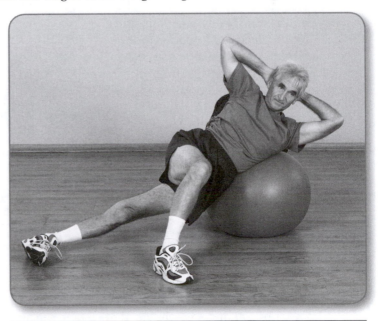

Figure 7.68   The side crunch performed on a stability ball.

size of your base of support. Place the hands behind the ears and extend the elbows out to the side. Then lift the top elbow toward the hip as far as possible while maintaining a stable position on the ball. Return to just past the starting position to create a slight stretch. To avoid using the ball or the rebound from the stretch to help perform the exercise, hesitate briefly at the bottom of the crunch before beginning a second repetition.

Safety Avoid locking the hands behind the neck and do not pull the head forward in an attempt to perform the exercise, as doing so may injure the cervical spine. Avoid bouncing up by using a ballistic movement of the back and buttocks to complete the movement, as this puts the low back at risk.

Side Plank

Environment This exercise can be performed in the gym or home.

Application The image of a wooden plank is a good visualization for this exercise. All planks are static exercises that engage the core while using the arms and legs as support. The side plank works the oblique, or side, muscles and the transverse abdominus, which is the deep band of muscles running across the abdominal area.

Position Lie on the floor on your side. Place the forearm and legs in a support position, but rest the majority of your weight on the hip. To increase your stability, place the forearm on the floor perpendicular to the body, and position the feet in front of and behind the body.

Execution Lift the hip off the floor and try to create a straight line from the head to the feet. Attempt to resemble the plank that gives this exercise its name (see figure 7.69).

Variations To increase the difficulty of the side plank, bring the feet closer together, straighten the upper arm to

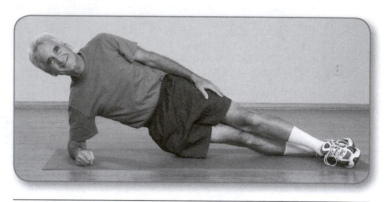

Figure 7.69 The side plank.

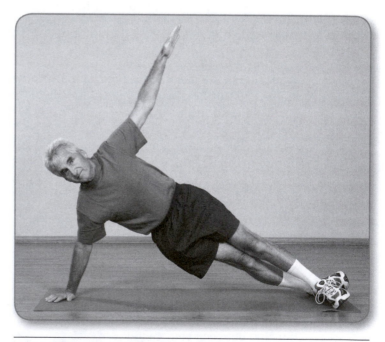

Figure 7.70 The side plank performed with the feet together and the arms extended.

raise your center of gravity, or use a straight arm for support (see figure 7.70). These variations all increase the need to engage the abdominal and back muscles to maintain stability. They can be employed separately or all at once.

Safety   Be careful not to progress to the advanced positions too quickly. The core muscles must have sufficient strength to stabilize the body and maintain balance. Loss of balance can lead to injury.

Bridge

Environment   This exercise can be performed in the gym or home.

Application   The bridge incorporates nearly all the core muscles. It uses dynamic rather than static contractions.

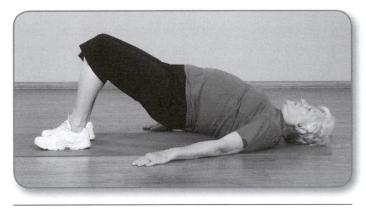

Position   Lie on the floor with the knees bent so that the feet are comfortably flat on the floor. The back should also feel comfortable against the floor.

Execution   Raise the hips so that the trunk is straight. Hold and then return to the starting position (see figure 7.71).

Figure 7.71   The bridge.

Safety   When you add this exercise to your core fitness routine, be sure to gradually progress to the fully extended position. Also, do not attempt to use a ballistic action to get into the final position.

Hip Rotator Exercise

Environment   This exercise can be performed in the gym or home.

Application   The hip rotator exercise targets the oblique muscles that are so important for transferring force from the hip to the shoulders. You use these muscles, for example, while reaching or moving an object from one counter or shelf to another with little or no movement of your feet.

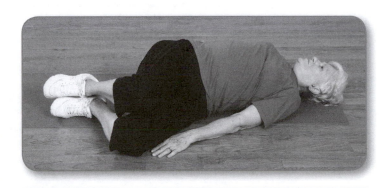

Position   To start the exercise, lie on your back with the knees bent.

Execution   While attempting to keep the shoulders on the floor, rotate the knees to one side and then back to the other side. Remember that this is not a simple stretch—rather, it's a

Figure 7.72   The hip rotator exercise.

movement performed by engaging the obliques. You can increase the resistance on this exercise by pushing against the top leg with your hand (see figure 7.72).

Safety   This exercise places considerable rotational stress on the low back. Be sure that you have enough flexibility to perform the exercise safely. Don't force the exercise beyond your comfortable ROM, and don't use ballistic movements to achieve a greater ROM.

Quadruped

Environment   This exercise can be performed in the gym or home.

Application   The quadruped exercise is named for our four-legged friends since it is performed on all fours. The idea behind the exercise is to apply different forces through the core by lifting different limbs to create different lines of force.

Position   To start this exercise, get down on your hands and knees (see figure 7.73*a*).

Execution   Once you are on your hands and knees, you can use numerous movements to overload the core musculature. The simplest is to lift one arm straight out. The next is to lift one leg straight out. The final pattern is to lift one arm and the opposite (contralateral) leg at the same time (see figure 7.73*b*). This position requires the highest level of core stability and core muscle activation.

Safety   The risk involved in this exercise is a loss of balance that can lead to a fall. When lifting the limbs, progress from low elevations to full elevations and remember that lifting the contralateral leg and arm together turns you into a human two-legged table. Be sure you're ready for it.

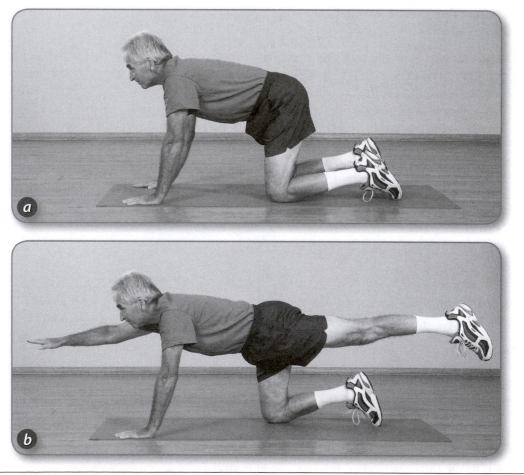

Figure 7.73   The quadruped exercise. *(a)* Starting position. *(b)* Ending position, with the opposing leg and arm lifted.

Superman

Environment   This exercise can be performed in the gym or home.

Application   Regardless of the name and the fact that this exercise is performed in a prone position, the superman requires only selective portions of the body to lose contact with the ground. The ability to fly is not a necessity.

Position   Lie facedown on the floor. Fully extend the arms and legs (see figure 7.74*a*).

Execution   Like the quadruped, the superman involves a number of options for working the core. You can raise one arm, one leg, the opposite arm and leg, both arms, both legs, or both arms and legs (see figure 7.74*b*).

Variation   To add difficulty, try performing the exercise on a stability ball (see figure 7.75).

Safety   While the superman is a wonderful exercise for the low back, remember that it can also put considerable stress on the low back. If you have low back problems or weakness, progress slowly until the back muscles can handle the stress.

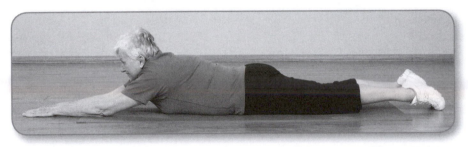

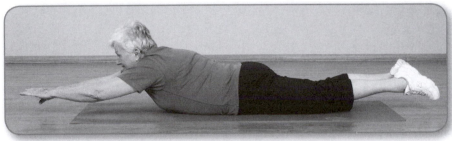

Figure 7.74   The superman. *(a)* The less challenging position. *(b)* The most challenging position is when both arms and legs are lifted.

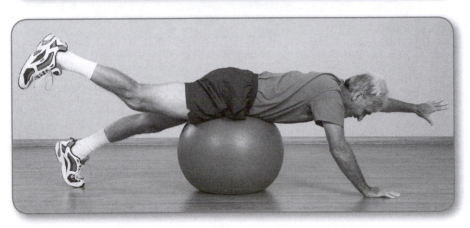

Figure 7.75   The superman performed on a stability ball.

SUMMARY

Resistance training is without a doubt one of the most important tools we have for addressing sarcopenia and the related loss in muscle strength, power, and endurance observed in older clients. Effective exercise prescriptions should use diagnostic tests to ensure that training brings muscle strength, power, and endurance to levels that are well beyond the critical thresholds necessary for minimal ADL performance (see figure 7.76). Doing this provides a buffer against future age-related declines and creates better efficiency and ease of performance during daily activities. Both research and practical application have demonstrated that proper cycling of training is necessary to maximize gains in power, strength, and endurance.

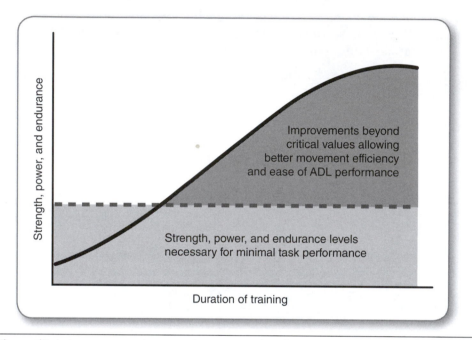

Figure 7.76 The goal is to increase muscle strength, power, and endurance beyond the critical levels needed for maintaining independence.

Topical Bibliography

Sarcopenia: What Makes It Happen?

Alshuaib, W.B., & Fahim, M.A. (1990). Effect of exercise on physiological age-related change at mouse neuromuscular junctions. *Neurobiol Aging* 11:555-561.

Aniansson, A., Grimby, G., Hedberg, M., & Krotkiewski, M. (1981). Muscle morphology, enzyme activity and muscle strength in elderly men and women. *Clinical Physiology* 1:73-86.

Baumgartner, R.N., Koehler, K.M., Gallagher, D., Romero, L., Heymsfield, S.B., Ross, R.R., Garry, P.J, & Lindeman, R.D. (1998). Epidemiology of sarcopenia among the elderly in New Mexico. *Am J Epidemiol* 147:755-763.

Baker, J.R., Bemben, M.G., Anderson, M.A., & Bemben, D.A. (2006). Effects of age on testosterone responses to resistance exercise and musculoskeletal variables in men. *J Strength Cond Res* 20:874-881.

Beccafico, S., Puglielli, C., Pietrangelo, T., Bellomo, R., Fano, G., & Fulle, S. (2007). Age-dependent effects on functional aspects in human satellite cells. *Ann N Y Acad Sci.* 1100:345-353.

Cai, D.Q., Li, M., Lee, K.K.H., Lee, K.M., Qin, L., & Chan, K.M. (2001). Parvalbumin expression is downregulated in rat fast-twitch skeletal muscles during aging. *Archives of Biochemistry and Biophysics* 387:202-208.

Cannon, J., Kay, D., Tarpenning, K.M., & Marino, F.E. (2007). Comparative effects of resistance training on peak isometric torque, muscle hypertrophy, voluntary activation and surface EMG between young and elderly women. *Clin Physiol Funct Imaging* 27:91-100.

Cardasis, C.A., & LaFontaine, D.M. (1987). Aging rat neuromuscular junctions: A morphometric study of cholinesterase-stained whole mounts and ultrastructure. *Muscle and Nerve* 10:200-213.

Delbono, O., Renganathan, M., & Messi, M. L. (1997). Excitation-Ca^{2+} release-contraction coupling in single aged human skeletal muscle fiber. *Muscle and Nerve* 5:S88S92.

Deschenes, M.R., Maresh, C.M., Crivello, J.F., Armstrong, L.E., Kraemer, W.J., & Covault, J. (1993). The effects of exercise training of different intensities on neuromuscular junction morphology. *Journal of Neurocytology* 22:603-615.

Doherty, T.J. (2003). Invited review: Aging and sarcopenia. *J Appl Physiol* 95:1717-1727.

Evans, W.J. (1997). Functional and metabolic consequences of sarcopenia. *J Nutr* 127:998S-1003S.

Fiatarone, M.A., O'Neill, E.F., Doyle-Ryan, N., Clements, K.M., Solares, G.R., Nelson, M.E., Roberts, S.B., Kehayias, J.J., Lipsitz, L.A., & Evans, W.J. (1994). Exercise training and nutritional supplementation for physical frailty in very elderly people. *New Eng J Med* 330:1769-1775.

Fiatarone, M.A., Marks, E.C., Ryan, N.D., Meredith, C.N., Lipsitz, L.A., & Evans, W.J. (1990). High intensity strength training in nonagenarians. *JAMA* 263:3029-3034.

Frontera, W.R., Hughes, V.A., Fielding, R.A., Fiatarone, M.A., Evans, W.J., & Roubenoff, R. (2000). Aging of skeletal muscle: A 12-yr longitudinal study. *J Appl Physiol* 88:1321-1326.

Frontera, W.R., Meredith, C.N., O'Reilly, K.P., Knuttgen, H.G., & Evans, W.J. (1988). Strength conditioning in older men: Skeletal muscle hypertrophy and improved function. *J Appl Physiol* 64:1038-1044.

Galvao, D.A., & Taaffe, D.R. (2005). Resistance training for the older adult: Manipulating training variables to enhance muscle strength. *Str Conditioning J* 27:48-54.

Herscovich, S., & Gershon, D. (1987). Effects of aging and physical training on the neuromuscular junction of the mouse. *Gerontology* 33:7-13.

Hikida, R.S., Staron, R.S., Hagerman, F.C., Walsh, S., Kaiser, E., Shell, S., & Hervey, S. (2000). Effects of high-intensity resistance training on untrained older men. II. Muscle fiber characteristics and nucleo-cytoplasmic relationships. *Journal of Gerontology: Biological Sciences* 55A: B347-B354.

Hinman, J.D., Peters, A., Cabral, H., Rosene, D.L., Hollander, W., Rasband, M.N., & Abraham, C.R. (2006). Age-related molecular reorganization at the node of Ranvier. *J Comp Neurol* 495:351-362.

Hunter, S.K., Thompson, M.W., Ruell, P.A., Harmer, A.R., Thom, J.M., Gwinn, T.H., & Adams, R.D. (1999). Human skeletal sarcoplasmic reticulum Ca + uptake and muscle function with aging and strength training. *Journal of Applied Physiology* 86:1858-1865.

Janssen, I., Heymsfield, S.B., Wang, Z., & Ross, R. (2000). Skeletal muscle mass and distribution in 468 men and women aged 18-88 yr. *Journal of Applied Physiology* 89:81-88.

Jejurikar, S.S., Henkelman, E.A., Cederna, P.S., Marcelo, C.L., Urbanchek, M.G., & Kuzon, Jr., W.M. (2006). Aging increases the susceptibility of skeletal muscle derived satellite cells to apoptosis. *Exp Gerontol* 41:828-836.

Kadi, F., Charifi, N., Denis, C., & Lexell, J. (2004). Satellite cells and myonuclei in young and elderly women and men. *Muscle Nerve* 29:120-127.

Kamen, G., & Knight, C.A. (2007). Training-related adaptations in motor unit discharge rate in young and older adults. *J Gerontol A Biol Sci Med Sci* 59:1334-1338.

Kenny, A.M., Dawson, L., Kleppingre, A., Iannuzzi-Sucich, M., & Judge, J.O. (2003). Prevalence of sarcopenia and predictors of skeletal muscle mass in nonobese women who are long-term users of estrogen-replacement therapy. *J Gerontol A Biol Sci Med Sci* 58:M436-M440.

Klitgaard, H., Ausoni, S., & Damiani, E. (1989). Sarcoplasmic reticulum of human skeletal muscle: Age-related changes and effect of training. *Acta Physiol Scand* 137:23-31.

Larsson, L. (1978). Morphological and functional characteristics of aging skeletal muscle in man. *Acta Physiol Scand* 457:S1-S36.

Latham, N.K., Bennett, D.A., Stretton, C.M., & Anderson, C.S. (2004). Systematic review of progressive resistance strength training in older adults. *J Gerontol A Biol Sci Med Sci* 59A: 48-61. Lexell, J. (1993). Aging and human muscle: Observations from Sweden. *Can J Appl Physiol* 18:2-18.

Lexell, J. (1997). Evidence for nervous system degeneration with advancing age. *J Nutr* 127:1011S-1013S.

Lexell, J., Taylor, C.C., & Sjostrom, M. (1988). What is the cause of the ageing atrophy? Total number, size and proportion of different fiber types studied in whole vastus lateralis muscle from 15- to 83-year-old men. *J Neurol Sci* 84:275-294.

Lexell, J. (1995). Human aging, muscle mass, and fiber type composition. *J Gerontol* 50A: 11-16.

Lexell, J., & Downham, D.Y. (1992). What is the effect of ageing on type II muscle fibers? *Neurolog.Sci* 107:250-251.

Lexell, J., Taylor, C.C., & Sjostrom, M. (1988). What is the cause of the ageing atrophy? *Journal of Neurological Sciences* 84:275-294.

Macaluso, A., & De Vito, G. (2004). Muscle strength, power and adaptations to resistance training in older people. *Eur J Appl Physiol* 91:450-472.

Mackey, A.L., Esmarck, B., Kadi, F., Koskinen, S.O., Kongsgaard, M., Sylvestersen, A., Hansen, J.J., Larsen, G., & Kjaer, M. (2007). Enhanced satellite cell proliferation with resistance training in elderly men and women. *Scand J Med Sci Sports* 17:34-42.

Nair, K.S. (2005). Aging muscle. *Am J Clin Nutr* 81:953-963.

Navarro, A., & Boveris, A. (2007). The mitochondrial energy transduction system and the aging process. *Am J Physiol Cell Physiol* 292:C670-C686.

O'Donnel, A., Travison, T., Harris, S., Tenover, L., & McKinlay, J. (2006). Testosterone, dehydroepiandrosterone, and physical performance in older men: Results from the Massachusetts Male Aging Study. *The Journal of Clinical Endocrinology and Metabolism* 91:425-431.

Patten, C., Kamen, G., & Rowland, D.M. (2001). Adaptations in maximal motor unit discharge rate to strength training in young and older adults. *Muscle Nerve* 24:542-550.

Plant, D.R., & Lynch, G.S. (2002). Excitation-contraction coupling and sarcoplasmic reticulum function in mechanically skinned fibres from fast skeletal muscles of aged mice. *Journal of Physiology* 543:169-176.

Rando, T.A. (2006). Stem cells, ageing and the quest for immortality. *Nature* 441:1080-1086.

Ribeiro, F., Mota, J., & Oliveira, J. (2007). Effect of exercise-induced fatigue on position sense of the knee in the elderly. *Eur J Appl Physiol* 99:379-385.

Staron, R.S., & Bumford, S.J. (1991). Correlation between myofibrillar ATPase activity and myosin heavy chain composition in single human muscle fibers. *Histochemistry* 96:21-24.

Thompson, L.V. (1994). Effects of age and training on skeletal muscle physiology and performance. *Physical Therapy* 74:71-81.

Toth, M.J., & Tchernof, A. (2006). Effect of age on skeletal muscle myofibrillar mRNA abundance: Relationship to myosin heavy chain protein synthesis rates. *Exp Gerontol* 41:1195-1200.

Trappe, S., Williamson, D., Godard, M., Porter, D., Rowden, G., & Costill, D. (2000). Effect of resistance training on single muscle fiber contractile function in older men. *Journal of Applied Physiology* 89:143-152.

Vandervoort, A.A. (2002). Aging of the human neuromuscular system. *Muscle Nerve* 25:17-25.

Vandervoot, A.A., & Symons, T.B. (2001). Functional and metabolic consequences of sarcopenia. *Can J Appl Physiol* 26:90-101.

Williams, G.N., Higgins, M.J., & Lewek, M.D. (2002). Aging skeletal muscle: Physiologic changes and the effects of training. *Phys Ther* 82:62-68.

Wilson, M.H., & Deschenes, M.R. (2005). The neuromuscular junction: Anatomical features and adaptations to various forms of increased, or decreased neuromuscular activity. *Intern J Neuroscience* 115:803-828.

Yamada, H., Masuda, T., & Okada, M. (2002). Age-related EMG variables during maximum voluntary contraction. *Percept Mot Skills* 95:10-14.

Effects of Resistance Training on the Causes of Sarcopenia

Abernethy, P.J., Jürimäe, J., Logan, P.A., Taylor, A.W., & Thayer, R.E. (1994). Acute and chronic response of skeletal muscle to resistance exercise. *Sports Med* 17:22-38.

Aniansson, A., Ljungberg, P., Rundgren, A., & Wetterqvist, H. (1984). Effect of a training programme for pensioners on condition and muscular strength. *Arch Gerontol Geriatr* 3:229-241.

Borst, S.E. (2004). Interventions for sarcopenia and muscle weakness in older people. *Age Ageing* 33:548-555.

Borst, S.E., De Hoyos, D.V., Garzarella, L., Vincent, K., Pollock, B.H., Lowenthal, D.T., & Pollack, M.L. (2001). Effects of resistance training on insulin-like growth factor-1 and IGF binding proteins. *Med Sci Sport Exerc* 33:648-653.

Coker, R.H., Hays, N.P., Williams, R.H., Brown, A.D., Freeling, S.A., Kortebein, P.M., Sullivan, D.H., Starling, R.D., & Evans, W.J. (2006). Exercise-induced changes in insulin action and glycogen metabolism in elderly adults. *Med Sci Sport Exerc* 38:433-438.

Craig, B.W., Brown, R., & Everhart, J. (1989). Effects of progressive resistance training on growth hormone and testosterone levels in young and elderly subjects. *Mechanisms of Ageing and Development* 49:159-169.

Fairey, A.S., Courneya, K.S., Field, C.J., Bell, G.J., Jones, L.W., & Mackey, J.R. (2003). Effects of exercise training on fasting insulin, insulin resistance, insulin-like growth factors, and insulin-like growth factor binding proteins in postmenopausal breast cancer survivors: A randomized controlled trial. *Cancer Epidemiol Biomarkers Prev* 12:721-727.

Fox, E., Bowers, R., & Foss, M. (1993). *The physiological basis for exercise and sport*. Madison, WI: Brown and Benchmark.

Häkkinen, K., Pakarinen, A., Kraemer, W.J., Häkkinen, A., Valkeinen, H., & Alen, M. (2001). Selective muscle hypertrophy, changes in EMG and force, and serum hormones during strength training in older women. *J Appl Physiol* 91:569-580.

Hameed, M., Lange, K.H., Andersen, J.L., Schjerling, P., Kjaer, M., Harridge, S.D., & Goldspink, G. (2004). The effect of recombinant human growth hormone and resistance training on IGF-I mRNA expression in the muscles of elderly men. *J Physiol* 555:231-240.

Jurimae, J., Abernethy, P.J., Blake, K., & McEniery, M.T. (1996). Changes in the myosin heavy chain isoform profile of the triceps brachii muscle following 12 weeks of resistance training. *Eur J Appl Physiol* 74:287-292.

Parkhouse, W.S., Coupland, D.C., Li, C., & Vanderhoek, K.J. (2000). IGF-1 bioavailability is increased by resistance training in older women with low bone mineral density. *Mech Ageing Dev* 113:75-83.

Reynolds IV, T.H., Supiano, M.A., & Dengel, D.R. (2004). Resistance training enhances insulin-mediated glucose disposal with minimal effect on the tumor necrosis factor-alpha system in older hypertensives. *Metabolism* 53:397-402.

Singh, M.A., Ding, W., Manfredi, T.J., Solares, G.S., O'Neill, E.F., Clements, K.M., Ryan, N.D., Kehayias, J.J., Fielding, R.A., & Evans, W.J. (1999). Insulin-like growth factor I in skeletal muscle after weight-lifting exercise in frail elders. *Am J Physiol* 277:E143.

Smilios, I., Pilianidis, T., Karamouzis, M., Parlavantzas, A., & Tokmakidis, S.P. (2006). Hormonal responses after a strength endurance resistance exercise protocol in young and elderly males. *Int J Sports Med* 28:401-406.

Staron, R.S., Malicky, E.S., Leonardi, M.J., Falkel, J.E., Hagerman, F.C., & Dudley, G.A. (1990). Muscle hypertrophy and fast fiber type conversions in heavy resistance-trained women. *Eur J Appl Physio Occup Physiol* 60:71-79.

Thorstensson, A., Hulten, B., von Dobeln, W., & Karlsson, J. (1976). Effect of strength training on enzyme activities and fibre characteristics in human skeletal muscle. *Acta Physiologica Scandinavia* 96:392-398.

Venojärvi, M., Puhke, R., Hämäläinen, H., Marniemi, J., Rastas, M., Rusko, H., Nuutila, P., Hänninen, O., & Aunola, S. (2005). Role of skeletal muscle-fibre type in regulation of glucose metabolism in middle-aged subjects with impaired glucose tolerance during a long-term exercise and dietary intervention. *Diabetes Obes Metab* 7:745-754.

Resistance Training to Reduce the Effects of Sarcopenia

Allen, T.J., & Proske, U. (2006). Effect of muscle fatigue on the sense of limb position and movement. *Exp Brain Res* 170:30-38.

Allman, B.L., & Rice, C.L. (2003). An age-related shift in the force-frequency relationship affects quadriceps fatigability in old adults. *J Appl Physiol* 96:1026-1032.

Allman, B.L., & Rice, C.L. (2002). Neuromuscular fatigue and aging: Central and peripheral factors. *Muscle and Nerve* 25:785-796.

Baechle, T.R., & Earle, R.W. (2008). *Essentials of strength training and conditioning, third edition*. Champaign, IL: Human Kinetics.

Bamman, M.M., Hill, V.J., Adams, G.R., Haddad, F., Wetzstein, C.J., Gower, B.A., Ahmed, A., & Hunter, G.R. (2003). Gender differences in resistance-training-induced myofiber hypertrophy among older adults. *Journal of Gerontology* 58A: 108-116.

Bassey, E.J., Fiatarone, M.A., O'Neill, E.F., Kelly, M., Evans, W.J., & Lipsitz, L.A. (1992). Leg extension power and functional performance in very old men and women. *Clinical Science* 82:321-327.

Bautmans, I., Gorus, E., Njemini, R., & Mets, T. (2007). Handgrip performance in relation to self-perceived fatigue, physical functioning and circulating IL-6 in elderly persons without inflammation. *BMC Geriatr* Mar 1;7:5.

Bazzucchi, I., Marchetti, M., Rosponi, A., Fattorini, L., Castellano, V., Sbriccoli, P., & Felici, F. (2005). Differences in the force/endurance relationship between young and older men. *Eur J Appl Physiol* 93:390-397.

Bean, J.F., Kiely, D.K., Herman, S., Leveille, S.G., Mizer, K., Frontera, W.R., & Fielding, R.A. (2002). The relationship between leg power and physical performance in mobility-limited older people. *Journal of American Geriatric Society* 50:461-467.

Behm, D.G., & Sale, D.G. (1993). Intended rather than actual movement velocity determines velocity-specific training response. *J Appl Physiol* 74:359-368.

Bellew, J.W., Yates, J.W., & Gater, D.R. (2003). The initial effects of low-volume strength training on balance in untrained older men and women. *J Strength Cond Res* 17:121-128.

Bellew, J.W., & Fenter, P.C. (2006). Control of balance differs after knee or ankle fatigue in older women. *Arch Phys Med Rehabil* 87:1486-1489.

Bonnefoy, M., Kostka, T., Arsac, L.M., Berthouze, S.E., & Lacour, J. (1998). Peak anaerobic power in elderly men. *Eur J Appl Physiol* 77:182-188.

Buchner, D., Larson, E.B., Wagner, E.H., Koepsell, T.D., & deLateur, B.J. (1996). Evidence for a non-linear relationship between leg strength and gait speed. *Age and Ageing* 25:386-391.

Carmel, M.P., Czaja, S., Morgan, R.O., Asfour, S., Khalil, T., & Signorile, J.F. (2000). The effects of varying training speed on changes in functional performance in older women. *The Physiologist* 43(4): 321.

Carpinelli, R.N., & Otto, R.M. (1998). Strength training. Single versus multiple sets. *Sports Med* 26:73-84.

Caserotti, P., Aagaard, P., Simonsen, E.B., & Puggaard, L. (2001). Contraction-specific differences in maximal muscle power during stretch-shortening cycle in elderly males and females. *Eur J Appl Physiol* 84:206-212.

Campos, G.E., Luecke, T.J., Wendeln, H.K., Toma, K., Hagerman F.C., Murray, T.F., Ragg, K.E., Ratamess, N.A., Krarmer, W.J., & Staron, R.S. (2002). Muscular adaptations in response to three different resistance-training regimens: Specificity of repetition maximum training zones. *Eur J Appl Physiol* 88:50-60.

Charette, S.L., McEvoy, L., Pyka, G., Snow-Harter, C., Guido, D., Wisell, P.A., & Marcus, R. (1991). Muscle hypertrophy response to resistance training in older women. *J Appl Physiol* 70:1912-1916.

Cheng, A., Ditor, D.S., & Hicks, A.L. (2003). A comparison of adductor pollicis fatigue in older men and women. *Can J Physiol Pharmacol* 81:873-879.

Cuoco, A., Callahan, D.M., Sayers, S., Frontera, W.R., Bean, J., & Fielding, R.A. (2004). Impact of muscle power and force on gait speed in disabled older men and women. *Journal of Gerontology* 59A: 1200-1206.

Curb, J.D., Ceria-Ulep, C.D., Rodriguez, B.L., Grove, J., Guralnik, J., Willcox, B.J., Donlon, T.A., Masaki, K.H., & Chen, R. (2006). Performance-based measures of physical function for high-function populations. *J Am Geriatr Soc* 54:737-742.

Clarkson, P.M., & Dedrick, M.E. (1988). Exercise-induced muscle damage, repair, and adaptation in old and young subjects. *J Gerontol* 43:M91-M96.

Cress, M.E., Buchner, D.M., Questad, K.A., Esselman, P.C., deLateur, B.J., & Schwartz, R.S. (1996). Continuous-scale physical functional performance in healthy older adults: A validation study. *Archives of Physical Medicine and Rehabilitation* 77:1243-1250.

Daubney, M.E., & Culham, E.G. (1999). Lower-extremity muscle force and balance performance in adults aged 65 years and older. *Phys Ther* 79:1177-1185.

De Vito, G., Bernardi, M., Forte, R., Pulejo, C., Macaluso, A., & Figura, F. (1998). Determinants of maximal instantaneous muscle power in women aged 50-75 years. *Eur J Appl Physiol Occup Physiol* 78:59-64.

de Vos, N.J., Singh, N.A., Ross, D.A., Stavrinos, T.M., Orr, R., & Singh, M.A.F. (2005). Optimal load for increasing muscle power during explosive resistance training in older adults. *Journal of Gerontology* 60A: 638-647.

de Vreede, P.L., Samson, M.M., van Meeteren, N.L., Duursma, S.A., & Verhaar, H.J. (2005). Functional-task exercise versus resistance strength exercise to improve daily function in older women: A randomized, controlled trial. *J Am Geriatr Soc* 53:2-10.

de Vreede, P.L., Samson, M.M., van Meeteren, N.L., van der Bom, J.G., Duursma, S.A., & Verhaar, H.J. (2004). Functional tasks exercise versus resistance exercise to improve daily function in older women: A feasibility study. *Arch Phys Med Rehabil* 85:1952-1961.

Earles, D.R., Judge, J.O., & Gunnarsson, O.T. (2000). Velocity training induces power-specific adaptations in highly functioning older adults. *Archives of Physical Medicine and Rehabilitation* 82:872-878.

Ferretti, G., Narici, M.V., Binzoni, T., Gariod, L., LeBas, J.F., Reutenauer, H., & Cerretelli, P. (1994). Determinants of peak muscle power: Effects of age and physical conditioning. *Eur J Appl Physiol* 68 :111-115.

Ferri, A., Narici, M., Grassi, B., & Pousson, M. (2006). Neuromuscular recovery after a strength training session in elderly people. *Eur J Appl Physiol* 97:272-279.

Fielding, R.A., LeBrasseur, N.K., Cuoco, A., Bean, J., Mizer, K., & Fiatarone Singh, M.A. (2002). High-velocity resistance training increases skeletal muscle peak power in older women. *J Am Geriatr Soc* 50:555-662.

Fleck, S.J., & Kraemer, W.J. (1997). *Designing resistance training programs.* Champaign, IL: Human Kinetics.

Flipse, D., Signorile, J.F., Wills, R., Perry, A., Lowensteyn, I., Caruso, J., Robertson, B., & Burnett, K. (1993). Increased muscular performance in the elderly with moderate speed isotonic training. *Med Sci Sport Exerc* 25:S130.

Foldvari, M., Clark, M., Iaviolette, L.C., Bernstein, M.A., Kaliton, D., Castaneda, C., Pu, C.T., Hausdorff, J.M., Fielding, R.A., & Fiatarone, M.A. (2000). Association of muscle power with functional status in community-dwelling elderly women. *J Gerontol A Biol Sci Med Sci* 55A: M192-M199.

Fry, R., Morton, A., & Keast, D. (1992). Periodisation and prevention of overtraining. *Canadian J Spt Sci* 17:241-248.

Galvao, D.A., & Taaffe, D.R. (2004). Single- vs multiple-set resistance training: Recent developments in the controversy. *J Str Cond Res* 18:660-667.

Gefen, A. (2001). Simulations of foot stability during gait characteristic of ankle dorsiflexor weakness in the elderly. *IEEE Trans Neural Syst Rehabil Eng* 9:333-337.

Gehlsen, G.M., & Whaley, M.H. (1990). Falls in the elderly: Part II. Balance, strength, and flexibility. *Archives of Physical Medicine and Rehabilitation* 71:739-741.

Givoni, N.J., Pham, T., Allen, T.J., & Proske, U. (2007). The effect of quadriceps muscle fatigue on position matching at the knee. *J Physiol* 584:111-119.

Gorelick, M., Brown, J.M., & Groeller, H. (2003). Short-duration fatigue alters neuromuscular coordination of trunk musculature: Implications for injury. *Appl Ergon* 34:317-325.

Gribble, P.A., & Hertel, J. (2004). Effect of hip and ankle muscle fatigue on unipedal postural control. *J Electromyogr Kinesiol* 14:641-646.

Gribble, P.A., & Hertel, J. (2004). Effect of lower-extremity muscle fatigue on postural control. *Arch Phys Med Rehabil* 85:589-592.

Hahn, M.E., Lee, H.J., & Chou, L.S. (2005). Increased muscular challenge in older adults during obstructed gait. *Gait Posture* 22:356-361.

Häkkinen, K., & Komi, P.V. (1985). The effect of explosive type strength training on electromyographic and force production characteristics of leg extensor muscles during concentric and various stretch shortening cycle exercises. *Scandanavian Journal of Sports Science* 7:65-76.

Hakkinen, K., Kraemer, W.J., Pakarinen, A., Triplett-McBride, N.T., McBride, J.M., Hakkinen, A., Alen, M., McGuigan, M.R., Bronks, R., & Newton, R.U. (2002). Effects of heavy resistance/power training on maximal muscle strength, muscle morphology, and hormonal response patterns in 60-75-year-old men and women. *Can J Appl Physiol* 27:213-231.

Henwood, T.R., & Taaffe, D.R. (2005). Improved physical performance in older adults undertaking a short-term programme of high-velocity resistance training. *Gerontology* 51:108-115.

Hortobagyi, T., Mizelle, C., Beam, S., & DeVita, P. (2003). Older adults perform activities of daily living near their maximal capacities. *J Gerontol A Biol Sci Med Sci* 58:M453-M460.

Hunter, G.R., Treuth, M.S., Weinsier, R.L., Kekes-Szabo, T., Kell, S.H., Roth, D.L., & Nichilson, C. (1995). The effects of strength conditioning on older women's ability to perform daily tasks. *Journal of the American Geriatrics Society* 43:756-760.

Hunter, G.R., Wetzstein, C.J., McLafferty, C.L., Zuckerman, P.A., Landers, K.A., & Bamman, M.M. (2001). High-resistance versus variable-resistance training in older adults. *Med Sci Sport Exerc* 33:1759-1764.

Hunter, S.K., Critchlow, A., & Enoka, R.M. (2004). Influence of aging on sex differences in muscle fatigability. *J Appl Physiol* 97:1723-1732.

Jankelowitz, S.K., McNulty, P.A., & Burke, D. (2007). Changes in measures of motor axon excitability with age. *Clin Neurophysiol* 118:1397-1404.

Jozsi, A.C., Campbell, W.W., Joseph, L., Davey, S.L., & Evans, W.J. (1999). Changes in power with resistance training in older and younger men and women. *J Gerontol A Biol Sci Med Sci* 54A: M591-M596.

Judge, J.O., Schechtman, K.B., & Cress, E. (1996). The relationship between physical performance measures and independence in instrumental activities of daily living. *JAGS* 44:1332-1341.

Kaczor, J.J., Ziolkowski, W., Antosiewicz, J., Hac, S., Tarnopolsky, M.A., & Popinigis, J. (2006). The effect of aging on anaerobic and aerobic enzyme activities in human skeletal muscle. *J Gerontol A Biol Sci Med Sci* 61:339-344.

Keogh, J.W., Morrison, S., & Barrett, R. (2007). Strength training improves the tri-digit finger-pinch force control of older adults. *Arch Phys Med Rehabil* 88:1055-1063.

Komi, P.V., Karlsson, J., Tesch, P.A., Suominen, H., & Heikkinen, E. (1982). Effects of heavy resistance and explosive type strength training on mechanical, functional, and metabolic aspects of performance. In P.V. Komi (Ed.), *Exercise and sports biology* (pp. 90-102). Champaign, IL: Human Kinetics.

Lamb, S.E., Morse, R.E., & Evans, J.G. (1995). Mobility after proximal femoral fracture: The relevance of leg extensor power, postural sway and other factors. *Age and Ageing* 24:308-314.

Landers, K.A., Hunter, G.R., Wetzstein, C.J., Bamman, M.M., & Weinsier, R.L. (2001). The interrelationship among muscle mass, strength, and the ability to perform physical tasks of daily living in younger and older women. *J Gerontol A Biol Sci Med Sci* 56:B443-B448.

Landgraff, N.C., Whitney, S.L., Rubinstein, E.N., & Yonas, H. (2006). Use of the physical performance test to assess preclinical disability in subjects with asymptomatic carotid artery disease. *Phys Ther* 86:541-548.

Lexell, J., Downham, D.Y., Larsson, Y., Bruhn, E., & Morsing, B. (1995). Heavy-resistance training in older Scandinavian men and women: Short- and long-term effects on arm and leg muscles. *Scand J Med Sci Sports* 5:329-341.

Lord, S.R., Ward, J.A., Williams, P., & Anstey, K.J. (1994). Physiological factors associated with falls in older community-dwelling women. *J Am Geriatr Soc* 42:1110-1117.

Lindstrom, B., Lexell, J., Gerdle, B., & Downham, D. (1997). Skeletal muscle fatigue and endurance in young and old men and women. *J Gerontol A Biol Sci Med Sci* 52A: B59-B66.

Lord, S.R., & Webster, I.W. (1990). Visual field dependence in elderly fallers and non-fallers. *Int J Aging Human Development* 31:267-277.

Lord, S.R., McLean, D., & Stathers, G. (1992). Physiological factors associated with injurious falls in older people living in the community. *Gerontology* 38:338-346.

Marigold, D.S., Eng, J.J., & Timothy Inglis, J. (2004). Modulation of ankle postural reflexes in stroke: Influence of weight-bearing load. *Clin Neurophysiol* 115:2789-2797.

McCarthy, E.K., Horvat, M.A., Holtsberg, P.A., & Wisenbaker, J.M. (2004). Repeated chair stands as a measure of lower limb strength in sexagenarian women. *J Gerontol A Biol Sci Med Sci* 59:1207-1212.

McCartney, N., Hicks, A.L., Martin, J., & Webber, C.E. (1995). Long-term resistance training in the elderly: Effects of dynamic strength, exercise capacity, muscle, and bone. *J Gerontol* 50A: B97-B104.

McCartney, N., Hicks, A.L., Martin, J., & Webber, C.E. (1995). Long-term resistance training in the elderly: Effects on dynamic strength, exercise capacity, muscle, and bone. *Journal of Gerontology* 50A: B97-B104.

McNeil, C.J., & Rice, C.L. (2007). Fatigability is increased with age during velocity-dependent contractions of the dorsiflexors. *J Gerontol A Biol Sci Med Sci* 62:624-629.

Metter, E.J., Conwit, R., Metter, B., Pacheco, T., & Tobin, J. (1998). The relationship of peripheral motor nerve conduction velocity to age-associated loss of grip strength. *Aging (Milano)* 10:471-478.

Miszko, T.A., & Cress, M.E. (2002).The effect of strength and power training on physical function in independent community-dwelling older adults. *Med Sci Sport Exerc* 34(5): S250.

Miszko, T.A., Cress, M.E., Slade, J.M., Convey, C.J., Agrawal, S.K., & Doerr, C.E. (2003). Effect of strength and power training on physical function in community-dwelling older adults. *Journal of Gerontology: Medical Sciences* 58A: 171-175.

Morganti, C.M., Nelson, M.E., Fiatarone, M.A., Dallal, G.E., Economos, C.D., Crawford, B.M., & Evans, W.J. (1995). Strength improvements with 1 yr of progressive resistance training in older women. *Med Sci Sport Exerc* 26:906-912.

Nelson, M.E., Fiatarone, M.A., Morganti, C.M., Trice, I., Greenberg, R.A., & Evans, W.J. (1994). Effects of high-intensity strength training on multiple risk factors for osteoporotic fractures. *JAMA* 272:1909-1914.

Orr, R., de Vos, N.J., Singh, N.A., Ross, D.A., Stavrinos, T.M., & Fiaterone-Singh, M.A. (2006). Power training improves balance in healthy older adults. *J Gerontol A Biol Sci Med Sci* 61:78-85.

Paasuke, M., Ereline, J., & Gapeyeva, H. (1999). Neuromuscular fatigue during repeated exhaustive submaximal static contractions of knee extensor muscles in endurance-trained, power-trained and untrained men. *Acta Physiol Scand* 166:319-326.

Petrella, J.K., Kim, J., Tuggle, S.C., Hall, S.R., & Bamman, M.M. (2005). Age differences in knee extension power, contractile velocity, and fatigability. *J Appl Physiol* 98:211-220.

Petrella, J.K., Kim, J., Tuggle, S.C., Hall, S.R., & Bamman, M.M. (2005). Age differences in knee extension power, contractile velocity, and fatigability. *Journal of Applied Physiology* 98(1):211-20

Petrella, J.K., Kim, J.S., Tuggle, S.C., & Bamman, M.M. (2007). Contributions of force and velocity to improved power with progressive resistance training in young and older adults. *Eur J Appl Physiol* 99:343-351.

Phillips, W.T., Benton, M.J., Wagner, C.L., & Riley, C. (2006). The effect of single set resistance training on strength and functional fitness in pulmonary rehabilitation patients. *J Cardiopulm Rehabil* 26:330-337.

Pruitt, L.A., Taaffe, D.R., & Marcus, R. (1995). Effects of a one-year high-intensity versus low-intensity resistance training program on bone mineral density in older women. *Journal of Bone and Mineral Research* 10:1788-1795.

Purser, J.L., Kuchibhatla, M.N., Fillenbaum, G.G., Harding, T., Peterson, E.D., & Alexander, K.P. (2006). Identifying frailty in hospitalized older adults with significant coronary artery disease. *J Am Geriatr Soc* 54:1678-1681.

Pyka, G., Taaffe, D.R., & Marcus, R. (1994). Effect of a sustained program of resistance training on the acute growth hormone response to resistance exercise in older adults. *Horm Metab Res* 26:330-333.

Rantanen, T., Guralnik, J.M., Izmirlian, G., Williamson, J.D., Simonsick, E.M., Ferrucci, L., & Fried, L.P. (1998). Association of muscle strength with maximum walking speed in disabled older women. *American Journal of Physical Medicine and Rehabilitation* 77:299-305.

Rhea, M.R., Alvar, B.A., & Burkett, L.N. (2002). Single versus multiple sets for strength: A meta-analysis to address the controversy. *Res Quar Exerc Sport* 73:485-488.

Rhea, M.R., Ball, S.D., Phillips, W., & Burkett, L. (2002). A comparison of linear and daily undulating periodized programs with equated volume and intensity for strength. *Journal of Strength and Conditioning Research* 16:250-255.

Rhea, M.R., Alvar, B.A., Burkett, L.N., & Ball, S.D. (2003). A meta-analysis to determine the dose response for strength development. *Med Sci Sport Exerc* 35:456-464.

Salavati, M., Moghadam, M., Ebrahimi, I., & Arab, A.M. (2007). Changes in postural stability with fatigue of lower extremity frontal and sagittal plane movers. *Gait Posture* 26:214-218.

Sayers, S.P., Bean, J., Cuoco, A., LeBrasseur, N., Jette, A., & Fielding, R.A. (2003). Changes in function and disability after resistance training:

Does velocity matter? *Am J Phys Med Rehabil* 82:605-613.

Sayers, S.P., Guralnik, J.M., Newman, A.B., Brach, J.S., & Fielding, R.A. (2006). Concordance and discordance between two measures of lower extremity function: 400 meter self-paced walk and SPPB. *Aging Clin Exp Res* 18:100-106.

Sayers, S.P. (2007). High-speed power training: A novel approach to resistance training in older men and women: A brief review and pilot study. *J Strength Cond Res* 21:518-526.

Schwendner, K.I., Mikeshy, A.E., Holt, W.S., Peacock, M., & Burr, D.B. (1997). Differences in muscle endurance and recovery between fallers and non-fallers, and between young and older women. *Journal of Gerontology: Medical Sciences* 52:M155-M160.

Seghers, J., Spaepen, A., Delecluse, C., & Colman, V. (2003). Habitual level of physical activity and muscle fatigue of the elbow flexor muscles in older men. *European Journal of Applied Physiology* 89:427-434.

Signorile, J.F., Sochet, L., Morgenstern, A., Caruso, J., Puhl, J., O'Keefe, S., & Perry, A. (1995). The superiority of high speed resistance training in an older population. *Med Sci Sport Exerc* 27:S233.

Signorile, J.F., Suidmak, P., Campbell, M.H., Miller, P., & Puhl, J. (1995). High speed training produces superior strength and functional capacity in an older population. *The Gerontologist* 35:91.

Signorile, J.F., Carmel, M.P., Czaja, S., Asfour, S., Morgan, R.O., Khalil, T., Ma, F., & Roos, B. (2002). Differential increases in average isokinetic power by specific muscle groups of older women due to variations in training and testing. *J Gerontol: Medical Science* 57A: M683-M690.

Signorile, J.F., Carmel, M.P., Lai, S., & Roos, B.A. (2005). Early plateaus of power and torque gains during high- and low-speed training in older women. *J Appl Physiol* 98:1213-1220.

Signorile, J.F., & Sandler, D. (2007). *Weight training everyone* (5th ed.). Winston-Salem, NC: Hunter Textbooks

Simons, R., & Andel, R. (2006). The effects of resistance training and walking on functional fitness in advanced old age. *J Aging Health* 18:91-105.

Skelton, D.A., Greig, C.A., Davies, J.M., & Young, A. (1994). Strength, power and related functional ability of healthy people aged 65-89 years. *Age and Ageing* 23:371-377.

Skelton, D.A., Kennedy, J., & Rutherford, O.M. (2002). Explosive power and asymmetry in leg muscle function in frequent fallers and non-fallers aged over 65. *Age and Ageing* 31:119-125.

Skelton, D.A., & Beyer, N. (2003). Exercise and injury prevention in older people. *Scandinavian Journal of Medicine and Science in Sports* 13:77-85.

Sonn, U., Frandin, K., & Grimby, G. (1995). Instrumental activities of daily living related to impairments and functional limitations in 70-year-olds and changes between 70 and 76 years of age. *Scandinavian Journal of Rehabilitative Medicine* 27:119-128.

Taaffe, D.R., Duret, C., Wheeler, S., & Marcus, R. (1999). Once-weekly resistance exercise improves muscle strength and neuromuscular performance in older adults. *J Am Geriatr Soc* 47:1208-1214.

Taaffe, D.R., Pruitt, L., Pyka, G., Guido, D., & Marcus, R. (1996). Comparative effects of high- and low-intensity resistance training on thigh muscle strength, fiber area, and tissue composition in elderly women. *Clinical Physiology* 16:381-392.

Tiedemann, A., Sherrington, C., & Lord, S.R. (2005). Physiological and psychological predictors of walking speed in older community-dwelling people. *Gerontology* 51:390-395.

Tomonaga, M. (1977). Histochemical and ultra-structural changes in senile human skeletal muscle. *Journal of the American Geriatrics Society* 25:125-131.

Van't Hul, A., Harlaar, J., Gosselink, R., Hollander, P., Postmus, P., & Kwakkel, G. (2004). Quadriceps muscle endurance in patients with chronic obstructive pulmonary disease. *Muscle Nerve* 29:267-274.

Vincent, K.R., Braith, R.W., Feldman, R.A., Magyari, P.M., Cutler, R.B., Persin, S.A., Lennon, S.L., Gabr, A.H., & Lowenthal, D.T. (2002). Resistance exercise and physical performance in adults aged 60 to 83. *J Am Geriatr Soc* 50:1100-1107.

Vincent, K.R., Vincent, H.K., Braith, R.W., Bratnagar, V., & Lowenthal, D.T. (2003). Strength training and hemodynamic responses to exercise. *Am J Geriatr Cardiol* 12:97-106.

Whipple, R.K., Wolfson, M.D., & Amerman, P.M. (1987). The relationship of knee and ankle weakness to falls in nursing home residents: An isokinetic study. *Journal of the American Geriatrics Society* 35:13-20.

Wickham, C., Cooper, C., Margetts, B.M., & Barker, D.J. (1989). Muscle strength, activity, housing and the risk of falls in elderly people. *Age and Ageing* 18:47-51.

Wolfson, L., Judge, J., Whipple, R., & King, M. (1995). Strength is a major factor in balance, gait, and the occurrence of falls. *Journal of Gerontology: Medical Sciences* 50:64-67.

Young, A., & Skelton, A. (1994). Applied physiology of strength and power in old age. *International Journal of Sports Medicine* 15:107-162.

Testing Neuromuscular Performance

Agarwal, S., & Kiely, P.D. (2006). Two simple, reliable and valid tests of proximal muscle function, and their application to the management of idiopathic inflammatory myositis. *Rheumat (Oxford)* 45:874-879.

Alexander, N.B., & Goldberg, A. (2006). Clinical gait and stepping performance measures in older adults. *Eur Rev Aging Phys Act* 3:20-28.

Costa, G., Miller, J., Wygand, J.W., Otto, R., & Perez, H.R. (1987). A modification of the Margaria-Kalamen power test. *Med Sci Sport Exerc* 19:574.

Cuoco, A., Callahan, D.M., Sayers, S., Frontera, W.R., Bean, J., & Fielding, R.A. (2004). Impact of muscle power and force on gait speed in disabled older men and women. *Journal of Gerontology* 59A: 1200-1206.

Csuka, M., & McCarty, D.J. (1985). Simple method of measuring lower extremity muscle strength. *Am J Med* 78:77-81.

De Vito, G., Bernardi, M., Forte, R., Pulejo, C., Macaluso, A., & Figura, F. (1998). Determinants of maximal instantaneous muscle power in women aged 50-75 years. *Eur J Appl Physiol Occup Physiol* 78:59-64.

Despres, J.P., Couillard, C., Gagnon, J., Bergeron, J., Leon, A.S., Rao, D.C., Skinner, J.S., Wilmore, J.H., & Bouchard, C. (2000). Race, visceral adipose tissue, plasma lipids, and lipoprotein lipase activity in men and women: The Health, Risk Factors, Exercise Training, and Genetics (HERITAGE) family study. *Arterioscler Thromb Vasc Biol* 20:1932-1938.

Després, J.P., & Lemieux, I. (2006). Abdominal obesity and metabolic syndrome. *Nature* 444:881-887.

Duncan, P.W., Weiner, D.K., Chandler, J., & Studenski, S. (1990). Functional reach: A new clinical measure of balance. *J Gerontol A Biol Sci Med Sci* 45:M192-M197.

Dusenberry, D.O. (2006). Evaluation of grasp-ability of handrails during falls on stairs. www. sgh.com/pdf/Effect-of-Handrail-Shape-on-Graspability.pdf

Eriksrud, O., & Bohannon, R.W. (2003). Relationship of knee extension force to independence in sit-to-stand performance in patients receiving acute rehabilitation. *Phys Ther* 83:544-551.

Feland, J.B., Hager, R., & Merrill, R.M. (2005). Sit to stand transfer: Performance in rising power, transfer time and sway by age and sex in senior athletes. *Br J Sports Med* 39:e39.

Guralnik, J.M., Simonsick, E.M., Ferrucci, L., Glynn, R.J., Berkman, L.F., Blazer, D.G., Scherr, P.A., & Wallace, R.B. (1994). A short physical performance battery assessing lower extremity function: Association with self-reported disability and prediction of mortality and nursing home admission. *J Gerontol* 49:M85-M94.

Helbostad, J.L., & Moe-Nilssen, R. (2003). The effect of gait speed on lateral balance control during walking in healthy elderly. *Gait and Posture* 18:27-36.

Hoeymans, N., Wouters, E.R.C.M., Feskens, E.J.M., van den Bos, G.A.M., & Kromhout, D. (1997). Reproducibility of performance-based and self-reported measures of functional status. *Journal of Gerontology* 52A: M363-M368.

Huskey, T., Mayhew, J.L., Ball, T.E., & Arnold, M.D. (1989). Factors affecting anaerobic power output in the Margaria-Kalamen test. *Ergonomics* 32:959-965.

Jones, C.J., Rikli, R.E., Max, J., & Noffal, G. (1998). The reliability and validity of a chair sit-and-reach test as a measure of hamstring flexibility in older adults. *Res Quar Exerc Sport* 69:338-344.

Jones, C.J., Rikli, R.E., & Beam, W.C. (1999). A 30-s chair-stand test as a measure of lower body strength in community-residing older adults. *Research Quarterly for Exercise and Sport* 70:113-117.

Judge, J.O., Schechtman, K.B., & Cress, E. (1996). The relationship between physical perfromance measures and independence in instrumental activities of daily living. *JAGS* 44:1332-1341.

Kalamen, J.L. (1968). *Measurement of maximum muscular power in man*. Ph.D. Ohio State University.

Kozak, K., Ashton-Miller, J.A., & Alexander, N.B. (2003). The effect of age and movement speed on maximum forward reach from an elevated surface: A study in healthy women. *Clinical Biomechanics* 18:190-196.

Lindemann, U., Claus, H., Stuber, M., Augat, P., Muche, R., Nikolaus, T., & Becker, C. (2003). Measuring power during the sit-to-stand transfer. *Eur J Appl Physiol* 89:466-470.

Lindemann, U., Najafi, B., Zijlstra, W., Hauer, K., Muche, R., Becker, C., & Aminian, K. (2008). Distance to achieve steady state walking speed in frail elderly persons. *Gait and Posture* 27(1):91-6.

Margaria, R., Aghemo, P., & Rovelli, E. (1966). Measurement of muscular power in man. *Journal of Applied Physiology* 21:1662-1664.

Mayhew, J.L., Hampton, B.K., & Armstrong, W. (1981). Task specificity among power tests in college males. *Kansas AAHPERD Journal* 49:5-7.

Metter, E.J., Talbot, L.A., Schrager, M., & Conwit, R.A. (2004). Arm-cranking muscle power and arm isometric muscle strength are independent predictors of all-cause mortality in men. *J Appl Physiol* 96:814-821.

Nagurney, J.T., Borczuk, P., & Thomas, S.H. (1998). Elderly patients with closed head trauma after a fall: Mechanisms and outcomes. *J Emerg Med* 16:709-713.

Netz, J., Ayalon, M., Dunsky, A., & Alexander, N. (2004). 'The multiple-sit-to-stand' field test for older adults: What does it measure? *Gerontology* 50:121-126.

Nevitt, M.C., Cummings, S.R., Kidd, S., & Black, D. (1989). Risk factors for recurrent nonsyncopal falls: A prospective study. *Journal of the American Medical Association* 261:2663-2668.

Rantanen, T., & Avela, J. (1997). Leg extension power and walking speed in very old people living independently. *Journal of Gerontology: Medical Sciences* 52:M225-M231.

Rikli, R.E., & Jones, C.J. (1999). Development and validation of a functional fitness test for community-residing older adults. *Journal of Aging and Physical Activity* 7:129-161.

Rikli, R.E., & Jones, C.J. (1999). Functional fitness normative scores for community residing older adults, ages 60-94. *Journal of Aging and Physical Activity* 7:162-181.

Rolland, Y.M., Cesari, M., Miller, M.E., Penninx, B.W., Atkinson, H.H., & Pahor, M. (2004). Reliability of the 400-m usual walk test as an assessment of mobility limitation in older adults. *J Am Geriatr Soc* 52:972-976.

Schwegler, T.M., Mayhew, J.L., & Piper, F.C. (1985). Effects of acceleration momentum on anaerobic power measurements. *Carnegie Research Papers* 1:23-26.

Schwendner, K.I., Mikeshy, A.E., Holt, W.S., Peacock, M., & Burr, D.B. (1997). Differences in muscle endurance and recovery between fallers and non-fallers, and between young and older women. *Journal of Gerontology: Medical Sciences* 52:M155-M160.

Seeman, T.E., Charpentier, P.A., Berkman, L.F., Tinetti, M.E., Guralnik, J.M., Albert, M., Blazer, D., & Rowe, J.W. (1994). Predicting changes in physical performance in a high-functioning elderly cohort: MacArthur studies of successful aging. *Journal of Gerontology: Medical Sciences* 49:M97-M108.

Signorile, J.F. (2007). Simple equations to predict concentric lower-body muscle power in older adults using the 30-second chair-rise test: a pilot study. *Clin Int Aging* 9;5:173-80.

Signorile, J.F., Carmel, M.P., Czaja, S., Asfour, S., Morgan, R.O., Khalil, T., Ma, F., & Roos, B. (2002). Differential increases in average isokinetic power by specific muscle groups of older women due to variations in training and testing. *J Gerontol: Medical Science* 57A: M683-M690.

Signorile, J.F., Sandler, D.J., Ma, F., Bamel, S.A., Stanziano, D.C., Smith, W., & Roos, B.A. (2007). The gallon jug shelf transfer test: An instrument to evaluate deteriorating function in older adults. *J Aging Phys Act* 15:56-74.

Signorile, J.F., Sandler, D., Kempner, L., Ma, F., & Roos, B. (2007). The ramp power test: A new method of power assessment for older individuals. *J Gerontol A Biol Sci Med Sci* 62(11):1266-73. .

Skelton, D.A., Greig, C.A., Davies, J.M., & Young, A. (1994). Strength, power and related functional ability of health people aged 65-89 years. *Age and Ageing* 23:371-377.

Skelton, D.A., Kennedy, J., & Rutherford, O.M. (2002). Explosive power and asymmetry in leg muscle function in frequent fallers and non-fallers aged over 65. *Age and Ageing* 31:119-125.

Smith, W.N., Rossi, G.D., Adams, J.B., Abderlarahman, K., Asfour, S.A., Roos, B.A., Suzuki,

T., Bean, J.F., & Fielding, R.A. (2001). Muscle power of the ankle flexors predicts functional performance in community-dwelling older women. *J Am Geriatr Soc* 49:1161-1167.

Widrick, J.J., Trappe, S.W., Costill, D.L., & Fitts, R.H. (1996). Force-velocity and force-power properties of single muscle fibers from elite master runners and sedentary men. *Am J Physiol* 271:C676-C683.

References

Aniansson, A., Ljungberg, P., Rundgren, A., & Wetterqvist, H. (1984). Effect of a training programme for pensioners on condition and muscular strength. *Arch Gerontol Geriatr* 3:229-241.

Campos, G.E., Luecke, T.J., Wendeln, H.K., Toma, K., Hagerman F.C., Murray, T.F., Ragg, K.E., Ratamess, N.A., Krarmer, W.J., & Staron, R.S. (2002). Muscular adaptations in response to three different resistance-training regimens: Specificity of repetition maximum training zones. *Eur J Appl Physiol* 88:50-60.

Carpinelli, R.N., & Otto, R.M. (1998). Strength training. Single versus multiple sets. *Sports Med* 26:73-84.

Fiatarone, M.A., Marks, E.C., Ryan, N.D., Meredith, C.N., Lipsitz, L.A., & Evans, W.J. (1990). High intensity strength training in nonagenarians. *JAMA* 263:3029-3034.

Flipse, D., Signorile, J.F., Wills, R., Perry, A., Lowensteyn, I., Caruso, J., Robertson, B., & Burnett, K. (1993). Increased muscular performance in the elderly with moderate speed isotonic training. *Med Sci Sport Exerc* 25:S130.

Frontera, W.R., Meredith, C.N., O'Reilly, K.P., Knuttgen, H.G., & Evans, W.J. (1988). Strength conditioning in older men: Skeletal muscle hypertrophy and improved function. *J Appl Physiol* 64:1038-1044.

Galvao, D.A., & Taaffe, D.R. (2004). Single- vs multiple-set resistance training: Recent developments in the controversy. *J Str Cond Res* 18:660-667.

Hunter, G.R., Wetzstein, C.J., McLafferty, C.L., Zuckerman, P.A., Landers, K.A., & Bamman, M.M. (2001). High-resistance versus variable-resistance training in older adults. *Med Sci Sport Exerc* 33:1759-1764.

Jones, C.J., Rikli, R.E., & Beam, W.C. (1999). A 30-s chair-stand test as a measure of lower body strength in community-residing older adults. *Research Quarterly for Exercise and Sport* 70:113-117.

Lindemann, U., Najafi, B., Zijlstra, W., Hauer, K., Muche, R., Becker, C., & Aminian, K. (2007). Distance to achieve steady state walking speed in frail elderly persons. *Gait and Posture* 27(1):91-96.

Rantanen, T., & Avela, J. (1997). Leg extension power and walking speed in very old people living independently. *Journal of Gerontology: Medical Sciences* 52:M225-M231.

Rhea, M.R., Alvar, B.A., & Burkett, L.N. (2002). Single versus multiple sets for strength: A meta-analysis to address the controversy. *Res Quar Exerc Sport* 73:485-488.

Rhea, M.R., Alvar, B.A., Burkett, L.N., & Ball, S.D. (2003). A meta-analysis to determine the dose response for strength development. *Med Sci Sport Exerc* 35:456-464.

Rikli, R.E., & Jones, C.J. (1999). Development and validation of a functional fitness test for community-residing older adults. *Journal of Aging and Physical Activity* 7:129-161.

Rolland, Y.M., Cesari, M., Miller, M.E., Penninx, B.W., Atkinson, H.H., & Pahor, M. (2004). Reliability of the 400-m usual walk test as an assessment of mobility limitation in older adults. *J Am Geriatr Soc* 52:972-976.

Roubenoff, R. (2000). Sarcopenia and its implications for the elderly. *Eur J Clin Nutr* 54(3): S40-S47.

Sayers, S.P., Guralnik, J.M., Newman, A.B., Brach, J.S., & Fielding, R.A. (2006). Concordance and discordance between two measures of lower extremity function: 400 meter self-paced walk and SPPB. *Aging Clin Exp Res* 18:100-106.

Signorile, J.F., Sandler, D.J., Ma, F., Bamel, S.A., Stanziano, D.C., Smith, W., & Roos, B.A. (2007). The gallon jug shelf transfer test: An instrument to evaluate deteriorating function in older adults. *J Aging Phys Act* 15:56-74.

Signorile, J.F., Sochet, L., Morgenstern, A., Caruso, J., Puhl, J., O'Keefe, S., & Perry, A. (1995). The superiority of high speed resistance training in an older population. *Med Sci Sport Exerc* 27:S233.

Signorile, J.F., Suidmak, P., Campbell, M.H., Miller, P., & Puhl, J. (1995). High speed training produces superior strength and functional capacity in an older population. *The Gerontologist* 35:91.

Skelton, D.A., Greig, C.A., Davies, J.M., & Young, A. (1994). Strength, power and related functional ability of health people aged 65-89 years. *Age and Ageing* 23:371-377.

Skelton, D.A., Kennedy, J., & Rutherford, O.M. (2002). Explosive power and asymmetry in leg muscle function in frequent fallers and non-fallers aged over 65. *Age and Ageing* 31:119-125.

Smith, W.N., Rossi, D.G., Adams, J.B., Abderlarahman, K.Z., Asfour, S.A., Roos, B.A., & Signorile, J.F. (2010). Simple equations to predict concentric lower-body muscle power in older adults using the 30-second chair-rise test: a pilot study. *Clinical Interventions in Aging* 5:173-180.

Taaffe, D.R., Duret, C., Wheeler, S., & Marcus, R. (1999). Once-weekly resistance exercise improves muscle strength and neuromuscular performance in older adults. *J Am Geriatr Soc* 47:1208-1214.

Whipple, R.K., Wolfson, M.D., & Amerman, P.M. (1987). The relationship of knee and ankle weakness to falls in nursing home residents: An isokinetic study. *Journal of the American Geriatrics Society* 35:13-20.

Cardiovascular Training

Since Kenneth Cooper published his landmark work *Aerobics* in 1968 cardiovascular (aerobic) training has been nearly synonymous with exercise. This chapter examines the declines in the cardiovascular system that occur with aging, the effects that those declines have on independence and well-being, and the most effective way to address those declines. I promise that developing a cardiovascular training program from the information provided in this chapter will improve your clients' hearts. Cross my heart.

INCREASING CARDIOVASCULAR FITNESS: BENEFITS AND METHODS

Numerous fitness and health benefits have been associated with cardiovascular exercise. Let's take a brief look at each benefit and then examine its importance to an aging population. Then we can look at the training methods that have been found to be the most effective in addressing performance and health concerns in older persons.

Benefits of Cardiovascular Exercise

The literature is rich with information concerning the performance and health benefits of cardiovascular training. Rather than concentrating on these benefits across all demographics, let's concentrate on the benefits of cardiovascular training for the population targeted in this text, older individuals.

Increased Oxygen Consumption

As we saw in chapter 1, an exponential drop in maximal oxygen consumption ($\dot{V}O_2max$) occurs with age. This drop is related to

1. the ability to ventilate (move air in and out of) the lungs,
2. the diffusion (transfer) of oxygen from the lungs to the bloodstream,
3. the extraction of blood by the working organs, and
4. the delivery of blood by the heart and circulatory system.

If this book had been written a decade or so ago, this section would have been very short. It would have said that persons older than age 60 lose their ability to adapt to cardiovascular training. We now know that the lack of improvement in cardiovascular capacity demonstrated by older persons in those early studies was due to the fact that the training programs lacked the intensity or volume to produce a training effect. When cardiovascular training is of sufficient intensity and volume, it can certainly improve oxygen consumption in older men and women. Let's look at the structural and functional changes that allow improvements in each of the four factors affecting $\dot{V}O_2max$.

Ventilation of the Lungs

The ability to ventilate the lungs is the first major factor affecting $\dot{V}O_2max$. With age, the ability to inflate the lungs decreases due to a weakening of the respiratory muscles and a drop in the elasticity of the rib cage. In the majority of the studies that have reported increases in $\dot{V}O_2$max there has been a complementary increase in minute ventilation ($\dot{V}O_E$), indicating an increased ability to ventilate the lungs. $\dot{V}O_E$ is the volume of air a person can move through the lungs in 1 minute.

Diffusion Capacity

The ability to move air in and out of the lungs is only the first step in oxygen utilization. The next step is diffusion. During diffusion, the oxygen from the air is passed from the lungs across the alveoli (air sacs) to the hemoglobin on the red blood cells. The red blood cells then carry it to the tissues of the body (see figure 8.1). It appears that training can improve diffusion capacity across the alveolar membrane.

Extraction of Oxygen by the Working Organs

The extraction of oxygen from the blood by the working organs can be measured as the difference in oxygen content between the delivery (arterial) side and the return (venous) side (see figure 8.2). This difference has been

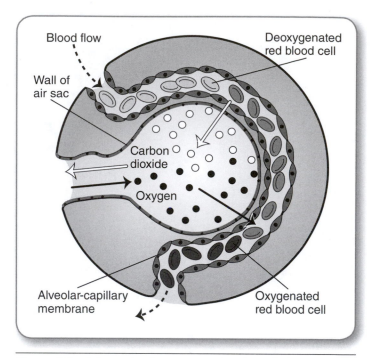

Figure 8.1 Schematic of oxygen passing from the lungs to the blood, where it is carried on the red blood cells. In addition, carbon dioxide passes from the blood to the lungs for removal during exhalation.

termed the *arteriovenous oxygen difference, or a-v(O₂)difference.* The extraction of oxygen from the blood is facilitated by capillary density and mitochondrial volume. Capillaries are the

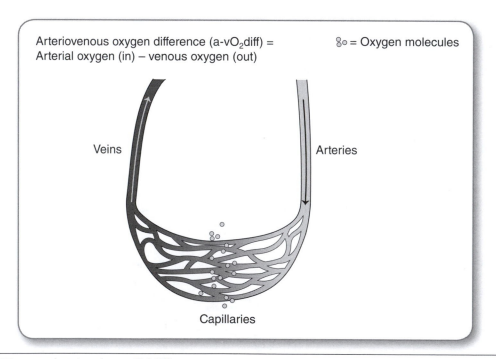

Figure 8.2 Diagram showing the a-v(O₂)difference.

small vessels that allow the transfer of oxygen to tissues of the body. Mitochondria are the little powerhouses within the cells that use oxygen to produce energy for the resynthesis of ATP. In fact, it is the exponential decline in the extraction of oxygen by tissues that dictates the shape of the $\dot{V}O_2$peak curve and, in your older clients, improvements in a-v(O_2)difference is the controlling factor for improvements in oxygen consumption.

Cardiovascular training can increase capillary density in the skeletal muscles of older clients, thereby improving the movement of oxygen from the blood to the working tissue. To match this change in capillary density, mitochondrial density also increases. As Terjung noted in his review article on the subject (Terjung, Zarzeczny, & Yang, 2002, p. 368),

> The increase in [mitochondria] appears essential to realize the increase in muscle $\dot{V}O_2$max with training and amplifies the rate-limiting influence of the muscles oxygen exchange capacity. Further, vascular remodeling induced by exercise in the elderly could be effective at improving flow capacity, if limited by peripheral obstruction.

To paraphrase, we may consider the aged muscle cell as a small, inactive, normal muscle cell that needs activity to get back to normal.

Delivery of Blood by the Heart and Circulatory System

Once oxygen has been transferred from the lungs to the red blood cells, there are two major variables responsible for increased oxygen consumption. These are the cardiac output ($\dot{Q}$) and the a-v(O_2)difference mentioned earlier.

$$\dot{V}O_2 = \dot{Q} \times \text{a-v}(O_2)\text{difference}$$

$\dot{Q}$ is the product of HR and stroke volume (SV). SV is the quantity of blood pushed out by a single contraction of the ventricles of the heart.

$$\dot{Q} = HR \times SV$$

One thing is obvious from the literature: Maximum heart rate (HR$_{max}$) drops a little less than 1 beat per minute for each year that a person passes after 45 years of age. Hirofumi Tanaka and colleagues (Tanaka, Monahan, &

Seals, 2001) have provided an exacting formula for this decline:

$$HR_{max} = 208 - 0.7 \times age$$

This formula was suggested in place of the old standard:

$$HR_{max} = 220 - age$$

Regardless of the equation used, one thing is clear: Age-related declines in HR are controlled predominantly by age and are independent of gender and habitual physical activity.

Given this fact, SV must compensate for the age-related decline in HR. The good news is that training can help older clients improve cardiac output. This improvement appears to be due to (1) an increase in the amount of blood in the ventricles (end diastolic volume), (2) an increase in the musculature (wall thickness) of the left ventricle, and (3) an improvement in the ability of the heart muscle to contract when stretched. This third factor is the result of what is termed the *Frank-Starling law of the heart*, which states that the force of contraction (end diastolic pressure) increases as the blood stretches the ventricles (see figure 8.3). In fact, long-term training studies have shown that moderate- to high-intensity training can increase end diastolic volume and SV as well as ejection fraction. Ejection fraction

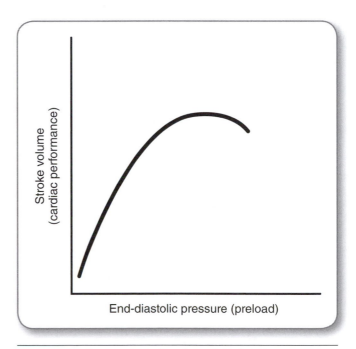

Figure 8.3 The Frank-Starling law of the heart.

is the percentage of the blood volume pumped from the ventricles in a single contraction. It can increase the volume of blood per beat even when SV stays the same.

Decreased Central Obesity

Central obesity is also called *apple-shaped* or *male-pattern obesity*. Central obesity refers to body fat deposits localized around the waistline (see figure 8.4). The reason why central obesity is so important is that it indicates the amount of visceral fat carried by an individual. Visceral fat surrounds the organs in the body's peritoneal cavity and is associated with metabolic syndrome. This metabolic syndrome (also known as *syndrome X)* is marked by the following:

- Central obesity: a waistline of 40 inches (102 cm) or more in men and 35 inches (89 cm) or more in women

- Hypertension: a blood pressure of 130/85 mmHg or higher or the use of blood pressure medications

- High triglycerides: levels greater than 150 mg/dl

- Low HDL (good) cholesterol: levels less than 40 mg/dl in men or 50 mg/dl in women

- Insulin resistance: a fasting blood glucose (sugar) level greater than 100 mg/dl or the use of glucose-lowering medications

A few studies have shown that exercise training can reduce central obesity in younger persons. However, there is limited evidence supporting the use of exercise to reduce central adiposity in older persons.

Reduced Insulin Resistance

Insulin resistance occurs when the cells of the body don't respond adequately to insulin (see figure 8.5). In muscle cells this leads to reduced glucose uptake, while in fat cells it leads to the breakdown of triglycerides and the release of fatty acids into the blood. In liver cells it leads to an inability to store glycogen that can lead to metabolic syndrome and type 2 diabetes. Cardiovascular exercise has been shown to improve insulin resistance, especially when high-intensity (greater than 70% $\dot{V}O_2$max) training is used. Both circuit resistance training and cardiovascular endurance training can benefit insulin resistance, and circuit training may have the edge when postponing the manifestations of non-insulin-dependent, or type 2, diabetes is the goal. However, although higher-intensity training has the edge when it comes to dealing with long-term changes, low-intensity training may have its place in improving insulin resistance. This mixed bag of intensities is actually quite convenient when considering the intensity changes that must occur across a properly designed periodized training cycle (see chapter 9).

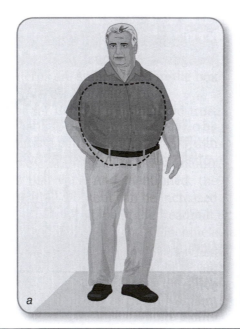 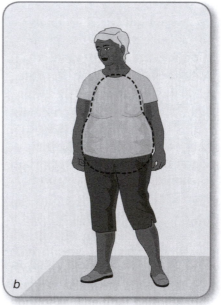

Figure 8.4   Illustration of *(a)* apple-shaped versus *(b)* pear-shaped distribution of body fat.

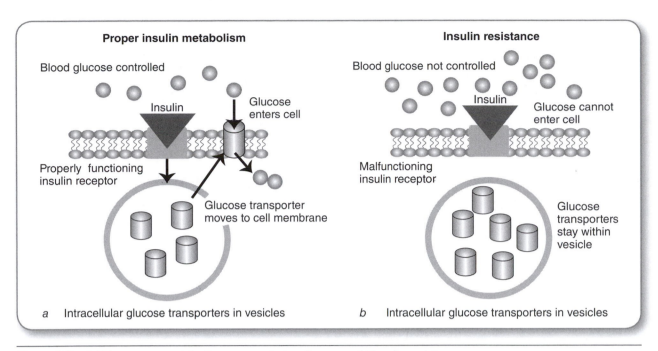

Figure 8.5 *(a)* The proper metabolic response to insulin versus *(b)* insulin resistance.

Better Lipid Profile

These days, we are all familiar with the increased risk of heart attack and stroke associated with high cholesterol levels. Additionally, we have all been formally introduced to the good lipoproteins (HDL), the bad lipoproteins (low-density lipoproteins, or LDL), and the intermediates.

Although aerobic training has been shown to have a positive effect on blood lipid profiles, many of the changes are small, and improvements don't reach the levels observed in many of the other variables improved by cardiovascular exercise. One of the reasons for this limited success appears to be the necessity to combine high-intensity exercise with a high work volume in order to achieve a significant improvement in total cholesterol or LDL cholesterol (especially small-particle LDL cholesterol). It also appears that a minimum weekly energy expenditure of 900 kilocalories is necessary to increase HDL cholesterol. Note that the concentration of the lipid-binding protein associated with LDL (apoprotein B) can be reduced while the level of apoprotein A, the vacuum cleaner protein that picks up lipids for disposal in the liver and other organs, can be increased by this level of training.

So what can we conclude? Certainly we have a good argument that aerobic training of sufficient volume and intensity has the potential to positively influence lipid profiles. We can expect the greatest improvements in blood lipids to occur in persons with the poorest blood profiles. This may explain the limited effects reported in many of the studies employing populations with good or marginal blood lipid profiles.

Lower Blood Pressure

Blood pressure increases with age. The major factor responsible for this age-related increase is a change in the compliance of the major and (to some extent) peripheral arteries. Other factors that may increase blood pressure include obesity, insulin resistance, high alcohol intake, high salt intake (in salt-sensitive patients), sedentary lifestyle, stress, low potassium intake, and low calcium intake.

According to the ACSM (Pescatello et al., 2004), a primary goal in dealing with hypertension is lifestyle modification, and at the forefront of this intervention is exercise. The ACSM adds that cardiovascular endurance activities are the principal training tool to prevent hypertension and to lower blood pressure in both hypertensive and normotensive adults. The ACSM also indicates that exercise has the greatest effect in people with high blood pressure. An acute exercise session lowers high blood pressure by 5 to 7 mmHg for up to 22 hours after exercise. Long-term training can lead to more pronounced effects. The ACSM statement makes it clear that a vigorous exercise program (60% $\dot{V}O_2max$) is appropriate for addressing hypertension. But remember, exercise prescriptions require the body to adapt over time. Beginning clients should start with moderate-intensity exercise (< 60% $\dot{V}O_2max$) that they can tolerate and should progress slowly while being monitored to confirm that they can tolerate increases in intensity or volume.

Better Heart Rate Variability

HR variability is a measure of the variation in HR across either a short or a long duration. It is of major concern since HR variability tends to decrease with age and this reduction is associated with an increased risk of cardiovascular morbidity and mortality. The age-associated decrease in HR variability seems to be due to reduced sympathetic and parasympathetic control. The sympathetic and parasympathetic nervous systems are the two divisions of the autonomic (or automatic) nervous system. The sympathetic division is responsible for the fight-or-flight response, which results in increased HR, sweating, breathing, and dry mouth during times of stress. In contrast, the parasympathetic division is responsible for slowing the HR. It produces more of a sit-down-and-have-a-nice-meal response. These two systems speak to the body's natural pacemaker (the sinoatrial node) and other components of the heart's conduction system in order to exert exacting control of HR across the wide range of activity and stress levels that occur during daily life (see figure 8.6). The good news is that training can restore autonomic response and positively affect HR variability.

APPLICATION POINT   As you can see from the above sections, there are a number of structural and functional changes that can occur from cardiovascular training. These changes will not only improve your clients' cardiovascular capacity, they will also have a positive effect on their metabolic health.

Training Methods

When choosing training methods for clients, you'll want to use the methods that are the most effective in addressing performance and health concerns in older persons. Providing the most effective exercise prescription requires us to ask some basic questions:

1. How much?
2. How hard?
3. What type?

Let's examine these questions in the context of the health parameters improved by cardiovascular training that we just discussed.

Maximal Oxygen Consumption

Researchers who examine training protocols to increase aerobic capacity consistently report that high-intensity exercises produce greater improve-

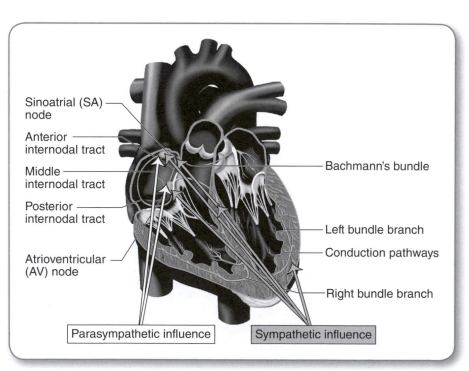

Figure 8.6 Sympathetic and parasympathetic influences on the heart.

Sinoatrial (SA) node
Anterior internodal tract
Middle internodal tract
Posterior internodal tract
Atrioventricular (AV) node
Bachmann's bundle
Left bundle branch
Conduction pathways
Right bundle branch
Parasympathetic influence
Sympathetic influence

ments in $\dot{V}O_2$max than low- or moderate-intensity exercises produce.

Recently high-intensity interval training has been examined as a training tool in older persons. One study compared moderate-intensity continuous training (70% peak HR) with aerobic interval training (95% peak HR) performed three times per week for 12 weeks. The subjects were 27 postinfarction heart failure patients and the average age was 75.7 years. $\dot{V}O_2$peak increased more than three times as much with the interval training than it did with the moderate continuous training. Additionally, only the interval training program caused the left ventricle to be remodeled so that end diastolic volume and ejection fraction (the filling and emptying capacities of the heart, respectively) actually increased. Also, the interval training program improved the function of the endothelium of the arteries. Improved endothelial function means that there is a better match between blood flow and the ability of the arteries to dilate. Finally, the interval training program decreased the amount of brain natriuretic peptide in the blood by 40%. Brain natriuretic peptide is released from the heart's ventricles and is increased in the blood during heart failure. Thus it is often used as a predictor of future cardiac incidents. The decrease seen in this study indicated improved cardiovascular health. The even better news is that clients can enjoy these cardiovascular benefits whether they train on land or in the pool.

APPLICATION POINT Let's make this simple. If improving a client's $\dot{V}O_2$max is the goal, then intensity is the name of the game.

Central Obesity

When it comes to eliminating central obesity, that annoyingly unhealthy fat beneath the belt buckle, it appears that overall calories burned is the controlling factor. In older persons, reductions in central obesity have been reported with both moderate-intensity, long-duration and high-intensity, short-duration training protocols. Additionally, mixed protocols of aerobic and resistance training have been equally successful at reducing central obesity, especially when combined with a dietary education program. A highly successful study at the Case Western Reserve University School of Medicine (O'leary et al., 2006) exam-

ined the effects of cycling and treadmill exercises performed 5 days per week for 12 weeks in older persons. Exercise intensity began at 60% and 65% of HR_{max} and gradually increased by the fourth week to 80% and 85% of HR_{max}. A significant decrease in both subcutaneous and visceral fat resulted from the training. Additionally, the decline in visceral fat was associated with a significant decrease in insulin resistance.

We should not leave this topic without discussing interval training. Talanian and colleagues (2007) showed that 2 weeks of high-intensity aerobic interval training could increase the capacity for fat oxidation during exercise in young women. While the exercise protocol may not have been appropriate for most of your older clients, nonetheless, the results demonstrate the effectiveness of these training protocols in addressing the problem of central obesity.

Insulin Resistance

Insulin resistance appears to be well addressed by even low-intensity exercise; however, long-term improvements in insulin sensitivity require high-intensity (80% $\dot{V}O_2$max) rather than moderate-intensity (65% $\dot{V}O_2$max) or low-intensity (50% $\dot{V}O_2$max) training. In addition, the results of the Insulin Resistance Atherosclerosis Study (Mayer-Davis et al., 1998) showed that increased energy expenditure, whether the result of vigorous or nonvigorous activity, is associated with significantly higher insulin sensitivity. This relationship is a dose–response relationship, meaning that the more frequently an individual exercises each week, the greater the improvement in insulin sensitivity (see figure 8.7).

As noted in previous sections, multiple short exercise bouts, or intervals, often have as good as an effect—if not a better effect—on health that continuous training has. This also seems to be true when it comes to insulin sensitivity. Eriksen, Dahl-Petersen, Haugaard, and Dela (2007) from the University of Copenhagen reported that three 10-minute sessions of moderate- to high-intensity training per day proved superior to one session of 30 minutes per day in improving glycemic (blood sugar) control. These authors also reported that the improvements in cardiorespiratory fitness were similar in each exercise group. They speculated that the energy expenditure associated with multiple short daily sessions was likely greater than that associated with a single daily session.

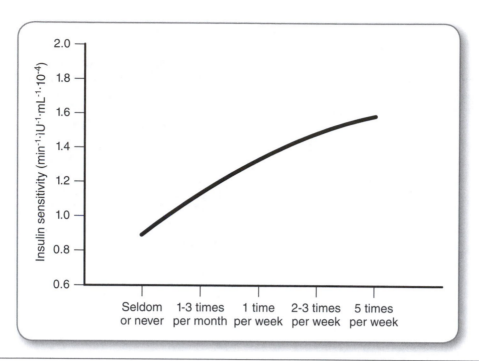

Figure 8.7   The dose–response relationship between insulin sensitivity and exercise volume.

Data from Mayer-Davis et al. 1998.

Blood Lipid Profile

Improvements in blood lipid profiles are related to the combined effects of exercise intensity and volume. If programs of moderate intensity (45%-50% of heart rate reserve, or HRR, which = 220 – age – resting HR × intensity + resting HR) and low frequency (3-4 days per week), programs of moderate intensity and high frequency (5-7 days per week), programs of high intensity (65%-75% HRR) and low frequency, and programs of high intensity and high frequency are compared, the high-intensity conditions, whether combined with low-frequency or high-frequency training, as well as the moderate-intensity, high-frequency condition produce significant increases in maximum oxygen uptake. However only high-intensity, high-frequency training significantly improves HDL cholesterol and the ratio of total cholesterol to HDL cholesterol. Additionally, combined lower-body cardiovascular endurance and upper-body resistance training can significantly improve blood lipid profiles and body composition. In contrast to exercise for improving oxygen consumption, for which land and aquatic exercise yield comparable results, only land training increases HDL cholesterol when equivalent

high-intensity training bouts are performed on land and in the water. The bottom line is that intensity, and to a lesser extent volume, is the major factor effecting positive changes in lipid profiles.

Before we leave the topic of blood lipids, let's take another look at interval training. Altena, Michaelson, Ball, and Thomas (2004) showed that a single bout of interval exercise is more effective than continuous exercise is for lowering circulating postprandial (postmeal) blood lipids in inactive individuals with normal lipid levels. In fact, a study by Miyashita, Burns, and Stensel (2006) suggested that both continuous and interval training can be used to deal with blood lipids. These authors reported that accumulating multiple short bouts of exercise (10 minutes each) throughout the day reduces postprandial plasma triglyceride concentrations to the same extent as a single 30-minute session of exercise in healthy young men does.

High Blood Pressure

In their review of the topic, Kokkinos, Narayan, and Papademetriou (2001) provided very specific guidelines to optimize exercise benefits for blood pressure. They recommended that the training program consist of 3 to 5 sessions per week and 30 to 60 minutes per session and that the intensity be at 50% to 80% of perceived HR_{max}. They also suggested that the program be individualized to meet the patient's needs and abilities, that both intensity and duration be progressed gradually until the final goal is reached, and that the progression be tailored to the individual's responses. And finally, they recommended that hypertensive patients who are overweight or obese employ a program that expends 300 to 500 kilocalories per day and 1,000 to 2,000 kilocalories per week in order to reduce body weight.

I would like to add two caveats to these recommendations. First, the program should employ a periodized progression as described in chapter 9 rather than follow a simple progression. Second, since part of the prescription targets caloric output, high-intensity training methods, which by nature are metabolically inefficient, should be used because they are excellent ways to burn a greater number of calories per unit of exercise time. However, the effectiveness of such programs compared with cardiovascular endurance training, which can affect blood pressure for up to 22 hours, has yet to be examined.

Heart Rate Variability

Both continuous and interval exercise training improve exercise capacity in cardiac patients. However, continuous training appears to have an edge in improving autonomic nervous system control over the heart.

APPLICATION POINT Although the training techniques presented in this chapter can be expected to have positive effects on most clients, you should pick and choose aspects of the exercise prescription to target the specific cardiovascular and metabolic issues facing your client.

Still Man's Best Friend

Per-Olof Åstrand, the father of work physiology, said one of my favorite quotes about cardiovascular training: "Take your dog for a walk every day . . . even if you don't have one." (American College of Sports Medicine, 2004). This humorous little tidbit is based on a significant number of studies showing the relationship between dog ownership and successful aging.

In a unique study from the School of Public Health and Community Medicine at the University of New South Wales, Roland Thorpe Jr. and coworkers (2006) examined whether dog ownership could translate into substantial disease prevention and health care cost savings. They found that increased mobility was seen in the older persons who actually walked their dogs but that many dog owners did not take their dogs out for a walk. The researchers recommended promoting dog walking through national strategies recommending dog walks for all by the year 2010. This study added further credence to a statement made by Adrian Bauman and coworkers several years earlier. They stated, "If all dog owners walked their dogs, substantial disease prevention and healthcare cost savings of $175 million per year might accrue" (Bauman et al., 2001, p. 632). In a study from western Canada, researchers found that people who do not own dogs walk an average of 168 minutes per week, while people who do own dogs walk an average of 300 minutes per week (Brown & Rhodes, 2006). The bottom line is that Fido can help clients improve their cardiovascular fitness—but not by sitting next to them on the couch.

I've often said that the average distance for a walk is about 52 miles (84 km). There's the 50 miles (80 km) from the couch to the front door, and then there's the 2-mile (3 km) walk that follows. This statement is actually supported by a women's health and aging study (Simonsick et al., 2005) that found that most women capable of walking at least eight blocks per week do not do so and that a major problem in increasing women's daily walking patterns is getting women out the door. Again, the responsibility of walking the dog may help increase that movement out the door. In fact, you might suggest to your clients that they train their dogs to bring them the leash to remind them when it's time to walk.

APPLICATION POINT What a great deal for you, having a personal trainer to fill in for you outside of your training sessions and to provide motivational puppy dog eyes to boot!

TESTING CARDIOVASCULAR FITNESS

Cardiovascular endurance is a strong independent predictor of ADL performance. To evaluate this fitness factor, I have chosen the 6-minute walk test. This test has been shown to be indicative of cardiovascular fitness in older persons.

6-Minute Walk Test

The 6-minute walk test was first developed by Kenneth Cooper in the 1960s. Individuals should wear walking or athletic shoes for the test. The tester should not walk with the individual during the test since it will most likely alter the subject's pace. In addition, having a number of persons walk together may alter an individual's results since it can promote competition. Therefore, be consistent when administering the test. Although the 6-minute test is often run as a shuttle test, the technique presented here is that described by Rikli and Jones (1999), and the norms presented reflect the Rikli and Jones version. The test has been shown to be a safe measure for the majority of persons aged 60 years and older. The variable measured is the total distance an individual can walk in 6 minutes.

Equipment Needed

- Four cones or similar position markers
- A stopwatch or other timing device

Protocol

- Place four orange pylons on a flat surface so that they form a rectangle measuring 20 × 5 yards (18.3 × 4.6 m).
- Demonstrate correct heel-to-toe walking, keeping at least one foot in contact with the ground at all times (to ensure no running).
- Give the signal to go while simultaneously starting the stopwatch.

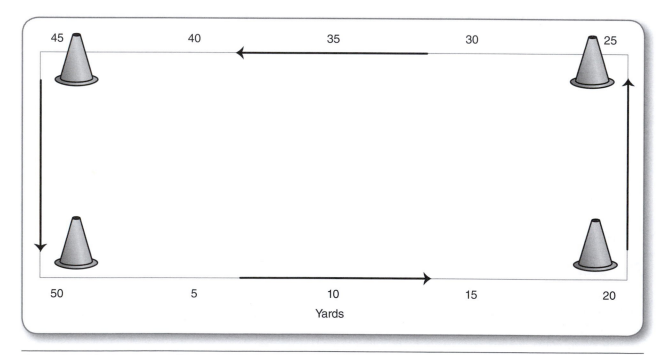

Figure 8.8   The 6-minute walk test.

- Have the subject walk continuously around the 50-yard (45.7 m) course (see figure 8.8) until the 6 minutes are up or until the subject decides to stop walking, whichever comes first.

By using the norms provided in the appendix (p. 299), or by typing the results of this test into the diagnostic testing battery included on the DVD, you can compare the percentile rank of this test to those of the other diagnostic tests presented in this book. In this way you can prioritize your client's need for cardiovascular training with other exercise interventions.

CARDIOVASCULAR TRAINING AND PROGRAM DESIGN

An accurate description of any cardiovascular training program should include three elements (see figure 8.9):

1. The type of exercise
2. The equipment used
3. The training protocol

The antiquated concept that aerobic exercise is limited to long, low-intensity walks or runs has been discredited by researchers, fitness organizations, and even governmental agencies. It's not the type of exercise or the equipment used that engages the cardiovascular system—rather, it's the

training protocol itself. In the following sections we'll scrutinize the strengths and shortcomings of the aerobic exercises available to us, look at the machines and environments for training, and, most importantly, examine specific training protocols and how they can be used in a periodized system to maximize gains in cardiovascular fitness and related health factors.

Type of Exercise

As professionals, most of us have a fairly good handle on the classic cardiovascular exercises such as walking, running, cycling, and swimming. When we picture using these exercises to improve fitness, we usually think of prolonged durations and target HR. We know that other types of exercise have been granted some level of cardiovascular benefit. These include recreational sports

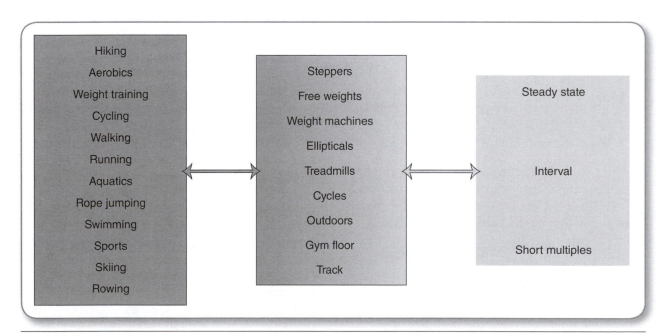

Figure 8.9 The types of exercise, equipment, and training protocols used for improving cardiovascular fitness.

such as tennis, skiing, kayaking, and softball. We understand that these are good for us, but their relationship to true cardiovascular exercise usually ranges from moderate to never really thought about it. Then there are the exercises that we all know are anaerobic, the most potent of which is weight training. These exercises are considered by many to have no effect at all on cardiovascular health because they only work the muscles and they don't keep the heart in its target training zone long enough to have any cardiovascular effect.

Let's get one thing straight so that you can continue to enjoy this chapter without further trepidation. There are no exercises that by definition are aerobic or anaerobic. For example, running can promote anaerobic changes during sprinting or aerobic changes during long-distance training. It's not the type of exercise performed but rather the way in which the exercise is performed that determines the metabolic system targeted.

When I am lecturing and I ask the audience to name a cardiovascular or an aerobic exercise, the number one answer I get is "running!" Once I receive this answer, I go to my whiteboard (how I miss chalk!) or flip chart and write the following list:

- 10-yard (10 m) sprint
- 50-meter sprint
- 100 meters
- 200 meters
- 400 meters
- 800 meters
- 1,600 meters
- 5K
- 10K
- Marathon

The remainder of the discussion follows a predictable pattern. It goes something like this and is more reflective of a Greek chorus response than a dialogue with a single member of the audience:

First they go: "I meant long-distance running."

Then I go: "How long is long? Where do I draw the line?"

Then they go: "Over a mile or a couple of kilometers."

Then I go: "So we don't use our hearts and lungs to deliver oxygen during a 400- or 800-meter run?"

Then they go: "To some extent!"

Then I go: "So those runs can be aerobic."

Then they go: "If they're done slow enough."

Then I go: "What about sprints?"

Then they go: "Not aerobic."

Then I go: "Then why are you breathing so hard at the end?"

Then they go: "To burn off the lactic acid."

Then I go: "Doesn't that take oxygen?"

Then they go: "Yes, but only after the exercise is over!"

Then I go: "So you could run 100 or 200 meters with a gag and a nose plug as long as you removed them after the race?"

At this point there is usually a significant division of thought between the majority of the audience and the "I know these are aerobic exercises" hard-liners. The final conversion usually requires a simple description of repeated sprints or of repeated high-intensity movements used all the time in step aerobics, aerobic dancing, and kickboxing classes. By the time I finish examining the changes in metabolic needs and cardiovascular responses across a series of so-called *anaerobic exercises,* everyone has at the very least modified their way of viewing exercise. Everyone, that is, except for a small minority who have left to buy rotten tomatoes or scour the city for tar and feathers for a surprise attack when I'm finally finished and stepping out into the hall, leaving the sanctuary of my whiteboard and PowerPoint presentation.

The message that you should derive from all this is that cardiovascular training is not limited to marathons or mall walking; it can be addressed by almost any type of exercise as long as the pattern of training is correct. There are, however, some considerations that should affect your choice of exercises.

The first, and most obvious, consideration is biomechanical specificity. If a client's test results indicate that fatigue is specific to a certain body part or movement pattern or indicate a need for upper-body strength in order to deal with a walking aid, you can choose a biomechanically specific exercise to address the client's particular need. You can also choose biomechanically specific exercises to address recreational activities such as sports, in which success is based on a particular kinetic chain (movement sequence). Common examples are tennis, golf, and skiing.

The second consideration is the performance environment. For example, swimming laps is not an effective choice for a person who can't swim and cycling is not a good idea for a person who doesn't ride a bike.

The third consideration is interaction with other goals. For example, increases in bone density are best addressed by weight-bearing or externally loaded exercises. Therefore, walking and circuit weight training are better choices than swimming or cycling for clients who want to improve bone density as well as cardiovascular health, because these exercises can address both concerns.

The fourth consideration is physical disability. A client with fibromyalgia or osteoarthritis might find a warm pool to be more comfortable than an air-conditioned workout room. Additionally, individuals who are obese may find supported exercises such as biking easier to tolerate, especially at the beginning of an exercise program.

Finally, keep diversity in mind. Remember that the diamond has many facets. Polishing one facet just because it's your or your client's favorite may not be the best way to go.

Equipment

When it comes to choosing an aerobic exercise machine, the options are as diverse as the aerobic exercise options. Let's look at some of the equipment options and consider the strengths and weaknesses of each type of machine.

Treadmills

The treadmill is the tried-and-true classic. Treadmills come with a variety of features, including programmable workouts, detailed displays, HR monitoring, and a host of other bells and whistles. When all is said and done, however, there are two basic factors that affect a client's treadmill workout: grade and speed. The grade is controlled by adjusting the angle of the treadmill. If you

remember your trigonometry, you may already know why the treadmill angle affects the grade. If you don't, pay attention to learn another incredible piece of information that you may be able to use at your next party or during an early *Jeopardy!* round. Perhaps the easiest way to understand the relationship between grade and angle is to look at it within the context of moving the body against gravity. At an angle of 0°, the treadmill grade equals 0. In other words, when we're walking on flat ground, we don't have to move any of our body weight against gravity. On the other hand, at an angle of 90°, which equates to walking up a wall, the grade is 100, meaning that we must move 100% of our body weight against gravity. This should give you a pretty good handle on why angles greater than 10° are so difficult to maintain or even attain. To determine the grades for angles between 0° and 90°, it is necessary to take the sine of the angle. Figure 8.10 shows the sines and grades for angles from 0° through 90°.

The second variable we can manipulate on the treadmill is the speed of the belt. The effects of manipulating this variable are a bit more obvious: The faster we go, the harder we work. The physiological changes that occur when speed is increased differ significantly depending on the variables being examined. Oxygen consumption tends to rise linearly with increases in speed until $\dot{V}O_2$max is approached, at which point the rate of oxygen consumption plateaus. The pattern of energy utilization reflects the interactions of all the energy systems and so behaves a little bit differently. As speed increases linearly, energy utilization goes up exponentially, especially as the anaerobic threshold is approached. This is because the faster we work, the lower our metabolic efficiency becomes and the more energy we must use to perform the work. This phenomenon holds true for all of the equipment described in this chapter and is covered in greater detail at the end of this chapter.

One of the strengths of treadmill training is that it closely resembles the patterns used during overland walking. Thus the treadmill is highly specific for mobility training. In addition, the controls are usually easy to master, and often it is possible to preset steady-state and interval programs. There are, however, shortcomings to the treadmill. The most obvious is the need for alertness and control. Unlike other machines, treadmills keep moving unless the user slows them down. Also, while on many exercise machines the user can punch a

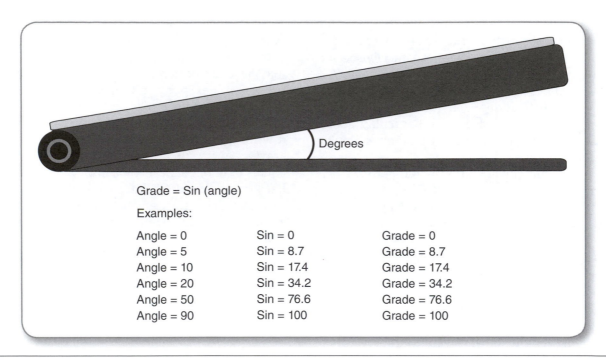

Grade = Sin (angle)

Examples:

Angle = 0	Sin = 0	Grade = 0
Angle = 5	Sin = 8.7	Grade = 8.7
Angle = 10	Sin = 17.4	Grade = 17.4
Angle = 20	Sin = 34.2	Grade = 34.2
Angle = 50	Sin = 76.6	Grade = 76.6
Angle = 90	Sin = 100	Grade = 100

Figure 8.10   The relationship between the grade of a treadmill and its angle of incline.

button to increase and decrease intensity at will, treadmills require the speed and incline to be manipulated to achieve the simple goal of altering the intensity. Another shortcoming is that running or walking on a treadmill is not biomechanically or bioenergetically the same as running or walking on the ground. Try to think of the last time the ground went backward while you walked in place! Even with these shortcomings, treadmill walking is an excellent alternative when the weather is inclement or the mall is too crowded.

APPLICATION POINT   Treadmills have the advantage of providing weight-bearing exercise while providing a cardiovascular overload.

Stationary Cycles

If treadmills are the most common cardiovascular exercise machines, then the second most common has to be the stationary cycle. There are numerous types of cycles, the most common being the upright and recumbent cycles. There are two ways to increase the intensity of the exercise when on the cycle. The first way is to increase the resistance on the pedals or the flywheel of the cycle. Most cycles increase the resistance by applying friction to the flywheel or by using an electromagnet to add drag to the flywheel.

The second way to increase intensity is to increase the pedaling speed. In rare cases the bike itself can be programmed to pedal faster, in which case the rider's job is simply to keep up. But more often speed changes are simply the product of how fast the user pedals.

Now let's look at the strengths and weaknesses of stationary cycling. Stationary cycling is not a weight-bearing exercise. So is this a strength or a weakness? The answer is both! It's a strength because it makes stationary cycling one of the safest cardiovascular exercises available. Clients are unlikely to twist an ankle or fall off the machine while riding a stationary cycle. However, it's a weakness because it means that stationary cycling has a limited effect on bone density.

A second strength of stationary cycling is that changing the intensity is simple. Additionally, the intensity levels can be reduced to nearly zero to accommodate individuals in poor cardiovascular condition or to facilitate recovery cycles during interval training. Weaknesses of stationary cycling include the following:

1. Stationary cycles target only the lower-body muscles and so provide limited cardiovascular overload when compared with treadmill training.

2. Stationary cycles use patterns of movement that do not easily translate into improvements in mobility.

Before leaving our discussion of stationary cycling, let's look at two alternatives to the stationary cycle: the upper-body cycle ergometer and the portable cycle exerciser. Upper-body cycle ergometers range from large freestanding machines to smaller portable machines that can be mounted to a table or other horizontal surface. Regardless of the machine's size or bells and whistles, all ergometers use the same concept: handles attached to a cycle crank that the user rotates to perform the exercise. We've all seen the small portable cycles that sit in front of a chair or sofa. Most have some type of friction device that allows the user to increase resistance. Each of these devices has somewhat restricted application for improving cardiovascular fitness due to the limited overloads that can be produced.

Stair-Climbers

The first generation of upright exercise machines to bridge the gap between the StepMill and the modern elliptical machine was the stair-climber. The name given to these machines pretty much describes their function. They use friction or pneumatic resistance to change the levels of work performed. There is an interesting interaction between speed of movement and resistance on these machines. The lower the resistance, the higher the movement speed. In effect, higher levels of resistance provide greater support and so reduce the intensity of the exercise, while lower levels of resistance require higher stepping speeds due to a lack of support. Watching a person climb at low resistance is almost like watching a cartoon character run at high speed just to stay in place on a slippery slope.

The benefits of stair-climbing are that it is a weight-bearing activity (except in the case of the recumbent climber), it simulates climbing, it uses speed rather than resistance to increase workload and thereby addresses the loss in movement speed associated with aging, and it is very safe with limited potential for injury when compared with using the treadmill or the StepMill. Additionally, there is an emphasis on the calf muscles (gastrocnemius and soleus) not seen in the other machines described in this section. The major

shortcoming of these machines is that many older persons are unable to maintain the speed necessary to use them.

Stair-climbers have lost popularity and have been supplanted by the elliptical trainers. One of the few models to survive this cultural switch is the recumbent. The recumbent model allows older persons to train the stepping pattern with the convenience and comfort of a recumbent cycle. Of course, the same limitations described for other recumbent exercises hold true for recumbent stepping.

Elliptical Trainers

The big winner for machine design in the past decade is the elliptical trainer. The name of the machine describes the movement pattern of the pedals. Among the strengths of the elliptical trainer is the ROM through which the body can work. The majority of these trainers produce relatively large stride lengths, which is helpful in improving ROM of the joints employed. Additionally, elliptical machines all but eliminate the ballistic forces that occur during running or even walking. This is not to say that these machines don't raise some concerns. Analyses of the forces around the joints have shown that forces at the hip flexors and knee extensors are greater during elliptical training than they are during walking, while forces at the plantar flexors and hip abductors are smaller than they are during walking. This profile presents two concerns. The first is that individuals with existing hip or knee problems should be cautious when choosing this machine as their primary mode of exercise. The second is that the lower leg is trained minimally by these machines, which means that elliptical trainers are less biomechanically specific to walking and improved mobility when compared with treadmill walking or stair-climbing.

Drag Devices

The pool is an excellent environment for cardiovascular training because it provides the opportunity to use the interactions between drag and movement speed to increase oxygen consumption. A variety of devices including paddles, webbed gloves, noodles, fins, and floating dumbbells can be used to increase drag when exercising in the water. And remember that in the pool, a linear increase in speed provides an exponential increase in resistance.

APPLICATION POINT Let's put all of this into perspective: While each cardiovascular exercise machine may have its own strengths and shortcomings, the truth is that when the volume and intensity of exercise are equal, all the machines presented here produce similar increases in maximum aerobic capacity.

Training Protocols

Now that we have examined the methods and equipment available for cardiovascular training, let's move on to the most important section of this chapter, which is examining the protocols that can be used to maximize clients' improvements. Earlier in this chapter, we examined the relative benefits of interval and steady-state training on cardiovascular fitness and health factors. We noted that rather than take a prolonged time slot out of the day, cardiovascular training can also be accumulated during the day. Now let's consider how these ideas can be used to structure a cohesive cardiovascular training cycle that incorporates work, recovery, overload, and periodization.

After reading the previous parts of this chapter, you may believe that interval training is the only way to go. While interval training certainly should be a substantial part of your client's training program, steady-state training definitely has its place. Additionally, modifying the lengths of the training periods and the durations of the recovery periods between them provides an even greater number of choices for developing training patterns.

Steady-State Training

Steady-state exercises are effective tools, especially at the beginning of training and when the training goals are to improve lipoprotein levels, blood sugar levels, or HR. True steady-state exercise is seldom accomplished without some type of feedback, such as that provided by an HR monitor or the speed and incline controls on a treadmill. Even exercises that are considered the epitome of steady state, such as mall walking, swimming, or overland running, often have work rates that vary throughout the training session. There are a number of variables that you can use to adjust clients' training. For steady-state training, the major variables are intensity and volume:

Intensity

- How fast is the workout performed?
- What is the speed or resistance provided during the workout?

Performance speed during steady-state exercise directly affects how much oxygen is used and how hard the cardiovascular system must work to deliver that oxygen. You can increase speed by increasing the velocity of the exercise device, as you might do when a client is using a motorized treadmill, or by having the client voluntarily adjust the speed, as the client can do when walking outside or pedaling on a stationary cycle.

Resistance can be manipulated in many ways. One way is to change from level walking or running to uphill walking or running. This can be done whether the exercise is performed outdoors or indoors on a treadmill. It also works for cycling outdoors. A second option is to increase the resistance on an exercise machine. This option is available on many stationary cycles and elliptical machines. The third possibility is to add external loading. External loads have been applied with backpacks, ankle weights, and hand weights. Note, however, that backpacks providing sufficient loads to affect oxygen consumption tend to put too much stress on the shoulders and back musculature. And as for ankle weights, the potential increase in oxygen consumption doesn't justify the stresses added to the knees and hips. The one set of weights that might be helpful are hand weights. Although holding hand weights can't significantly increase oxygen consumption during walking, actively moving the hand weights through a substantial ROM (approximately 30°) can significantly increase oxygen consumption. Another way to increase resistance is to exercise in the pool. In fact, I would be remiss if I were to leave the topic of resistance and oxygen consumption without mentioning pool walking. In the pool, the faster you walk, the greater the level of resistance and the more oxygen you use. Finally, you should recognize that oxygen utilization is directly affected by the volume of muscle being used. Exercises such as walking and running, which alternate movements of the arms and legs, use more oxygen than the exercises that engage only the upper or lower body use.

Volume

- How long is each workout?
- How many workouts are to be done per week?

Controlling workout duration is a simple matter of deciding how long a workout will last. Important here are the results suggesting that multiple training sessions of short duration are as effective as a single long-duration session in improving cardiovascular fitness. In addition, multiple short training sessions may be more effective in controlling blood glucose levels (Eriksen et al., 2007). Recommendations vary from 3 to 5 sessions per week and 30 to 60 minutes per session (or using between 1,000 and 2,000 kcal per week). These can be expected to vary due to your client's fitness level and where the client is in the periodized training cycle. Additionally, remember that volume can be cumulative so you do not need to overdo it in any single session; this is especially true when you are dealing with an untrained or detrained individual.

When planning a steady-state aerobic training program, remember the cardinal rule: Start easy at 40% to 50% HRR and increase gradually. Concentrate on increasing volume during the initial stages and on increasing intensity toward the end of the training cycle. Also note that cardiovascular programs usually find their top end at 70% to 80% HRR.

Interval Training

As you have seen earlier in the chapter, if increasing aerobic capacity, reducing high blood pressure, or weight loss (especially around the waistline) is the goal, then interval training is one of the most effective tools you possess to reach that goal. If you are recommending aerobics classes, spinning, or aquatic exercise programs as part of the client's cardiovascular training program, you are recommending interval training. Land-based interval techniques can also include performing walking routines, stair-climbing, using an elliptical trainer, stationary cycling, and circuit resistance training. Let's look at the controlling factors for designing interval workouts and then put it all together so you can design the best interval workout for your clients.

The two factors that are manipulated during steady-state exercise, intensity and volume, are also effective modulators of interval exercise. However, other variables are also in play during interval workouts.

Work–Recovery Ratios

Let's start by discussing work–recovery ratios. These ratios are simply the amount of time spent working compared with the amount of time spent recovering from work. They are commonly referred to as duty cycles. For example, spending 10 seconds working at a high-intensity bout and 30 seconds working at a low-intensity recovery gives a work–recovery ratio of 10 seconds to 30 seconds, or a 1:3 duty cycle. An important factor that is seldom discussed in interval design is the absolute cycle length. Take, for example, a series of intervals with the same 1:2 work–recovery duty cycles. Plugging base values of 10, 20, 30, 60, 120, or 300 seconds into that 1:2 ratio produces very different metabolic overloads. Table 8.1 shows the drastic differences among these interval protocols that occur when different values are plugged into this same ratio. So when you read informative articles that make work–recovery ratios sound like the only thing to be considered when developing an interval program, remember that at one time it sounded like a good idea to think of only Bernie Madoff when you invested your money . . . and we all know how that came out!

So what are the other factors to consider in interval training? The first, as you have seen, is the absolute length of the cycle. The second is how hard to work during the work and recovery intervals. The third is how many intervals to do. The fourth is how to vary the work–recovery cycles during a workout, and the fifth is how to vary the workout structure across a periodization cycle. Let's address these one at a time.

Cycle Length

The length of the work cycle is often associated with the energy system that is targeted; longer cycles target aerobic fitness and shorter cycles target anaerobic fitness. However, this is true only if the work cycle is done at maximal effort every time. Once the level of exercise is voluntarily reduced there is a significant shift toward the aerobic systems regardless of the cycle length. As for the length of the recovery cycle, remember that the shorter the recovery cycle, the less time the body has to recover its anaerobic systems. This means that each subsequent cycle is performed

Table 8.1 Interval Protocols and Metabolic Overload: Variations on a 1:2 Work–Recovery Ratio

Work cycle	Recovery cycle	Metabolic impact
10 s	20 s	Short work cycle allows the highest intensity. Short recovery times allow only partial recovery. Cycles are at a feasible length. Most effective for increasing rate of oxygen consumption typical of higher-intensity daily activities.
20 s	40 s	
30 s	60 s (1 min)	Moderately short work cycle allows for fairly high intensity. The somewhat longer recovery times allow more complete recovery. Cycles are still at a feasible length. Any number of studies have shown these cycles to be more effective than longer-distance steady-state programs.
60 s (1 min)	120 s (2 min)	Longer work cycles require the most difficult mix of work and recovery. The length of the recovery allows a more complete recovery of the anaerobic systems. A very difficult cycle to complete, perhaps too difficult to be feasible for a nonathletic population.
120 s (2 min)	240 s (4 min)	Work cycles of very low intensity with extremely long recovery times and ridiculously long overall cycle lengths. The cycle lengths make it more beneficial to just perform a steady-state exercise.
300 s (5 min)	600 s (10 min)	

at a lower intensity with a greater and greater contribution by the aerobic systems.

Intensity

How hard a person works is dictated by the difficulty of the movement, the speed at which the movement is performed, and the amount of resistance against which the exercise is performed. There are any number of ways to assess how hard a client is working during exercise; the most common are assessing HR and rating of perceived exertion (RPE). For interval training, HR is probably the least effective way to assess intensity, especially during high-intensity training. When considering the use of HR to assess intervals, recognize that increases in HR do not occur until the work interval has ended. Therefore using HR to assess intensity during a workout always places you in an assessment time warp. Also, increases in HR are cumulative across multiple cycles (see figure 8.11), but these accumulated effects can never be assessed accurately due to the ever-changing nature of interval design. So what is the best way to measure the intensity of exercise during interval training cycles? The answer is RPE. There are two derivations of the Borg RPE scale that are commonly used to evaluate exercise intensity: the 10-point and 20-point

scales. It really doesn't matter which one you use with clients, although the 10-point scale may be easier for most exercisers to understand. RPE can also be assessed by using a verbal rather than numerical scale. In our book *The South Beach Diet Supercharged* (Agaston & Signorile, 2008), Arthur Agatston and I developed a four-level scale and called the four levels *easy, moderate, revved up,* and *supercharged.* We defined these as being able to hold a conversation while exercising, being able to talk with some effort, being able to talk with great difficulty, and exercising as hard as possible. Regardless of the scale used, RPE is the best way to maintain proper intensity during interval training.

Number of Intervals

The number of intervals also affects the nature of the cardiovascular benefit the client receives. Figure 8.12 illustrates a series of alternating work–recovery cycles (10 seconds:20 seconds) that show two patterns that demonstrate the effect of interval training on oxygen consumption. First, notice that the greatest increases in oxygen consumption occur during the recovery cycle (light gray) rather than the work cycle (dark gray). Second, notice that the levels of oxygen consumption rise gradually and then plateau between the sixth interval and the eighth interval. This pattern demonstrates

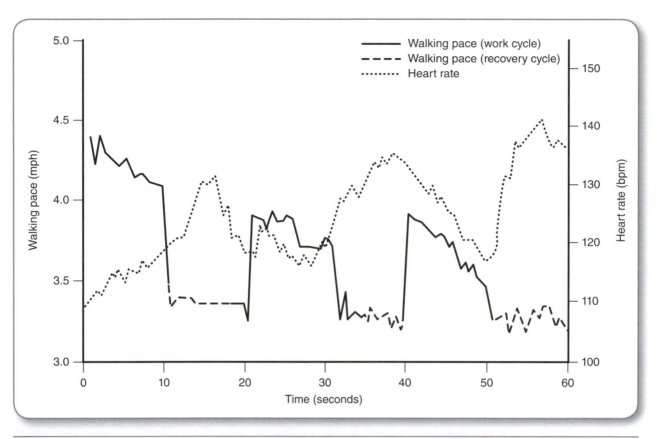

Figure 8.11   The relationship between pace (black line) and HR response (dotted line) across multiple work and recovery cycles.

that the belief that interval training is anaerobic and has no effect on the cardiovascular system has no basis in reality.

Variations in Work–Recovery Cycles

The only real question that remains is what duty cycle most efficiently trains the cardiovascular system. And the winner is . . . the old 2:1 standby composed of 20 seconds of work and 10 seconds of recovery. This is not to say that a work–recovery duty cycle of 20 seconds to 10 seconds is the panacea of cardiovascular training. In fact, the best idea is to use a diverse mix of work–recovery cycles depending on the desired work intensity, the desired $\dot{V}O_2$max, and the need to use reduced-intensity cycles for recovery.

The concepts underlying the cycle patterns for an interval training session follow some basic rules. First, at the beginning of the workout, long, low-intensity work cycles with short recoveries should be used to warm up the muscles and connective tissues. Then the work should build slowly, with intermediate-duration to long-duration

work cycles (20-30 seconds) alternating with shorter (15-20 seconds) recovery cycles. Finally, toward the end of the workout, the work cycles should be shortened (10-15 seconds) and the recovery cycles lengthened (20-30 seconds). If this pattern seems familiar, it's because it reflects both the long-term pattern seen in periodized training and the pattern evident in most of the aerobic training classes you have ever taken (see figure 8.13)—which, by the way, were interval training workouts. In fact, the pattern used to develop most interval programs is to nest different patterns of exercise within specific sections of the workout in order to maximize exercise effectiveness. I have coined the term *nested intervals* to describe this structuring since it reminds me of the nesting tables prominent in the 1960s and 1970s.

Periodization

The structuring of periodized programs can be addressed most effectively through the combined use of steady-state and interval workouts to create higher-volume and higher-intensity sessions.

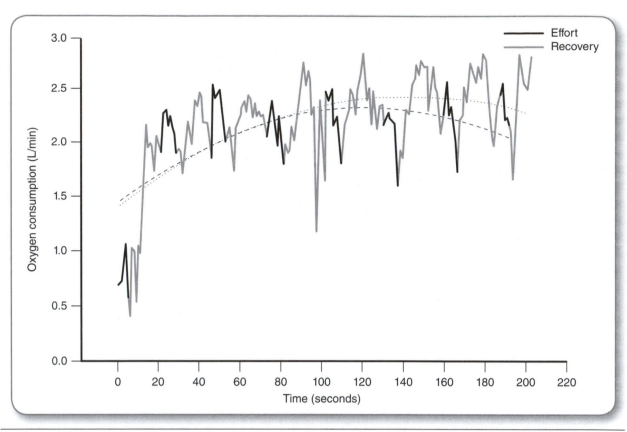

Figure 8.12 Patterns of oxygen consumption during eight work cycles (black lines) and recovery cycles (gray lines). The dotted and dashed lines represent the overall patterns as change for the effect and recovery portions of the workout.

When we examine structured periodization programs in chapter 9, we will expand upon these mixes.

Putting It All Together

You can now see that specific patterns should be followed when designing interval training sessions. These patterns are summarized in the box titled *Designing Interval Workouts.*

These patterns for interval training hold true, regardless of the environment in which the workout is performed. It is only the methods by which the volume and intensity of the workouts are manipulated that vary. As I mentioned, the intensity of a treadmill workout can be increased by increasing the speed or grade of the treadmill, while a client's movement speed and a machine's resistance levels can modify intensity on a cycle or stair-climber. In an aerobics class, intensity can be varied by increasing or decreasing the pitch (beat), varying the complexity of the movement, or changing the volume of muscle used (for example, using the lower body versus the upper body).

Designing Interval Workouts

1. The workout should increase in volume at the beginning and then later decrease in volume in favor of increasing intensity.

2. Within the overall pattern there should be cyclical changes in intensity and volume so that an increase in one is offset by a decrease in the other.

3. Intervals should be mixed in such a way that higher-intensity intervals are preceded and followed by lower-intensity intervals.

4. Higher-intensity intervals should be followed by recovery periods that are longer than those following the low-intensity intervals, especially as the workout progresses toward the end, when intensity should dominate.

5. Every workout should be preceded and followed by a warm-up and cool-down, respectively.

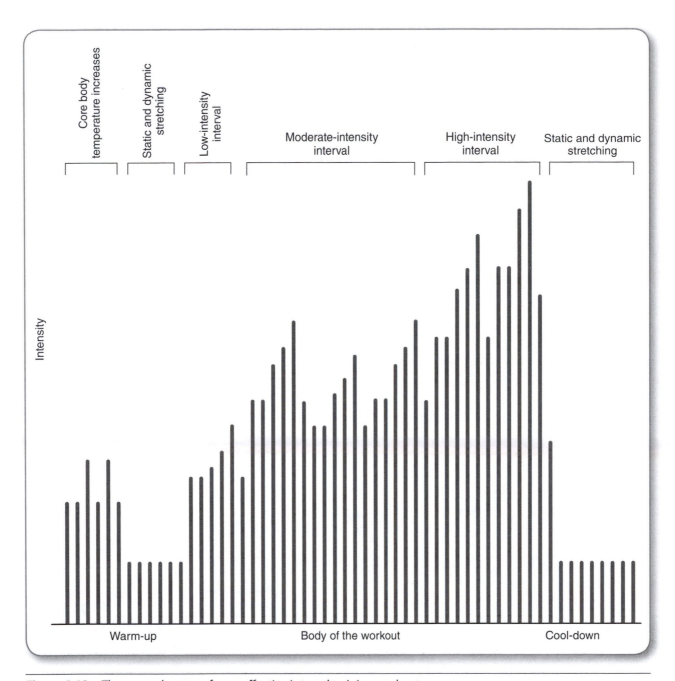

Figure 8.13   The general pattern for an effective interval training workout.

The resistance training classes that have the greatest effect on cardiovascular fitness are those that employ circuit training. However, low- to moderate-intensity programs don't appear to improve cardiovascular fitness except in individuals at low fitness levels, such as those just beginning a program or those returning to exercise after a prolonged layoff. High loads and high lifting speeds have been shown to be most effective. Additionally, shorter rest periods have

been shown to be more effective than longer rest periods when the goal is to target the cardiovascular system. Consider, however, that these higher-intensity protocols may not be safe for individuals rehabilitating after a cardiovascular incident.

So what are the numbers for resistance training that benefits cardiovascular health? Resistance levels should max out at 70% to 80% 1RM and can begin as low as 40% 1RM. Repetitions should be performed at near-maximum speed with a recovery period of approximately 20 seconds between sets. Some words of caution, however: Don't begin a program at either this load or this training speed. Also, if you incorporate high training speeds, try to limit them to the concentric portions of the lifts. Overall, given the positive effects that high-speed training has on power development and balance, you will be getting a two-for-one special with these training methods.

The aquatic training programs that have the greatest effect on cardiovascular fitness in older persons are high-intensity programs performed in shoulder-deep water or higher. When interval work is done in the pool, the speed of movement and resistance are interrelated due to the nature of water. This relationship has to do with the formula for the drag force in water:

$$F_D = (1/2) \cdot C_d \cdot p \cdot A \cdot v^2$$

where F_D = drag force, C_d = coefficient of drag, p = fluid density, A = frontal area exposed to flow, and v = velocity relative to the water.

As speed increases linearly, the drag force increases exponentially. Also, an increase in surface area and a change in shape can have a dramatic effect on the drag force. For example, changing the position of the hand relative to the flow of water affects the frontal surface area. Figure 8.14 shows a progression of hand positions providing increasingly greater drag forces. The level of drag can be increased further by adding paddles, webbed gloves, or other devices that increase frontal surface area. Other tools that can be used to increase oxygen consumption are flotation devices such as aquatic dumbbells, which require the user to exert continuous force if they are to be held beneath the water surface. Finally, one of the most important controlling factors dictating the level of work done in the pool is the depth of the water. The general rule is that deeper water means harder work. Applying these concepts in conjunction with a properly designed interval workout facilitates cardiovascular conditioning in an environment that is both safe and nurturing.

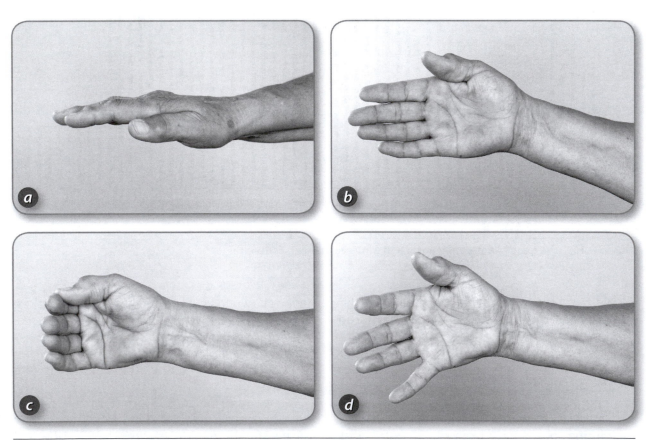

Figure 8.14   The (a) knife, (b) flat, (c) cupped, and (d) spread hand positions provide increasingly greater drag forces during pool exercises.

SUMMARY

Cardiovascular training is an effective tool for addressing the declines in oxidative capacity associated with the aging process. It also provides an intervention for dealing with the myriad of symptoms known as *metabolic syndrome.* Needless to say, heart attack and stroke are two of the major killers associated with aging, and the specters of diabetes and obesity materialize all too often in our sedentary fast-food society.

Periodized cardiovascular training using an undulating mix of high- to moderate-intensity exercise can successfully address these problems. It appears that in order to be the most effective, training methods should burn 2,000 kilocalories a week. This can be accomplished by incorporating interval training into the schedule. And finally, if your clients need a training partner, that furry little character that sits next to them can always be depended on when it comes time to go for a walk.

Topical Bibliography

Increasing Cardiovascular Fitness: Benefits and Methods

Baster, T., & Baster-Brooks, C. (2005). Exercise and hypertension. *Aust Fam Physician* 34:419-424.

Carretero, O.A., & Oparil, S. (2000). Essential hypertension: Part I: Definition and etiology. *Circulation* 101:329-335.

Cooper, K.H. (1968). *Aerobics.* New York: Bantam Books.

Coudert, J., & Van Praagh, E. (2000). Endurance exercise training in the elderly: Effects on cardiovascular function. *Curr Opin Clin Nutr Met Care* 3:479-483.

DiPietro, L., Dziura, J., Yeckel, C.W., & Neufer, P.D. (2006). Exercise and improved insulin sensitivity in older women: Evidence of the enduring benefits of higher intensity training. *J Appl Physiol* 100:142-149.

Ehsani, A.A., Ogawa, T., Miller, T.R., Spina, R.J., & Jilka, S.M. (1991). Exercise training improves left ventricular systolic function in older men. *Circulation* 83:96-103.

Evans, E.M., Racette, S.B., Peterson, L.R., Villareal, D.T., Greiwe, J.S., & Holloszy, J.O. (2005). Aerobic power and insulin action improve in response to endurance exercise training in healthy 77-87 yr olds. *J Appl Physiol* 98:40-45.

Frank, L.L., Sorensen, B.E., Yasui, Y., Tworoger, S.S., Schwartz, R.S., Ulrich, C.M., Irwin, M.L., Rudolph, R.E., Rajan, K.B., Stanczyk, F., Bowen, D., Weigle, D.S., Potter, J.D., & McTiernan, A. (2005). Effects of exercise on metabolic risk variables in overweight postmenopausal women: A randomized clinical trial. *Obesity Res* 13:615-625.

Harris, B.A. (2005). The influence of endurance and resistance exercise on muscle capillarization in the elderly: A review. *Acta Physiol Scand* 185:89-97.

Hautala, A., Torkkell, S., Raty, K., Junnari, T., Kantola, J., Mantsala, P., Hakala, J., & Ylihonko, K. (2003). Cardiovascular autonomic function correlates with the response to aerobic training in healthy sedentary subjects. *Am J Physiol Heart Circ Physiol* 285:H1747-H1752.

Huang, G., & Osness, W.H. (2005). Changes in pulmonary function response to a 10-week controlled exercise program in sedentary elderly adults. *Percept Mot Skills* 100:394-402.

Kay, S.J., & Fiatarone Singh, M.A. (2006). The influence of physical activity on abdominal fat: A systematic review of the literature. *Obes Rev* 7:183-200.

Kelly, G.A., & Kelly, K.S. (2007). Effects of aerobic exercise on lipids and lipoproteins in adults with type 2 diabetes: A meta-analysis of randomized-controlled trials. *Public Health* 121:643-655.

Kodama, S., Shu, M., Saito, K., Murakami, H., Tanaka, K., Kuno, S., Ajisaka, R., Sone, Y., Onitake, F., Takahashi, A., Shimano, H., Kondo, K., Yamada, N., & Sone, H. (2007). Even low-intensity and low-volume exercise training may improve insulin resistance in the elderly. *Intern Med* 46:1071-1077.

Kodama, S., Tanaka, S., Saito, K., Shu, M., Sone, Y., Onitake, F., Suzuki, E., Shimano, H., Yamamoto, S., Kondo, K., Ohashi, Y., Yamada, N., &

Sone, H. (2007). Effect of aerobic exercise training on serum levels of high-density lipoprotein cholesterol: A meta-analysis. *Arch Intern Med* 167:999-1008.

Kraus, W.E., Houmard, J.A., Duscha, B.D., Knetzger, K.J., Wharton, M.B., McCartney, J.S., Bales, C.W., Henes, S., Samsa, G.P., Otvos, J.D., Kulkarni, K.R., & Slentz, C.A. (2002). Effects of the amount and intensity of exercise on plasma lipoproteins. *N Engl J Med* 347:1483-1492.

Lavie, C.J., & Milani, R.V. (2007). Aerobic and resistance exercise training in the elderly. *Am J Geriatr Cardiol* 16:36-37.

Malfatto, G., Branzi, G., Riva, B., Sala, L., Leonetti, G., & Facchini, M. (2002). Recovery of cardiac autonomic responsiveness with low-intensity physical training in patients with chronic heart failure. *Eur J Heart Fail* 4:159-166.

McGuire, D.K., Levine, B.D., Williamson, J.W., Snell, P.G., Blomqvist, C.G., Saltin, B., & Mitchell, J.H. (2001). A 30-year follow-up of the Dallas Bedrest and Training Study: II. Effect of age on cardiovascular adaptation to exercise training. *Circulation* 104:1358-1366.

Pardo, Y., Merz, C.N., Velasquez, I., Paul-Labrador, M., Agarwala, A., & Peter, C.T. (2000). Exercise conditioning and heart rate variability: Evidence of a threshold effect. *Clin Cardiol* 23:615-620.

Pescatello, L.S., Franklin, B.A., Fagard, R., Farquhar, W.B., Kelley, G.A., Ray, C.A., & American College of Sports Medicine (2004). American College of Sports Medicine position stand. Exercise and hypertension. *Med Sci Sports Exerc* 36:533-553.

Pickering, G.P., Fellmann, N., Morio, B., Ritz, P., Amonchot, A., Vermorel, M., & Coudert, J. (1997). Effects of endurance training on the cardiovascular system and water compartments in elderly subjects. *J Appl Physiol* 83:1300-1306.

Poehlman, E.T., Dvorak, R.V., DeNino, W.F., Brochu, M., & Ades, P.A. (2000). Effects of resistance training and endurance training on insulin sensitivity in nonobese, young women: A controlled randomized trial. *J Clin Endocrinol Metab* 85:2463-2468.

Pogliaghi, S., Terziotti, P., Cevese, A., Balestreri, F., & Schena, F. (2006). Adaptations to endurance training in the healthy elderly: Arm cranking versus leg cycling. *Eur J Appl Physiol* 97:723-731.

Seals, D.R., Monahan, K.D., Bell, C., Tanaka, H., & Jones, P.P. (2001). The aging cardiovascular system: Changes in autonomic function at rest and in response to exercise. *International Journal of Sport Nutrition and Exercise Metabolism* 11:S189-S195.

Spina, R.J., Turner, M.J., & Ehsani, A.A. (1997). Exercise training enhances cardiac function in response to an afterload stress in older men. *Am J Physiol* 272:H995-H1000.

Teramoto, S., Fukuchi, Y., Nagase, T., Matsuse, T., Orimo, H. (1995). A comparison of ventilation components in young and elderly men during exercise. *J Gerontol A Biol Sci Med Sci* 50A(1): B34-39.

Terjung, R.L., Zarzeczny, R., & Yang, H.T. (2002). Muscle blood flow and mitochondrial function: Influence of aging. *Int J Sport Nutr Exerc Metab* 12:368-378.

Wilmore, J.H., Green, J.S., Stanforth, P.R., Gagnon, J., Rankinen, T., Leon, A.S., Rao, D.C., Skinner, J.S., & Bouchard, C. (2001). Relationship of changes in maximal and submaximal aerobic fitness to changes in cardiovascular disease and non-insulin-dependent diabetes mellitus risk factors with endurance training: The HERITAGE Family Study. *Metabolism* 50:1255-1263.

Yataco, A.R., Fleisher, L.A., & Katzel, L.I. (1997). Heart rate variability and cardiovascular fitness in senior athletes. *Am J Cardiol* 80:1389-1391.

Cardiovascular Fitness Testing

American Thoracic Society Board of Directors. (2002). ATS statement: Guidelines for the six-minute walk test. *Res Crit Care Med* 166:111-117.

Enright, P.L. (2003). The 6-minute walk test. *Respir Care* 48:783-785.

Enright, P.L., McBurnie, M.A., Bittner, V., Tracy, R.P., McNamara, R., Arnold, A., & Newman, A.B. (2003). The 6 minute walk test: A quick measure of functional status in elderly adults. *CHEST* 123:387-398.

Rikli, R.E., & Jones, C.J. (1999a). Development and validation of a functional fitness test for community-residing older adults. *Journal of Aging and Physical Activity* 7:129-161.

Rikli, R.E., & Jones, C.J. (1999b). Functional fitness normative scores for community residing older adults, ages 60-94. *Journal of Aging and Physical Activity* 7:162-181.

Roomi, J., Johnson, M.M., Waters, K., Yohannes, A., Helm, A., & Connolly, M.J. (1996). Respiratory rehabilitation, exercise capacity and quality of life in chronic airways disease in old age. *Age Ageing* 25:12-16.

Cardiovascular Training and Program Design

Agaston, A., & Signorile, J.F. (2008) The South Beach diet supercharged. New York: Rodale.

Ahmaidi, S., Masse-Biron, J., Adam, B., Choquet, D., Freville, M., Libert, J.P., & Prefaut, C. (1998). Effects of interval training at the ventilatory threshold on clinical and cardiorespiratory responses in elderly humans. *Eur J Appl Physiol Occup Physiol* 78:170-176.

Altena, T.S., Michaelson, J.L., Ball, D., & Thomas, T.R. (2004). Single sessions of intermittent and continuous exercise and postprandial lipemia. *Med Sci Sport Exerc* 36:1364-1371.

American Thoracic Society Board of Directors. (2002). ATS statement: Guidelines for the six-minute walk test. *Res Crit Care Med* 166:111-117.

Atlantis, E., Chin-Moi, C., Kirby, A., & Fiaterone-Singh, M.A. (2006). Worksite intervention effects on physical health: A randomized controlled trial. *Health Promotion International* 21:191-200.

Bauman, A.E., Russell, S.J., Furber, S.E., & Dobson, A.J. (2001). The epidemiology of dog walking: An unmet need for human and canine health. *Med J Aust* 175:632-634.

Beckham, S.G., & Earnest, C.P. (2000). Metabolic cost of free weight circuit weight training. *J Sports Med Phys Fitness* 40:118-125.

Bermingham, M.A., Mahajan, D., & Neaverson, M.A. (2004). Blood lipids of cardiac patients after acute exercise on land and in water. *Arch Phys Med Rehabil* 85:509-511.

Branch, J.D., Pate, R.R., & Bourque, S.P. (2000). Moderate intensity exercise training improves cardiorespiratory fitness in women. *J Womens Health Gend Based Med* 9:65-73.

Branch, J.D., Pate, R.R., Bourque, S.P., Convertino, V.A., Durstine, J.L., & Ward, D.S. (1999). Exercise training and intensity does not alter vascular volume responses in women. *Aviat Space Environ Med* 70:1070-1076.

Brentano, M.A., Cadore, E.L., Da Silva, E.M., Ambrosini, A.B., Coertjens, M., Petkowicz, R., Viero, I., & Kruel, L.F. (2008). Physiological adaptations to strength and circuit training in postmenopausal women with bone loss. *J Strength Cond Res* 22:1816-1825.

Broman, G., Quintana, M., Lindberg, T., Jansson, E., & Kaijser, L. (2006). High intensity deep water training can improve aerobic power in elderly women. *Eur J Appl Physiol* 98:117-123.

Brown, S.G., & Rhodes, R.E. (2006). Relationships among dog ownership and leisure-time walking in Western Canadian adults. *Am J Prev Med* 30:131-136.

Chu, K.S., Eng, J.J., Dawson, A.S., Harris, J.E., Ozkaplan, A., & Gylfadóttir, S. (2004). Water-based exercise for cardiovascular fitness in people with chronic stroke: A randomized controlled trial. *Arch Phys Med Rehabil* 85:870-874.

DeGroot, D.W., Quinn, T.J., Kertzer, R., Vroman, N.B., & Olney, W.B. (1998). Circuit weight training in cardiac patients: Determining optimal workloads for safety and energy expenditure. *Journal of Cardiopulmonary Rehabilitation* 18:145-152.

Dimopoulosa, S., Anastasiou-Nanab, M., Sakellarioua, D., Drakosb, S., Kapsimalakoua, S., Maroulidisb, G., Roditisa, P., Papazachoua, O., Vogiatzisa, I., Roussosa, C., & Nanasa, S. (2006). Effects of exercise rehabilitation program on heart rate recovery in patients with chronic heart failure. *Eur J Cardiovasc Prev Rehabil* 13:67-73.

Duncan, G.E., Anton, S.D., Sydeman, S.J., Newton Jr, R.L., Corsica, J.A., Durning, P.E., Ketterson, T.U., Martin, A.D., Limacher, M.C., & Perri, M.G. (2005). Prescribing exercise at varied levels of intensity and frequency: A randomized trial. *Arch Intern Med* 165:2362-2369.

Duncan, J.J., Gordon, N.F., & Scott, C.B. (1991). Women walking for health and fitness. How much is enough? *JAMA* 266:3295-3299.

Egaña, M., & Donne, B. (2004). Physiological changes following a 12 week gym based stair-climbing, elliptical trainer and treadmill running program in females. *J Sports Med Phys Fitness* 44:141-146.

Eriksen, L., Dahl-Petersen, I., Haugaard, S.B., & Dela, F. (2007). Comparison of the effect of multiple short-duration with single long-duration exercise sessions on glucose homeostasis in type 2 diabetes mellitus. *Diabetologia* 50:2245-2253.

Eriksson, J., Tuominen, J., Valle, T., Sundberg, S., Sovijärvi, A., Lindholm, H., Tuomilehto, J., & Koivisto, V. (1998). Aerobic endurance exercise or circuit-type resistance training for individuals with impaired glucose tolerance? *Horm Metab Res* 30:37-41.

Gaesser, G.A., & Rich, R.G. (1984). Effects of high- and low-intensity exercise training on aerobic capacity and blood lipids. *Med Sci Sports Exerc* 16:269-274.

Gettman, L.R., Ayres, J.J., Pollock, M.L., & Jackson, A. (1978). The effect of circuit weight training on strength, cardiorespiratory function, and body composition of adult men. *Med Sci Sports* 10:171-176.

Gettman, L.R., Ward, P., & Hagan, R.D. (1982). A comparison of combined running and weight training with circuit weight training. *Med Sci Sports Exerc* 14:229-234.

Gossard, D., Haskell, W.L., Taylor, C.B., Mueller, J.K., Rogers, F., Chandler, M., Ahn, D.K., Miller, N.H., & DeBusk, R.F. (1986). Effects of low- and high-intensity home-based exercise training on functional capacity in healthy middle-aged men. *Am J Cardiol* 57:446-449.

Graves, J.E., Martin, A.D., Miltenberger, L.A., & Pollock, M.L. (1988). Physiological responses to walking with hand weights, wrist weights, and ankle weights. *Med Sci Sports Exerc* 20:265-271.

Haennel, R., Teo, K.K., Quinney, A., & Kappagoda, T. (1989). Effects of hydraulic circuit training on cardiovascular function. *Med Sci Sports Exerc* 21:605-612.

Haltom, R.W., Kraemer, R.P., Sloan, R.A., Hebert, E.P., Frank, K., & Tryniecki, J.L. (1999). Circuit weight training and its effects on excess postexercise oxygen consumption. *Medicine and Science in Sports and Exercise* 31:1613-1618.

Huffman, K.M., Samsa, G.P., Slentz, C.A., Duscha, B.D., Johnson, J.L., Bales, C.W., Tanner, C.J., Houmard, J.A., & Kraus, W.E. (2006). Response of high-sensitivity C-reactive protein to exercise training in an at-risk population. *Am Heart J* 152:793-800.

Jürimäe, T., Jürimäe, J., & Pihl, E. (2000). Circulatory response to single circuit weight and walking training sessions of similar energy cost in middle-aged overweight females. *Clin Physiol* 20:143-149.

Kokkinos, P.F., Narayan, P., & Papademetriou, V. (2001). Exercise as hypertension therapy. *Cardiol Clin* 19:507-516.

Maiorana, A.J., Briffa, T.G., Goodman, C., & Hung, J. (1997). A controlled trial of circuit weight training on aerobic capacity and myocardial oxygen demand in men after coronary artery bypass surgery. *J Cardiopulmonary Rehabil* 17:239-247.

Mayer-Davis, E.J., D'Agostino Jr, R., Karter, A.J., Haffner, S.M., Rewers, M.J., Saad, M., & Bergman, R.N. (1998). Intensity and amount of physical activity in relation to insulin sensitivity: The Insulin Resistance Atherosclerosis Study. *JAMA* 279:669-674.

Miyashita, M., Burns, S.F., & Stensel, D.J. (2006). Exercise and postprandial lipemia: Effect of continuous compared with intermittent activity patterns. *Am J Clin Nutr* 83:24-29.

Monteiro, A.G., Alveno, D.A., Prado, M., Monteiro, G.A., Ugrinowitsch, C., Aoki, M.S., & Piçarro, I.C. (2008). Acute physiological responses to different circuit training protocols. *J Sports Med Phys Fitness* 48:438-442.

Motoyama, M., Sunami, Y., Kinoshita, F., Kiyonaga, A., Tanaka, H., Shindo, M., Irie, T., Urata, H., Sasaki, J., & Arakawa, K. (1998). Blood pressure lowering effect of low intensity aerobic training in elderly hypertensive patients. *Med Sci Sport Exerc* 30:818-823.

O'Leary, V.B., Marchetti, C.M., Krishnan, R.K., Stetzer, B.P., Gonzalez, F., & Kirwan, J.P. (2006). Exercise induced reversal of insulin resistance in obese elderly is associated with reduced visceral fat. *J Appl Physiol* 100:1584-1589.

Oja, P. (2001). Dose response between total volume of physical activity and health and fitness. *Med Sci Sport Exerc* 33:S428-S437.

Owens, S.G., al-Ahmed, A., & Moffatt, R.J. (1989). Physiological effects of walking and running with hand-held weights. *J Sports Med Phys Fitness* 29:384-387.

Park, S.K., Park, J.H., Kwon, Y.C., Yoon, M.S., & Kim, C.K. (2003). The effect of long-term aerobic exercise on maximal oxygen consumption, left ventricular function and serum lipids in elderly women. *J Physiol Anthropol* 22:11-17.

Petersen, S., Miller, G., Quinney, H.A., & Wenger, H.A. (1988). The influence of high-velocity resistance training on aerobic power. *Journal of Orthopedic Sports Physical Therapy* 9:339-344.

Petersen, S.R., Haennel, R.G., Kappagoda, C.T., Belcastro, A.N., Reid, D.C., Wenger, H.A., & Quinney, H.A. (1989). The influence of high-velocity circuit resistance training on V̇O₂max and cardiac output. *Can J Sport Sci* 14:158-163.

Pichot, V., Roche, F., Denis, C., Garet, M., Duverney, D., Costes, F., & Barthélémy, J.C. (2005). Interval training in elderly men increases both heart rate variability and baroreflex activity. *Clin Auton Res* 15:107-115.

Simonsick, E.M., Guralnik, J.M., Volpato, S., Balfour, J., & Fried, L.P. (2005). Just get out the door! Importance of walking outside the home for maintaining mobility: Findings from the Women's Health and Aging Study. *J Am Geriatr Soc* 53:198-203.

Tabata, I., Irisawa, K., Kouzaki, M., Nishimura, K., Ogita, F., & Miyachi, M. (1997). Metabolic profile of high intensity intermittent exercises. *Med Sci Sports Exerc* 29:390-395.

Tabata, I., Nishimura, K., Kouzaki, M., Hirai, Y., Ogita, F., Miyachi, M., & Yamamoto, K. (1996). Effects of moderate-intensity endurance and high-intensity intermittent training on anaerobic and V̇O₂max. *Medicine and Science in Sports and Exercise* 28:1327-1330.

Takeshima, N., Tanaka, K., Kobayashi, F., Watanabe, T., & Kato, T. (1993). Effects of aerobic exercise conditioning at intensities corresponding to lactate threshold in the elderly. *Eur J Appl Physiol* 67:138-143.

Talanian, J.L., Galloway, S.D., Heigenhauser, G.J., Bonen, A., & Spriet, L.L. (2007). Two weeks of high-intensity aerobic interval training increases the capacity for fat oxidation during exercise in women. *J Appl Physiol* 102:1439-1447.

Tanaka, H., Monahan, K.D., & Seals, D.R. (2001). Age-predicted maximal heart rate revisited. *J Am Coll Cardiol* 37:153-156.

Taunton, J.E., Rhodes, E.C., Wolski, L.A., Donelly, M., Warren, J., Elliot, J., McFarlane, L., Leslie, J., Mitchell, J., & Lauridsen, B. (1996). Effect of land-based and water-based fitness programs on the cardiovascular fitness, strength and flexibility of women aged 65-75 years. *Gerontology* 42:204-210.

Thorpe Jr, R.J., Simonsick, E.M., Brach, J.S., Ayonayon, H., Satterfield, S., Harris, T.B., Garcia, M., & Kritchevsky, S.B. (2006). Dog ownership, walking behavior, and maintained mobility in late life. *J Am Geriatr Soc* 54:1419-1424.

Verney, J., Kadi, F., Saafi, M.A., Piehl-Aulin, K., & Denis, C. (2006). Combined lower body endurance and upper body resistance training improves performance and health parameters in healthy active elderly. *Eur J Appl Physiol* 97:288-297.

Vincent, K.R., Braith, R.W., Feldman, R.A., Kallas, H.E., & Lowenthal, D.T. (2002). Improved cardiorespiratory endurance following 6 months of resistance exercise in elderly men and women. *Arch Intern Med* 162:673-678.

Vogiatzis, I., Terzis, G., Nanas, S., Stratakos, G., Simoes, D.C., Georgiadou, O., Zakynthinos, S., & Roussos, C. (2005). Skeletal muscle adaptations to interval training in patients with advanced COPD. *CHEST* 128:3838-3845.

Wisløff, U., Støylen, A., Loennechen, J.P., Bruvold, M., Rognmo, Ø., Haram, P.M., Tjønna, A.E., Helgerud, J., Helgerud, J., Slørdahl, S.A., Lee, S.J., Bye, A., Smith, G.L., Najjar, S.M., Ellingsen, Ø., & Skjaerpe, T. (2007). Superior cardiovascular effect of aerobic interval training versus moderate continuous training in heart failure patients: A randomized study. *Circulation* 115:3086-3094.

References

Agaston, A., & Signorile, J.F. (2008) The South Beach diet supercharged. New York: Rodale.

Altena, T.S., Michaelson, J.L., Ball, D., & Thomas, T.R. (2004). Single sessions of intermittent and continuous exercise and postprandial lipemia. *Med Sci Sport Exerc* 36:1364-1371.

Bauman, A.E., Russell, S.J., Furber, S.E., & Dobson, A.J. (2001). The epidemiology of dog walking: An unmet need for human and canine health. *Med J Aust* 175:632-634.

Brown, S.G., & Rhodes, R.E. (2006). Relationships among dog ownership and leisure-time walking in Western Canadian adults. *Am J Prev Med* 30:131-136.

Cooper, K.H. (1968). *Aerobics.* New York: Bantam Books.

Eriksen, L., Dahl-Petersen, I., Haugaard, S.B., & Dela, F. (2007). Comparison of the effect of multiple short-duration with single long-duration exercise sessions on glucose homeostasis in type 2 diabetes mellitus. *Diabetologia* 50:2245-2253.

Kokkinos, P.F., Narayan, P., & Papademetriou, V. (2001). Exercise as hypertension therapy. *Cardiol Clin* 19:507-516.

Mayer-Davis, E.J., D'Agostino Jr, R., Karter, A.J., Haffner, S.M., Rewers, M.J., Saad, M., & Bergman, R.N. (1998). Intensity and amount of physical activity in relation to insulin sensitivity: The Insulin Resistance Atherosclerosis Study. *JAMA* 279:669-674.

Miyashita, M., Burns, S.F., & Stensel, D.J. (2006). Exercise and postprandial lipemia: Effect of continuous compared with intermittent activity patterns. *Am J Clin Nutr* 83:24-29.

O'Leary, V.B., Marchetti, C.M., Krishnan, R.K., Stetzer, B.P., Gonzalez, F., & Kirwan, J.P. (2006). Exercise induced reversal of insulin resistance in obese elderly is associated with reduced visceral fat. *J Appl Physiol* 100:1584-1589.

Pescatello, L.S., Franklin, B.A., Fagard, R., Farquhar, W.B., Kelley, G.A., Ray, C.A., & American College of Sports Medicine (2004). American College of Sports Medicine position stand. Exercise and hypertension. *Med Sci Sports Exerc* 36:533-553.

Rikli, R.E., & Jones, C.J. (1999). Development and validation of a functional fitness test for community-residing older adults. *Journal of Aging and Physical Activity* 7:129-161.

Simonsick, E.M., Guralnik, J.M., Volpato, S., Balfour, J., & Fried, L.P. (2005). Just get out the door! Importance of walking outside the home for maintaining mobility: Findings from the Women's Health and Aging Study. *J Am Geriatr Soc* 53:198-203.

Talanian, J.L., Galloway, S.D., Heigenhauser, G.J., Bonen, A., & Spriet, L.L. (2007). Two weeks of high-intensity aerobic interval training increases the capacity for fat oxidation during exercise in women. *J Appl Physiol* 102:1439-1447.

Tanaka, H., Monahan, K.D., & Seals, D.R. (2001). Age-predicted maximal heart rate revisited. *J Am Coll Cardiol* 37:153-156.

Terjung, R.L., Zarzeczny, R., & Yang, H.T. (2002). Muscle blood flow and mitochondrial function: Influence of aging. *Int J Sport Nutr Exerc Metab* 12:368-378.

Thorpe Jr, R.J., Simonsick, E.M., Brach, J.S., Ayonayon, H., Satterfield, S., Harris, T.B., Garcia, M., & Kritchevsky, S.B. (2006). Dog ownership, walking behavior, and maintained mobility in late life. *J Am Geriatr Soc* 54:1419-1424.

Putting the
Program Together

Part III of this book shows you how to apply the previously learned concepts to real-life situations. In chapter 9 you will learn how to design targeted training cycles based on the periodization model, which uses the proper mix of work and recovery to maximize improvements and reduce the potential for overtraining and injury. Chapter 10 addresses the question of what to do during the scheduled recovery periods that will still contribute to clients' progress. The answer is the translational periods exclusive to this book. These periods allow you to convert clients' physical gains into performance patterns that they will use in daily activities. In this way, you can continuously modify your clients' training programs to match their evolving needs.

Periodized Training

Organizing your client's program into logical training cycles is the final step in successfully bending the aging curves. But doing this involves much more than just slapping together a critical mass of exercises in some sort of workout smorgasbord. Instead, it involves creating a carefully orchestrated banquet with each course designed to maximize the benefit to the client and reduce the possibility for exercise indigestion. Periodizing training by combining specific training cycles that target individual needs with the proper pattern of work and recovery allows you to construct the most effective program with the lowest risk for overtraining or overuse injury. This chapter shows how specific cycles associated with different physiological needs can be constructed and then applied within an overall program.

In this chapter, we'll look at periodization theory and application. Then we'll examine why periodization may be of special importance to older individuals both when training is just beginning for them and when exercise has become a part of their lives.

PERIODIZATION: THE UNDERLYING THEORIES

Periodization is the development and application of a training calendar that uses targeted work and recovery cycles to maximize gains and reduce the incidence of overtraining and overuse injuries. To understand how periodization works, let's look at the supercompensation curve and the two theories that explain its shape.

The Supercompensation Curve

The classic supercompensation curve, which illustrates changes in performance resulting from training, has four phases (see figure 9.1). These phases are as follows:

1. The fatigue or depletion phase, during which performance level declines
2. The compensation or restitution phase, during which performance level increases
3. The supercompensation or overcompensation phase, during which the performance level increases above the original baseline level
4. The involution or detraining phase, during which performance level drops to baseline due to a cessation of training

To this supercompensation curve I have added an additional component, which is represented by the dashed line in figure 9.1. This line illustrates a phase of prolonged fatigue that occurs due to continued training and that is known as *overtraining* or *staleness*. Exercise is a stress, and the body will adapt to that stress. But like any stress, exercise can be applied at too high a level or for too long a time, in which case it ultimately produces a negative result. That result may be as transient as a sore muscle group the day after a workout or as final as death.

APPLICATION POINT Since training is a stressor, it is not surprising that recovery is a necessary component of the supercompensation concept.

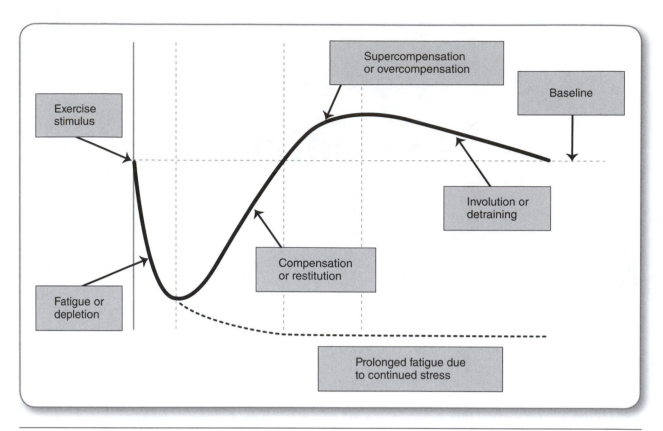

Figure 9.1   The phases of the supercompensation curve.

Shape of the Supercompensation Curve

Originally, the shape of the supercompensation curve was attributed to a single factor, fatigue. It was believed that fatigue caused the downward or depletion portion of the curve and that the removal of fatigue through rest or recovery caused the upward swing to supercompensation. However, this theory did not actually explain the shape of the curve since removal of fatigue, with no other influences, should result only in a return to baseline. A more recent and prevalent model is the fitness–fatigue model presented by Edward Bannister (Chiu & Barnes, 2003). This model holds that fitness and fatigue are two opposing effects that coexist during training. Their additive effects dictate the shape of the supercompensation curve. While some scientists and practitioners see this model as incompatible with classic supercompensation theory, most see it as a viable explanation for the shape of the curve (see figure 9.2).

The difference between the two theories is subtle but may have considerable effect on the application of periodization to training. Modern training theory encourages strategies that maximize fitness effect and minimize fatigue. You might ask, "Why not just give my client the minimal amount of work and avoid all of the potential problems associated with overtraining?" The reply is that fatigue is an inevitable consequence of training overload, and overload leads to adaptation. The optimal balance between fitness and fatigue is shown in figure 9.3. The solid line depicts the ideal overload that leads to maximum training response. The dashed line shows what occurs when the overload is too low to generate a maximal response. The dotted line shows what happens when the overload is so great that the fatigue response dominates and there is little or no supercompensation. So the training strategies you use *should* cause fatigue, but they should also maximize the fitness effect. This is especially important in older, nonathletic populations for which undue fatigue can cause overtraining, overuse injuries, and noncompliance.

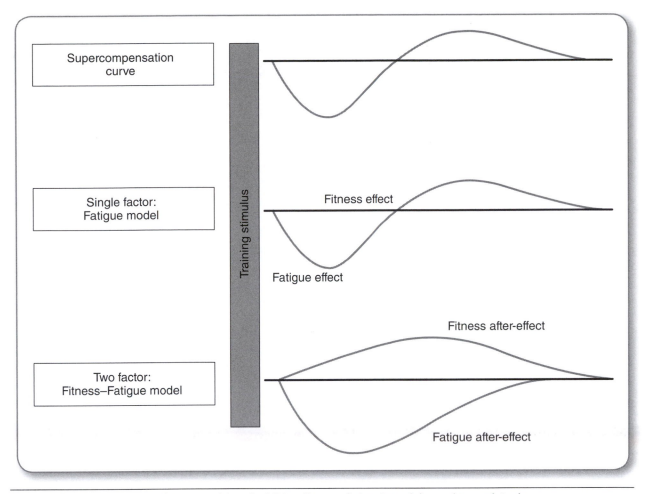

Figure 9.2 The sequential (fatigue-only) and additive (fitness–fatigue) models used to explain the supercompensation curve.

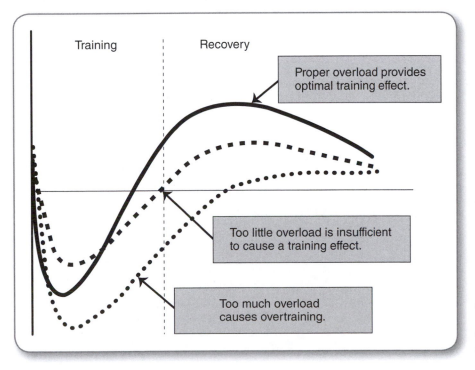

Figure 9.3 The relationships among overload, depletion, and training response.

APPLICATION POINT   You are likely familiar with the positive "feeling" that often follows your shower after a tiring workout. This is a rudimentary example of the fitness–fatigue model in action.

FATIGUE DURING TIME-BASED TRAINING CYCLES

Before we address proper strategies to optimize training and reduce the potential for overtraining and overuse injuries, let's look at the time-based cycles associated with periodized training. Table 9.1 shows the three major periodization cycles (the microcycle, mesocycle, macrocycle), the event and daily cycles, and the factors associated with fatigue during each cycle. The fatigue factors are arranged in order of importance for each cycle. These cycles are like building blocks in that the microcycles are used to build the mesocycles and the mesocycles are used to construct the macrocycles (see figure 9.4).

As shown in table 9.1, the event cycle is the smallest building unit (like a particle of clay within a single brick). It is a single workout or training session. During this single training session, fatigue results from depletion of creatine phosphate stores and possibly from muscle and liver glycogen depletion during training bouts of long duration. Other contributing factors include waste product buildup, diminished calcium flux within the muscle fiber, and a reduced capacity of the motor nerve to fire muscle fibers.

The daily training cycle (the single brick) is the workout schedule for a day. Fatigue within this time frame is most likely the result of reduced glycogen stores, muscle damage, peripheral nervous system fatigue, and central nervous system fatigue (an inability to send adequate neural messages to the working muscles).

The microcycle is the weekly planning schedule (seven bricks). Fatigue during this cycle results from reductions in longer-term fuel sources such as muscle and liver glycogen and from increases in muscle damage. Additionally, decrements in the ability of the central and peripheral nervous systems to drive the muscles and other tissues can accumulate across training days.

The mesocycle (multiweek) fatigue aftereffect is based on the fatigue accumulated across multiple microcycles (multiple sets of seven bricks). The factors involved include central nervous system

Table 9.1   Training Cycles

Cycle	Exercise stimulus	Source of fatigue aftereffect
Event cycle	Single training bout	Fuel source depletion Waste product buildup Peripheral neuromuscular fatigue
Daily cycle	Repeated training bouts on a single day	Fuel source depletion Microscopic muscle damage Peripheral nervous system fatigue
Microcycle	Specific overload applied on a daily basis	Fuel source depletion Microscopic muscle damage Central nervous system fatigue Peripheral nervous system fatigue
Mesocycle	Weekly training bouts continued over a number of weeks	Central nervous system fatigue Fuel source depletion Microscopic muscle damage Connective tissue damage Neuroendocrine disruption
Macrocycle	Combined effects of individual mesocycles	Central nervous system fatigue Neuroendocrine disruption Muscle and connective tissue injury

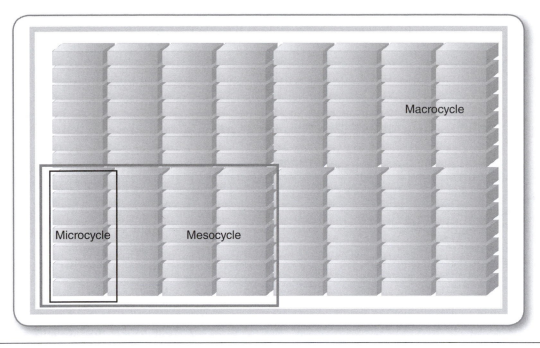

Figure 9.4 A brick wall analogy of periodization cycles.

fatigue, glycogen depletion, and muscle damage. Additionally, connective tissue damage due to accumulated overuse may become apparent at this point. The effects of training also manifest in the neuroendocrine system. Stress hormones begin to increase and the anabolic (tissue-building) hormones are stunted. These factors are the major markers of overtraining syndrome.

The largest cycle is the macrocycle (the entire wall), which may be a seasonal, annual, or even multiyear cycle. In this text, we will look at it as a yearly plan. This plan will change from year to year as the competing effects of aging and training selectively affect the different systems of the body. Fatigue during the macrocycle is once again a cumulative effect, but this time it accumulates over multiple mesocycles. The major responses are overuse injuries, central nervous system fatigue, and neuroendocrine (nerve and hormone) disruption.

CONTROLLING THE FITNESS–FATIGUE BALANCE DURING TRAINING

The goal of a properly designed periodization program is to offer sufficient overload to produce change while avoiding levels of fatigue that can lead to overtraining or overuse injuries. By using targeted training cycles you can address your clients' specific needs within the framework of the periodized model.

The Event Cycle

For a single workout, or event cycle, the balance between fitness and fatigue is accomplished by using a properly designed work–recovery duty cycle. This is the same concept of matching work and recovery that we discussed for resistance training. If you look back at table 7.1 (p. 138), you'll notice that the lifting patterns that require the greatest effort (those targeting maximal strength) are matched with the longest recoveries. At the same time, the lifting patterns that require less effort, such as those targeting muscular endurance and hypertrophy, are coupled with shorter recoveries. Part of the need for this work–recovery balancing act can be attributed to the conflicting effects of acute fatigue and postactivation potentiation (the increase in performance seen after conditioning contractions). Within the event cycle, these effects can be compared with the fitness and fatigue aftereffects responsible for the shape of the supercompensation curve (see figure 9.5). A properly designed interval training workout employs the same strategies that the longer micro- and

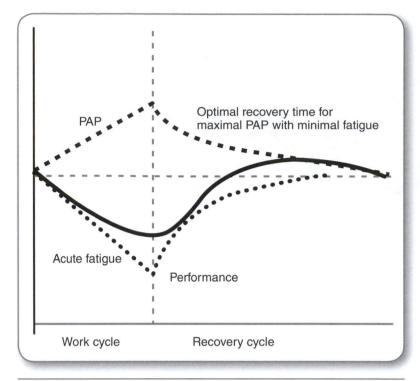

Figure 9.5   Acute responses to training showing the additive effects of fatigue and postactivation potentiation (PAP).

I'm still having a hard time squatting down to pick things up!" It is clear from the scientific literature that the pain felt a day or two after a workout, or DOMS, is the result of microscopic damage to muscles and connective tissues. DOMS can take as long as 2 weeks to repair and in extreme cases can even lead to a condition called *rhabdomyolysis* in which enzymes, other proteins, and cell by-products leak through the damaged membrane of the muscle cell into the bloodstream and cause kidney damage or even kidney failure. In untrained older adults the potential for this problem is prevalent, especially at the beginning of a training program. So proceed gradually, avoid the temptation to perform multiple high-intensity workouts in a day, and don't try to work through the pain. Remember, you can either give the body the recovery it needs today or spend months recovering after an overuse injury.

mesocycles employ. At the beginning of the interval workout there is a warm-up that prepares the tissues for work. Then there is the body of the workout, in which work–recovery duty cycles rise and fall, always building toward an increase in intensity (increases in intensity dictate decreases in duration). Finally, the workout ends with a cool-down, during which the intensity and duration of the work taper to allow recovery as the workout is completed.

The Daily Cycle

We can address fatigue during the daily cycle by logically planning the patterns of training within a day. There are two concepts that usually destroy these plans:

- No pain, no gain.
- More is better.

These two myths still guide many of us when we train. We know intellectually that they are incorrect, and yet we still talk about effective workouts by using statements such as, "What a great workout—when I finished I could hardly walk!" and "I had a fabulous workout yesterday—

Microcycles and Mesocycles

Structuring microcycles to maximize the fitness aftereffect while still providing sufficient overload to bring about a training effect across a mesocycle is a challenge. There are several different periodization strategies that have been used to maximize benefits. Among the most prevalent are classic linear periodization, nonlinear periodization, and block periodization. Classic linear periodization uses opposing curvilinear changes in volume and intensity and an increase in technique practice across its preparatory, competition, and transition phases (see figure 9.6a). The nonlinear or undulating strategy adds waves of change to the linear model. Volume and intensity follow the same overall patterns, but the levels rise and fall within the patterns (see figure 9.6b). In fact, it has been suggested that hypertrophy, strength, and power can each be addressed on separate days during a single training week. It should be recognized, however, that many coaches and exercise scientists argue that all periodization is nonlinear. The final periodization strategy, block periodization, uses targeted blocks to concentrate

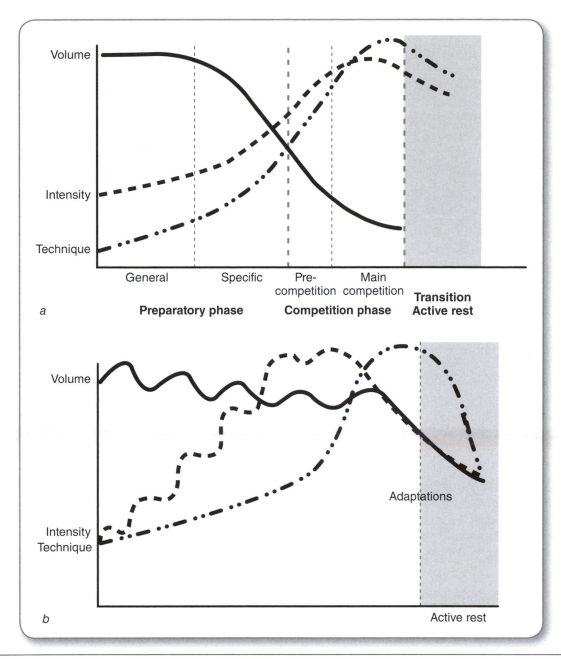

Figure 9.6 *(a)* The classic linear training cycle illustrating a gradual increase in intensity and decrease in volume across the training period. *(b)* An undulating, or nonlinear, mesocycle. Note the fluctuations in intensity and volume and the reciprocating nature of this undulation, in which increases in intensity are associated with decreases in volume and vice versa.

on specific factors. Since the training effects of these blocks have a certain residual or carryover effect, the order of training can be designed to maximize efficiency (see figure 9.7). Examples of these carryovers are provided in table 9.2.

So which is the correct strategy? My answer is . . . they are all correct. Figure 9.8 shows how the linear, undulating, and block concepts can all

come together seamlessly. Note that I have divided the mixed periodization scheme in figure 9.8 into two major contextual areas or phases, targeted training and translation. The targeted training phase is dictated by the diagnosis of the client's needs and the translation phase is used to translate the improvements made during training into motor patterns applicable to daily performance.

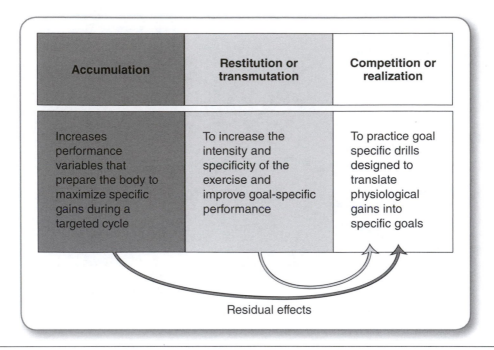

Figure 9.7   The blocks associated with the block periodization method.

The targeted training is further subdivided into accumulation (building) and transfer (peaking) blocks. Within the context of block periodization, we can apply training with longer hangover times, such as strength or aerobic endurance training, during the accumulation block and combine this training with more specific goals such as speed or more anaerobic-based endurance during the transfer block. The realization block is synonymous with the translational phase. During realization, or translation, the gains from the first two training blocks are translated into real-life function. If you examine the volume and intensity lines in figure 9.8 you'll notice the combined influences of the linear and undulating periodization models. There is a general pattern of increase throughout the initial portion of the targeted training phase, and then volume decreases to allow further increases in intensity. This is followed by a decrease in intensity to allow a taper containing the motor pattern train-

Table 9.2	Carryover Effects From Training	
Motor ability	**Residual duration (days)**	**Physiological background**
Aerobic endurance	30 ± 5	Increase in aerobic enzymes, number of mitochondria, muscle capillaries, hemoglobin capacity, glycogen storage, and fat metabolism
Maximum strength	30 ± 5	Improvement of neural mechanism and muscle hypertrophy due mainly to muscle fiber enlargement
Aerobic glycolytic endurance	18 ± 4	Increase in anaerobic enzymes, buffering capacity, and glycogen storage and lactate accumulation
Strength endurance	15 ± 5	Muscle hypertrophy, mainly in slow-twitch fibers, improved aerobic and anaerobic enzymes, better local blood circulation and lactic acid tolerance
Maximum speed (alactic)	5 ± 3	Improved neuromuscular interactions and motor control, increased creatine phosphate storage

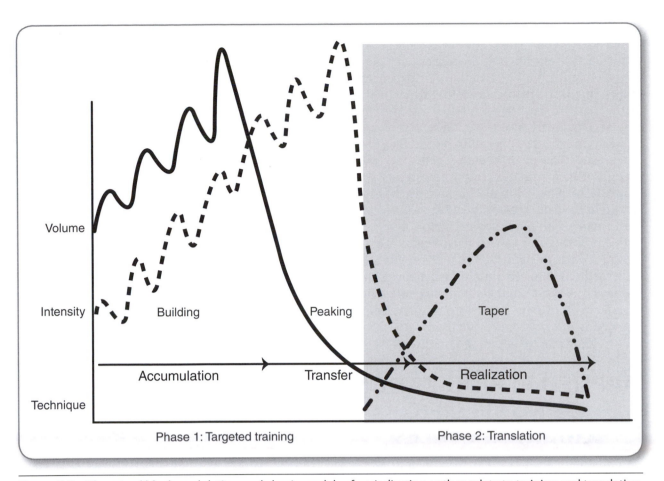

Figure 9.8 The mixed block, undulating, and classic models of periodization as they relate to training and translation.

ing. Lastly, you'll notice there is a wavelike pattern of volume and intensity. This pattern illustrates harder and easier days within microcycles.

The Translational Taper

During the fluctuating increases in intensity and volume at the beginning of the targeted training cycle, the level of skill (ADL-simulated) training is very low. Look at the patterns of decline in each component in figure 9.8 as the transition takes place from the targeted training phase to the translation phase. The rapid decreases in intensity and volume are known to athletes as a *taper*. This taper allows significant recovery, maximization of the fitness effect, and supercompensation. It also allows us to switch our concentration from fitness to skill training.

So what's the best way to taper? In a review paper on the topic, Inigo Mujika and Sabino Padilla (2003) presented the common patterns of taper and examined their effectiveness. These authors looked at three major factors: (1) the duration of the taper,

(2) the volume decline during the taper, and (3) the optimal pattern to use for the taper. Although the duration of the taper producing the best performance varied due to the nature of the activity and the training status of the participant, the average length was 2 weeks. Individuals using longer durations of training or very high intensities required longer tapers than individuals training at a more moderate level. Additionally, well-conditioned individuals responded more quickly to a taper when compared with individuals at a lower level of conditioning. For older clients, there is clear evidence that recovery takes longer for older versus younger athletes, all other things being equal. But since all things aren't equal, and older clients often work at considerably lower levels than a young athlete works at, a 2-week taper is recommended.

The volume change that produced the best performance across a 2-week taper was a decrease between 50% and 75%. This included a decrease of 50% in the frequency of training. The last variable that Mujika and Padilla examined was the pattern of the taper. There were four patterns studied.

The first was an immediate drop in training load called a *step taper*. The second was a linear taper in which load declined at a constant rate across the tapering period. The last two were exponential tapers, one fast and one slow, that began rapidly at the start of the 2-week period and then plateaued. Obviously, the faster taper used a more rapid decline in training volume than the slower taper used. The most effective pattern of taper seemed to be to maintain intensity at a high level while decreasing volume. This strategy has been shown to have the greatest positive effect on both performance and physiological factors associated with cardiovascular as well as strength training.

Also notice in figure 9.8 that there is a rapid increase in skill-based training occurring during the taper. Since formalized training targeting a specific need usually occurs 3 days per week on alternating days, secondary goals and ADL-based skill training can be addressed on the off days.

APPLIED PERIODIZATION USING SPECIFIC TRAINING CYCLES

Now that we have examined the concepts underlying periodization, let's look at some specific examples of how periodization may be applied to clients. To that end I provide three examples. I begin each example with the description of a client and the results of the testing battery. I then recommend specific exercises from those described in this book and present the concepts supporting their use. Next, I discuss the changes in training patterns that should occur across the building (accumulation) and peaking (realization) stages of the specific training block. Finally, I present translational training recommendations. You can examine the descriptions of the exercises recommended for each translational cycle in chapter 10. Let's get started.

Client 1

The results of client 1's diagnostic tests are shown in table 9.3. Client 1 is a 61-year-old woman who is 61 inches (155 cm) tall and weighs 110 pounds (50 kg). She has not trained in the past 10 years. She states that she has problems climbing multiple flights of stairs, walking long distances, and grocery shopping. However, she has very little difficulty getting up off the floor or out of bed. As you can see by looking at the diagnostic chart (table 9.3), client 1 shows low performance values for the 6-minute walk and sit-and-reach tests. To ascertain if the problem with the 6-minute walk test is due to lower-body strength and power, let's look at the 30-second chair stand test, 15-foot (4.6 m) walk test, and the modified ramp power test. While none of these tests produced very high values, their results were still not as low as the 6-minute walk test. Therefore we can come to the logical conclusion that the client's primary goal should be to increase cardiovascular fitness. Also, given the client's BMI, we know that the performance level is being affected minimally by body composition. So what should the prescription be?

Let's begin with a building (accumulation) block that employs a mixture of steady-state and interval training. Given the untrained nature of the client, let's use a 6-week block. The first 3 weeks can be used to adapt the tissues to a training stimulus (tissue adaptation period), and the following 3 weeks can address the need to increase cardiovascular fitness. The initial 3 weeks should employ short steady-state walks (durations of 5-10 minutes) that increase to 20 to 25 minutes at low to moderate intensities. During the following 3 weeks interval training cycles can be used to increase intensity. The pattern should begin with prolonged work and recovery cycles. During the succeeding weeks the duration of the work cycle should decline (remember to undulate) as the intensity increases and the recovery cycle lengthens to allow sufficient regeneration of energy sources (remember that intensity requires recovery). The number of cycles should increase through weeks 4 and 5 and then decrease sharply during week 6 in preparation for the translational phase. Because client 1's flexibility scores are so low, the translational phase should concentrate on repetitive drills that increase ROM. For example, repeated ladder drills using higher and longer stepping patterns can address both flexibility and cardiovascular fitness. Additionally, reaching drills such as the pickup drills featured in chapter 10 are also advisable. And certainly speed and stride drills and step drills are appropriate. As you will read in chapter 10 and can observe on the translational exercise section of the DVD, each of these drills will cause your client to increase her range of motion.

Table 9.3   Test Results for Client 1

Name or ID Number	11	Date	7/7/2010
Age (years)	61	Gender	F
Height (in.)	61	Weight (lb)	110
Height (m)	1.55	Weight (kg)	50.00

Note: The *Test* column shows the name of the test and the units you should use when entering each trial's result.

Test	Trial 1	Trial 2	Average	Percentile
Chair Sit-and-Reach, Left (in.)	-1	-1.5	-1.25	10-25
Chair Sit-and-Reach, Right (in.)	-1	-1	-1.00	10-25
Back Scratch, Left (in.)	0.5	1	0.75	50-75
Back Scratch, Right (in.)	1	1	1.00	50-75
Modified Trunk Rotation (in.)	27	26	26.50	50-75
Single-Leg Stance Balance (s)	27	26	26.50	50-75
Functional Reach (in.)	11	12	11.50	50-75
8-Foot (2.4 m) Up-And-Go (s)	5.25	5.5	5.38	25-50
30-Second Chair Stand (reps)	18	19	18.50	75-90
Modified Ramp Power (s)	1.5	1.5	1.50	5-25
30-Second Arm Curl (reps)	17	19	18.00	50-75
Gallon Jug Shelf (s)	11.03	9.86	10.45	25-50
6-Minute Walk (yards)	450		450.00	<10
15-Foot (4.6 m) Walk, Usual (s)	3.1	3.93	3.52	25-50
15-Foot (4.6 m) Walk, Maximal (s)	2.5	2.3	2.40	50-75
% Body Fat	33.56	33.54	33.55	25-50
BMI			20.78	75-90
Modified Ramp Power Test				
Ramp Height (m)	0.33			
Ramp Power (absolute)	107.98			
Ramp Power (per kg bw)	2.16			

In addition, repeated performance of these drills constitutes lower intensity interval training, which will further address her cardiovascular needs.

Client 2

Client 2 is a 71-year-old man with a BMI of 23.85. He has been training informally using a mix of resistance and cardiovascular training (plate machines and treadmill work) for the past 8 months. As you can see in table 9.4, he scored quite well on all the assessments except for the gait speed, functional reach, single-leg stand and modified ramp power tests, each of which fell below the 25th percentile. Although he also scored in the 25th to 50th percentile on the 6-minute

Table 9.4   Test Results for Client 2

Name or ID Number	12	Date	7/7/2010
Age (years)	71	Gender	M
Height (in.)	71.1	Weight (lb)	171
Height (m)	1.81	Weight (kg)	77.73

Note: The *Test* column shows the name of the test and the units you should use when entering each trial's result.

Test	Trial 1	Trial 2	Average	Percentile
Chair Sit-and-Reach, Left (in.)	2	2.5	2.25	75-90
Chair Sit-and-Reach, Right (in.)	2	2	2.00	75-90
Back Scratch, Left (in.)	2	1.5	1.75	>90
Back Scratch, Right (in.)	2.5	3	2.75	>90
Modified Trunk Rotation (in.)	27	26	26.50	50-70
Single-Leg Stance Balance (s)	4	3	3.5	10-25
Functional Reach (in.)	9	8.5	8.75	10-25
8-Foot (2.4 m) Up-And-Go (s)	6	6.5	6.25	25-50
30-Second Chair Stand (reps)	18	19	18.50	75-90
Modified Ramp Power (s)	1.5	1.5	1.50	5-25
30-Second Arm Curl (reps)	19	19	19.00	75-90
Gallon Jug Shelf (s)	8	8.25	8.13	75-90
6-Minute Walk (yards)	495		495.00	25-50
15-Foot (4.6 m) Walk, Usual (s)	4	4.5	4.25	10-25
15-Foot (4.6 m) Walk, Maximal (s)	2.6	2.6	2.60	10-25
% Body Fat	22.60	22.62	22.61	50-75
BMI			23.85	50-75
Modified Ramp Power Test				
Ramp Height (m)	0.33			
Ramp Power (absolute)	167.85			
Ramp Power (per kg bw)	2.16			

walk test, his overall test results indicate that this performance decrement is most likely due to neuromuscular rather than cardiovascular limitations. Given his low scores in the gait speed, functional reach, and modified ramp power tests and his relatively high score in the 30-second chair stand test, it appears that his needs center around speed-based power and balance. Given these results, let's

develop a training program targeting speed-based power and balance.

Since this client already has a significant background in strength training, we can most likely forego a formal tissue adaptation period. Therefore, let's begin with a load-dominated power training program that uses loads of 70% to 75% 1RM. For the first (accumulation) block, let's start with 2 to 3 sets of 8 to 12 repetitions at 75% 1RM performed three times per week during the first week. On days 1 and 3, let's provide two sets, and on day 2 let's prescribe three sets. During week 2, we can reverse the pattern, with days 1 and 3 using three sets and day 2 using two. All sets should be performed by using maximal speed during the concentric phase and controlled speed (1-2 seconds) during the eccentric phase. During week 3 we can decrease volume by reducing load (from 70% 1RM to 50% 1RM) or sets (from 2 or 3 to 1 or 2). This drop in volume and load will allow for a goal-specific increase in lifting speed that can serve as a further increase in intensity (this is a velocity- rather than load-based increase). Suggested exercises include the leg press, knee extension and flexion, plantar flexion, dorsiflexion, hip abduction, hip adduction, and hip flexion and extension. Depending on the client's previous training, we can also include a limited number of upper-body exercises. Also, all warm-ups and cool-downs should concentrate on flexibility training, and achieving full ROM should be emphasized throughout the exercises.

The second block, or transfer block, should target the prescribed focus of the training even more. Therefore, this 3 to 4 week phase should concentrate on velocity-specific power training. Let's reduce the loads to 40% 1RM and begin the volume at three sets of 8 to 12 repetitions performed three times per week. Across the first week or two of this training period, let's gradually decrease the volume as the training velocity increases. By the last week workouts should occur twice per week and consist of one set per exercise. During this week, the first week of the translational (motor training) phase should begin. Motor training should become the dominant training modality by the next week.

During the translational phase, the client should perform drills that specifically target speed and balance. There are a number of translational drills that can be used to increase movement speed, such as the short and intermediate distance interval ladder and cone drills presented in the next chapter and on the DVD. Given the decrements detected in balance, let's also prescribe drills that target balance and agility. Remember that the increases in movement speed we have already worked on are important components in stumble recovery and dynamic

balance. Possible drills include the pillow stands, triple-line drill, lateral shuffle, forward and backward cone drill, zigzag drill, and heel walk. Additionally, use ladder drills concentrating on both lateral and backward movements such as the between-every-other-rung; two-in, two-out; and in-and-out-the-window drills. Cone drills concentrating on fast changes in direction are also appropriate, such as the lateral shuffle, forward and backward cone, cone-touch, in-and-out agility, and skating drills. And let's not forget truckin'! Once again, these drills are presented in chapter 10 and on the DVD.

Client 3

Table 9.5 presents the test battery results for client 3. Client 3 is an 89-year-old man who works out sporadically and concentrates mainly on resistance training. His flexibility tests all fall between the 75th and the 90th percentile. He demonstrates excellent upper-body strength and power, as indicated by his performances on the 30-second arm curl test and the gallon jug shelf test. His lower-body strength and power values are also above average. However, his balance and cardiovascular endurance are a little weak, as evidenced by his performances on the 8-foot (2.4 m) up-and-go test and the functional reach test, for which he falls into the 25th to 50th percentile, and especially on the 6-minute walk test, for which his performance level is below the 10th percentile. Finally, he is in the 25th to 50th percentile for body composition. The three interrelated concerns of cardiovascular endurance, balance, and body composition may best be addressed by a combined cardiovascular and resistance training program designed to deal with both the cardiovascular and the body composition needs. The balance component could then be addressed during the translational period.

Given the fact that this client has some training background, let's start right in with a training program. As you will recall from chapters 4 and 8, interval training is one of the most effective ways to deal with both cardiovascular conditioning and body composition. Additionally, circuit resistance training, especially training using high-velocity movements, is highly effective at increasing lean body mass and decreasing adipose tissue. Given the client's training background, let's begin the training program with a minimum concern for tissue adaptation. While we might employ a number of strategies for this client, let's begin the accumulation block with low to moderate intervals (1:2 to 1:4 work–recovery duty cycles based on 60-second units) and gradually increase the training volume and intensity across the first 2 weeks by increasing the number of intervals from 5 to 20 cycles. As the client progresses, the third week should show a reduction in the number

of cycles, a shortening of the work cycle, and a lengthening of the recovery cycle in order to allow higher-intensity training. During the last week of the accumulation block, the number of cycles and training intensity can be reduced in preparation for the transfer block.

The transfer block should use circuit resistance training to further affect changes in body composition. The circuit training in the transfer block

Table 9.5 Test Results for Client 3

Name or ID Number	13	Date	7/7/2010
Age (years)	89	Gender	M
Height (in.)	70	Weight (lb)	220
Height (m)	1.78	Weight (kg)	100.00

Note: The *Test* column shows the name of the test and the units you should use when entering each trial's result.

Test	Trial 1	Trial 2	Average	Percentile
Chair Sit-and-Reach, Left (in.)	2	2.5	2.25	75-90
Chair Sit-and-Reach, Right (in.)	2	2	2.00	75-90
Back Scratch, Left (in.)	0	0.5	0.25	>90
Back Scratch, Right (in.)	0	0	0.00	>90
Modified Trunk Rotation (in.)	21	22	21.50	50-70
Single-Leg Stance Balance (s)	5	6	5.5	25-50
Functional Reach (in.)	12.5	12.5	12.5	25-50
8-Foot (2.4 m) Up-And-Go (s)	7.8	8	7.9	25-50
30-Second Chair Stand (reps)	13	13	13	50-75
Modified Ramp Power (s)	2.6	2.5	2.55	50-75
30-Second Arm Curl (reps)	19	19	19.00	75-90
Gallon Jug Shelf (s)	8	8.25	8.13	75-90
6-Minute Walk (yards)	285	■	285.00	<10
15-Foot (4.6 m) Walk, Usual (s)	3	2.5	2.75	50-75
15-Foot (4.6 m) Walk, Maximal (s)	2.5	2.6	2.55	50-75
% Body Fat	28.75	28.75	28.75	25-50
BMI	■	■	31.75	<10
Modified Ramp Power Test				
Ramp Height (m)	0.33			
Ramp Power (absolute)	127.03			
Ramp Power (per kg bw)	3.24			

should concentrate on lower-body exercises (leg press, knee extension and flexion, plantar flexion, dorsiflexion, hip abduction, hip adduction, and hip flexion and extension) but should also include core and limited upper-body exercises. Loads will be between 45% and 55% 1RM. The progression across the transfer block will be to increase from one circuit to three circuits across the first 3 weeks and then drop drastically. Throughout the training block the client should increase his lifting speeds during the concentric portions of the exercises and perform controlled eccentric phases. As the training volume decreases, the client should become capable of faster lifting speeds during this portion of the training block. The use of speed rather than load has two purposes: First, it increases the caloric output during each session, and second, it addresses the need to improve balance.

The translational block should concentrate on speed endurance and balance. Speed and stride drills incorporating intervals and a distance of 98 feet (30 m) are appropriate to translate the training cycles into increased walking capacity. Additionally, balance and agility drills such as the

triple-line drill, lateral shuffle, forward and backward cone drill, zigzag drill, cone-touch drill, heel walk, ladder drills, and pillow stands presented in chapter 10 are feasible choices.

SUMMARY

This chapter brings together three important concepts. The first of these is exercise specificity. The prescriptions provided for clients are based on the diagnostic tests and other information provided by the clients. The second concept is periodization. Periodization provides a training timetable that uses the durations of specific training residuals and changes in training intensity and volume to maximize gains across a targeted training cycle. The third and final concept is translation. This chapter mentions a number of translational drills designed to convert the client's improved physical capacity into practical motor patterns applicable to daily living. Chapter 10 presents these translational drills and explains how they fit into the overall blueprint for bending the aging curves.

Topical Bibliography

Periodization: The Underlying Theories

Chiu, L.Z.F., & Barnes, J.L. (2003). The fitness-fatigue model revisited: Implications for planning short- and long-term training. *National Strength and Conditioning Association Journal* 25:42-51.

Fry, A.C., & Kraemer, W.J. (1997). Resistance exercise overtraining and overreaching. Neuroendocrine responses. *Sports Medicine* 23:106-129.

Plisk, S.S., & Stone, M.H. (2003). Periodization strategies. *National Strength and Conditioning Association Journal* 25:19-37.

Controlling the Fitness–Fatigue Balance During Training

Gibala, M., MacDougall, J.D., & Sale, D.G. (1994). The effects of tapering on strength performance in trained athletes. *Int J Sports Med* 15:492-497.

Kraemer, W.J., Hakkinen, K., Newton, R.A., McCormick, M., Nindl, B.C., Volek, J.S., Gotshalk, L.A., Fleck, S.J., Campbell, W.W., Gordon, S.E., and others. (1998). Acute hormonal responses to heavy resistance exercise in younger and older men. *Eur J Appl Physiol* 77:206-211.

McGuire, D.K., Levine, B.D., Williamson, J.W., Snell, P.G., Blomqvist, C.G., Saltin, B., & Mitchell, J.H. (2001). A 30-year follow-up of the Dallas bed rest and training study. II. Effect of age on cardiovascular adaptation to exercise training. *Circulation* 104:1358-1366.

Mujika, I., & Padilla, S. (2003). Scientific bases for precompetition tapering strategies. *Med Sci Sport Exerc* 35:1182-1187.

Oliveto, N. (2004). Establishing volume load parameters: A different look in designing a strength training periodization for throwing athletes. *Str Conditioning J* 26:52-55.

Rhea, M.R., Ball, S.D., Phillips, W., & Burkett, L. (2002). A comparison of linear and daily undulating periodized programs with equated volume and intensity for strength. *Journal of Strength and Conditioning Research* 16:250-255.

Rhea, M.R., Phillip, W.T., Burkett, L.N., Stone, W.J., Ball, S.D., Alvar, B.A., & Thomas, A.B. (2003). A comparison of linear and daily undulating periodized programs with equated volume and intensity for local muscular endurance. *Journal of Strength and Conditioning Research* 17: 82-87.

Shepley, B., MacDougall, J.D., Cipriano, N., Sutton, J.R., Tarnopolsky, M.A., & Coates, G. (1992). Physiological effects of tapering in highly trained athletes. *J Appl Physiol* 72:706-711.

Stone, M.H., O'Bryant, H.S., Schilling, B.K., Johnson, R.L., Pierce, K.C., Haff, G.G., Koch, A.J., & Stone, M. (1999). Periodization: Effects of manipulating volume and intensity. Part 1. *Str Conditioning J* 21:56-63.

Wiswell, R.A., Hawkins, S.A., Jaque, S.V., Hyslop, D., Constantino, N., Tarpenning, K., Marcell, T., & Schroeder, E.T. (2001). Relationship between physiological loss, performance decrement, and age in master athletes. *J Gerontol A Biol Sci Med Sci* 56:M618-M626.

References

Chiu, L.Z.F., & Barnes, J.L. (2003). The fitness-fatigue model revisited: Implications for planning short- and long-term training. *National Strength and Conditioning Association Journal* 25:42-51.

Mujika, I., & Padilla, S. (2003). Scientific bases for precompetition tapering strategies. *Med Sci Sport Exerc* 35:1182-1187.

The Translational Cycle: Active Recovery Meets Functional Practice

To this point we have discussed strengthening the muscles, improving the heart and lungs, enhancing flexibility, and changing body composition. Now let's talk about restructuring the most important organ of the body: the brain. Training the brain requires a completely different strategy than training the other systems in the body requires. The research clearly shows that restructuring the brain and nervous system requires the use of complex movement patterns. Simple overloads such as weight training or walking have little or no effect on the intricate wiring of the nervous system. As Gene Wilder stated in *Young Frankenstein,* "Hearts and kidneys are tinker toys! I am talking about the central nervous system!"

So what is the best way to proceed? One thing known for sure is that the central nervous system remaps itself in patterns called *kinetic movement chains.* For clients to get good at an activity, they must practice the kinetic movement chain on which that activity depends. Once a client does this, all the structures in the cerebral cortex, midbrain, spinal column, and peripheral nervous system are rewired to make that movement easier to perform.

But let's not stop at remapping a movement. To truly accomplish the purpose of translational training, we must match the motor pattern training of the translational period to the improvements made in physical performance during the preceding training cycle. While the link between physical performance improvements and motor pattern training is not absolute, there are a number

of logical decisions that allow us to choose one drill over another. Additionally, we can often incorporate tests as part of our training portfolio. A simple example illustrating the link between testing and training is the way music was added to the classic Harvard step test to create step aerobics. So let's put on our thinking caps and restructure clients' nervous systems to maximize the benefits of training.

Many physical therapy clinics and fitness facilities incorporate exercises simulating ADLs as part of rehabilitation after acute injury or surgery. Occupational therapists commonly have their patients practice everyday activities to improve function and increase independence. Additionally, several laboratories and clinics have compared ADL-specific training to standard resistance training protocols and have shown similar or greater improvements with ADL-based training. Additionally, ADL-based training alone is highly effective at improving independence in older persons. However, no one has matched ADL-specific drills to a standard training program using the periodized training cycles described in chapter 9.

Martin Ginis and colleagues (2006) compared a standard resistance training program with that same program combined with an educational component that explained the association between resistance training and improved ADL performance. The people in the combined program indicated that they could perform ADLs better as a result of the resistance training, and they had a greater belief in their capacity to perform ADL tasks when compared with the people who only performed the resistance training.

This chapter shows the ADL-based motor learning cycles that provide recovery and translate the physiological gains produced during training cycles into improvements in ADL performance. These translational cycles match the diagnosed needs of the client and therefore expand on the physiological improvements made during the training cycles to which they are linked. In this way the training and translational cycles combine to address the unique physiological and motor pattern needs of the individual.

> **APPLICATION POINT** To benefit fully from any training program, at least some portion of the program should concentrate on training motor patterns associated with your client's daily activities.

BASIC CONCEPT OF THE TRANSLATIONAL CYCLE

The use of translational cycles mirrors a basic concept employed for decades by sport coaches and strength and conditioning specialists. These coaches and specialists understand that increasing the physical capacities of an athlete provides little advantage during competition if these improvements do not translate into better performances on the field or court. They also recognize that the way in which translation occurs is through the use of drills specifically designed to improve the motor skills applied in the particular sport being practiced. The training methods and motor learning drills used for each sport differ depending on the physiological and biomechanical factors that dictate success in the specific sport environment. For example, the physiological goals and associated motor training patterns of a tennis player and a football lineman differ drastically.

In most sports, skill practice occupies a larger percentage of the athlete's training than resistance or cardiovascular training occupies, especially during the season. Given the relentless comparisons between life and sport in the media, it is surprising that we who work with older adults have failed to provide training interventions that reflect these comparisons. That is, we have failed to include translational training as part of a well-

structured training program designed to address the needs of older citizens.

> **APPLICATION POINT** In the game of life practicing the skills necessary for success is as important as in any sport if you wish to win.

TRANSLATIONAL CYCLES AND PERIODIZATION

In chapter 9, I presented periodization models that focus on specific fitness variables such as strength, power, and cardiovascular conditioning and spoke briefly about translational cycles. Although these models can effectively address clients' needs, there are factors involved that may reduce their effectiveness as tools to enhance successful aging.

The first factor is that once clients develop the habit of training, they are often reluctant to accept recovery periods, even though such periods are necessary to optimize fitness effects and to reduce the potential for overtraining and overuse injuries. The second factor is that the training techniques used to address physiological declines often lack the biomechanical and neuromuscular specificity needed to improve independence, reduce fall probability, and increase mobility. If we wish to address functional decline and physical frailty, we must address both of these concerns, and translational cycles can do just that.

Despite the efforts of many scientists and practitioners, our profession still works in a no pain, no gain environment in which any reduction in training is seen as a failure in compliance. In an attempt to neutralize this environment of failure and to help people understand that recovery periods are not a time for exercising the remote control or couch muscles but instead are a time for improving motor performance, I like to use the more palatable and descriptive term *translational cycle* in place of the term *recovery period*. The challenge is to link targeted physiological overload and translational motor skill training with diagnosed weaknesses, thereby making interventions both beneficial and meaningful to clients. Once this is accomplished, clients will be prepared for the most important competition of all: playing against Father Time for personal independence on the field of life. Let's look at the strategies that we can use to link physiological overloads and translational drills with diagnosed needs of individuals.

Translational cycles are your training double whammy: They provide recovery and ADL-specific motor training.

TIMING OF TRANSLATIONAL CYCLES

In the training scheme, the most effective time to administer the diagnostic battery is after the translational cycle. In this way, testing occurs during a taper period when the fitness aftereffect is maximized and the fatigue aftereffect is minimized. The recurrent pattern of training, translation, and reassessment is shown in figure 10.1. This model increases exercise adherence because it not only allows clients to see their own progress but also demonstrates how their progress is linked to the exercise prescription, since their improvements typically mirror the intervention. Additionally, as a client reaches the 90th percentile in specific tests, you can target norms for persons who are years, if not decades, younger. In this way, clients begin to perceive that the training is changing their functional age. And now the added bonus: When clients realize that they are being compared with younger persons, they also recognize that they are, in effect, getting younger. This provides tremendous motivation and maximizes adherence to the program.

MOTOR LEARNING DRILLS: THE NEED FOR PROGRESSION

Figure 10.2 shows a triplanar (three-dimensional) graph first presented in the *Journal on Active Aging* in 2005 (Signorile, 2005). It shows the

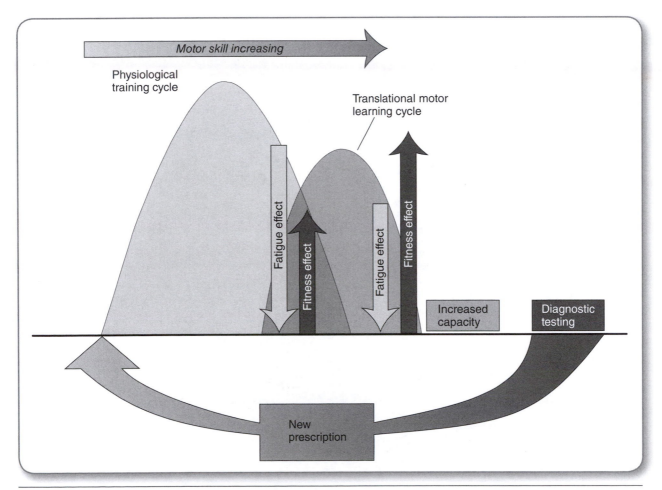

Figure 10.1   The overall pattern of targeted training and translational periods showing the positive effects of a translational recovery period on the fitness and fatigue effects of a training cycle.

factors that should be considered in designing a translational cycle. These factors include the following:

1. *Factors associated with independence, fall probability, and mobility (y-axis).* Notice that these factors are linked to increased physical vulnerability and frailty. Clearly losses in mobility, the ability to rise from a chair or bed, or the capacity to manipulate objects signal a decline in independence and an increased potential for falls and associated injuries.

2. *Specific needs (z-axis).* We have already discussed meeting specific physical needs extensively in this text. If the term *translational cycle* is to have meaning, the patterns of motor training must be related to the physiological goal of the preceding training cycle.

3. *Logical progression (x-axis).* The progression for the translational cycle mirrors that of the classic mesocycle, in which there is a gradual undulating increase in volume and intensity during the initial portion of the cycle, followed by a steep decline in volume and then in intensity. Accompanying these changes is a constantly

increasing concentration on skill and performance enhancement.

Figure 10.3 presents the three components that can be manipulated during a translational cycle: intensity, volume, and complexity. In figure 10.4 you can see the general pattern for each of these components. Note the fluctuating patterns inherent in nonlinear periodization.

Component 1: Intensity

As shown in figure 10.3, you can manipulate the intensity of training by varying the speed at which the drill is performed, the loading pattern associated with the drill, or the mechanical efficiency of the movement pattern used in the drill. At first glance, movement speed may seem the easiest variable to manipulate; however, remember that movement speed may be affected by the joints included in the movement, the skill level of the person performing the movement, the potential for injury, and, most importantly, the goal of the training cycle.

Changes in load can be achieved in a number of ways. The most obvious way is to change the

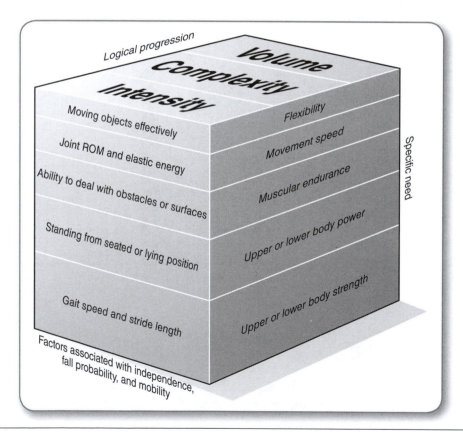

Figure 10.2   Three-dimensional diagram of factors that should be considered when designing a translational cycle.

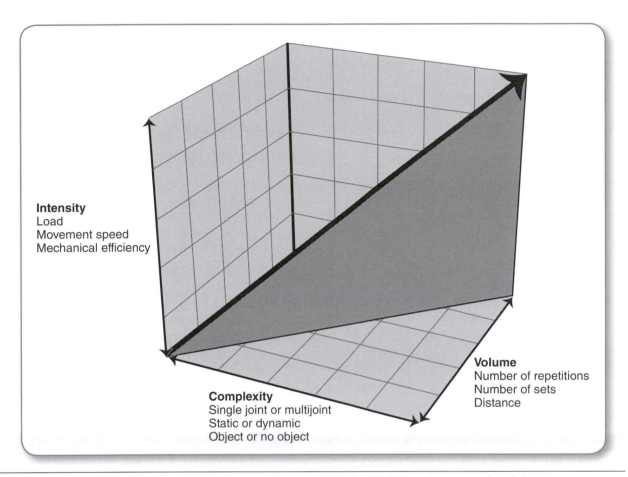

Figure 10.3 The three components (intensity, volume, and complexity) that can be manipulated during a translational cycle.

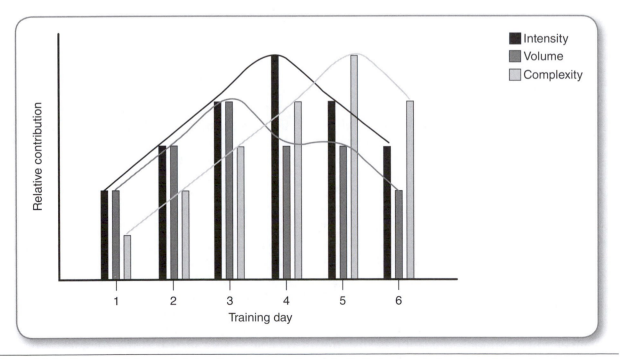

Figure 10.4 Patterns of change in intensity, volume, and complexity that occur during a translational cycle.

weight of an object being used in the drill. For example, you might increase or decrease the amount of water in a jug. Another method is to manipulate the effect of gravity on an object or on the body. The most obvious example of this is changing the incline on a treadmill—it takes more work to walk up a hill than it does to walk on level ground.

Mechanical efficiency may be the most subtle, yet most elegant, variable that you can manipulate. We all recognize that we can perform tasks the easy way or the hard way, and for the most part we like to choose the easy way. If, however, the objective is to provide motor pattern training that leads to better efficiency when a movement is performed during everyday life, one of the best ways to accomplish the objective is to force the body to perform the movement inefficiently. One caution here: Do not disrupt motor patterns so much that the movement is no longer recognizable or increases the probability of injury. Simple and safe examples of manipulating mechanical efficiency are asking a person to move an object when in a sitting versus a standing position (doing so reduces the capacity of the lower body to aid in the movement) and asking someone to rise from a chair while holding the arms crossed against the chest.

Component 2: Volume

The volume of work the client performs can be manipulated easily (see figure 10.3) by increasing the number of drills performed or the number of repetitions performed for a particular drill. Increasing the number of sessions per week also increases volume. Some of the latest training studies have indicated that performing a number of sessions of shorter duration may be as effective as performing longer training sessions, depending on the goal of the training. Volume can also be manipulated by changing the amount of time dedicated to a task. For example, a balance or standing drill might last anywhere from 10 seconds to 60 seconds. Changing the distance over which the client performs a drill can also affect the total volume of work. A 10-foot (3 m) gait or agility drill is a much smaller volume than that of a 50-foot (15 m) drill. There are two things to remember when manipulating volume. First, the distances and durations chosen should reflect both the goal of the training cycle and the time point within the training cycle. Second, volume and intensity are interactive. Increases in volume should be accompanied by decreases in intensity and vice versa.

Component 3: Movement Complexity

Motor tasks associated with ADLs usually involve the sequential firing of a number of joints and muscle groups within a kinetic chain. Firing those groups in the necessary sequence requires skill and practice. The first strategy for manipulating movement complexity (see figure 10.3) is to vary the number of joints (and related muscle groups) used by modifying a drill. The greater the number of muscle groups and joints used and the more intricate the pattern in which they are used, the greater the complexity of the task. The second strategy is to shift between static tasks and dynamic tasks. For example, while a static balance drill such as standing on one leg may be difficult, dynamic balance drills such as walking around cones or other objects are more biomechanically complex. Another way to make a task more dynamic is to perform a static task such as standing with the feet in a tandem position in an unstable environment such as on a rubber mat, pillow, or BOSU ball. The third strategy for increasing task complexity is to add object manipulation to an activity. For example, you might begin a movement sequence with a shallow lunge, progress to a full lunge, and then add the movement of telephone books to the lunge. You can complicate the object manipulation by making it multidirectional (see figure 10.5), and then you can complicate things further by increasing the level of fine motor control involved in the object manipulation. For example, the telephone books can be replaced with a tennis ball that must be cradled in the hole on the top of a cone.

The final strategy for adding complexity to a task is multitasking. For decades researchers and clinicians have recognized that adding a cognitive skill to a motor skill can significantly increase the complexity of a task. For example, reciting a multiplication table while negotiating an obstacle course greatly increases the complexity of both skills.

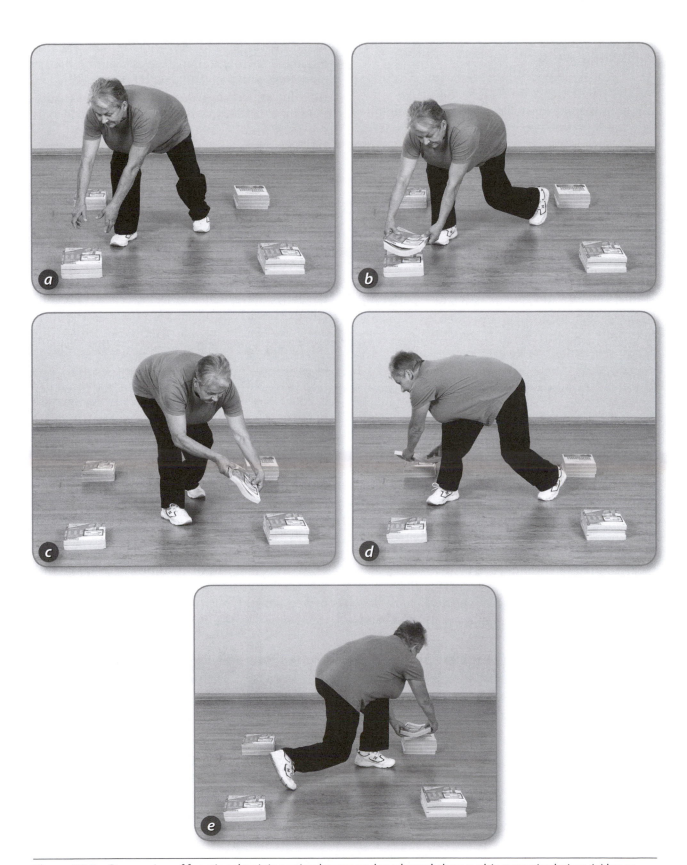

Figure 10.5 Progression of functional training using lunges and moderately heavy object manipulation: *(a)* lunge with no object, *(b)* forward lunge with a telephone book, *(c)* lateral lunge with a telephone book, *(d)* backward lunge with a telephone book, and *(e)* diagonal movement of the telephone book.

Manipulating intensity, volume, and complexity to maximize both overload and recovery is as important during motor training as it is during fitness training cycles.

MATCHING TRANSLATIONAL AND TRAINING CYCLES

One of the concepts that is central to the periodized training programs presented in this book is that the motor learning drills should be related either biomechanically or conceptually to the training cycles they are intended to translate into daily performance. Mismatching the drills between training cycles and translational cycles is like trying to match a purple striped shirt with green checkered pants.

Many drills can be used to translate power, strength, flexibility, and cardiovascular training into everyday performance. But let's make some generalizations on how to make effective matches. Translational drills that are related to both static and dynamic balance are best matched with cycles designed to increase leg strength and power. Object movement drills including ball drills can be used in conjunction with upper-body and core training. Mobility drills and ladder drills often have their greatest effects when linked to cardiovascular and speed training cycles. This is especially true when the performance patterns are specifically matched to duration (short recovery and multiple repeats)

or speed (long recovery and limited repeats). Finally, flexibility training cycles work best when combined with translational drills that incorporate reaching or bending as part of their skill set. Additionally, drills designed to amplify stride length are good fits with flexibility training cycles.

The translational cycle should reflect the established goal of the training cycle. For example, if a client demonstrates poor balance scores on the diagnostic battery, the translational drills should target balance rather than another factor such as strength or cardiovascular endurance. Table 10.1 presents a chart to demonstrate how to match goals to translational cycles. The three columns in table 10.1 represent three different goals a cycle can target: (1) power, balance, and speed; (2) strength, balance, and control; and (3) both. These three goals are closely related neuromuscularly—I did this intentionally to illustrate that specific drills can be associated with seemingly similar training goals.

As you read through the drills outlined in this chapter, look back on this table. Note that the drills in the power, balance, and speed column increase movement speed by using dynamic agility and balance drills that require high-speed movements in a horizontal plane. The strength, balance, and control column, by comparison, contains drills that concentrate on controlled tasks that require vertical movements in which working against gravity dictates a higher loading condition. Also consider the middle column. This column features drills that can be modified to fit into either the strength, balance, and control column or the power, balance, and speed column. For example, the two-in-every-rung drill is designed to increase

Table 10.1 Training and Translational Matching

Power, balance, and speed	Both	Strength, balance, and control
Functional reach drill	Heel stand	Skating drill
Pillow stands	Heel walk	Lateral advances
Triple-line drill	Lateral throw	Back-to-back handoff
Lateral shuffle drill	Forward and backward passes	Chest pass
Forward and backward cone drill	Truckin' drill	Overhead and lateral throw
Zigzag drill	Dual tasking	Soccer kicks
Cone-touch drill	8-foot (2.4 m) up-and-go drill	Broom hockey
Speed and stride drill	Ladder drills	Step drill
Hexagon drill	Chair drills	Scarf drill
Star excursion drill	Coin pickup drill	Book drills
	Gallon jug drill	Ball-and-pylon drills
	Dot drills	Floor coin pickup drill

foot speed, while the one-in-every-other-rung drill requires longer steps and a prolonged single-leg stance and therefore increases strength. With a bit of ingenuity and an eye toward caution, you can easily modify most drills to match the goals for a particular cycle. Just remember to keep your eye on the goal that's being targeted and don't get lost in the fun of exploring variations for their own sake.

TRANSLATIONAL EXERCISES

Although I have concentrated thus far on the links between training cycles and diagnosis of physiological declines, the functional connection between decreased independence and increased fall probability and motor pattern training is equally, if not more, important. This section presents a number of drills that have specific goals. As we go through the drills, we'll look at those goals and how they relate to the diagnosed needs of the client. And then we'll look beyond that and see how to modify certain drills by changing their speed, ROM, or complexity so that they more closely match the diagnosed needs of the client. The instructions in the following exercises speak directly to the client so that you can read them to the client if desired.

Balance Drills   264
Heel Stand and Heel Walk   264
Functional Reach Drill   265
Pillow Stands With Changes in Center of Gravity   266
Triple-Line Drill   268
Line Drills   269
Lateral Line Drill   269
Forward and Backward Passes   270
Truckin' Drill   271
Dual Tasking   271
Agility Drills   272
Skating Drill   272
Zigzag Drill   273
8-Foot (2.4 m) Up-and-Go Drill   273
Cone-Touch Drill   274
In-and-Out Agility Drill   274
Lateral Shuffle Drill   275
Forward and Backward Cone Drill   275
Ladder Drills   276
Between-Every-Rung Drill   277
Two-Between-Every-Rung Drill   277
Between-Every-Other-Rung Drill   278
Two-In, Two-Out Drill   278
In-and-Out-the-Window Drill   279
Lateral Advances   280

Drills Based on Activities of Daily Living   281
Chair Stand Drill   281
Chair Drills   281
Broom Hockey   283
Step Drill   284
Lateral Step-Up   287
Speed and Stride Drill   287
Drills Based on Instrumental Activities of Daily Living   288
Scarf Drill   288
Book Drills   288
Ball-and-Pylon Drills   290
Coin Pickup Drill   290
Gallon Jug Drill   291
Eye–Foot Coordination Drills   292
Dot or Grid Drills   292
Hexagon Drill   293
Star Excursion Drill   293
Ball Drills   294
Back-to-Back Handoff   294
Chest Pass   294
Overhead Throw   295
Lateral Throw   295
Soccer Kick   296
Dance Movements   296

BALANCE DRILLS

The balance drills included here are designed to help you train balance under both dynamic and static conditions.

Heel Stand and Heel Walk

The relationship between our center of gravity and base of support varies throughout the performance of daily activities. Shifting backward onto the heels is one of the most challenging balance disruptions. Begin this drill by holding onto a chair, counter, or other stable object. Then rock back on the heels and attempt to maintain balance in this position (see figure 10.6a). Once you have mastered this skill, you can attempt to walk on the heels along a selected and progressively more difficult course (see figure 10.6b). It is best to have a safety rail and spotter available at all times to ensure safety during the drill. Start by using shorter distances.

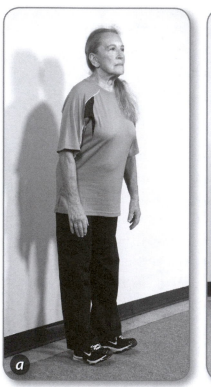
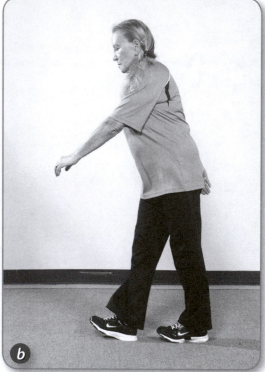

Figure 10.6 *(a)* Heel standing and *(b)* heel walking.

Functional Reach Drill

This drill is a spin-off of the functional reach balance test. To perform the drill, stand next to a wall with the feet shoulder-width apart and the arm closest to the wall extended at shoulder level. Reach forward as far as possible, keeping the heels in contact with the floor (see figure 10.7). Regain your balance and perform the drill again, attempting to reach farther this time. You can increase the difficulty level of this drill by bringing the feet closer together, switching from a single-arm reach to a double-arm reach, or alternating reaching arms.

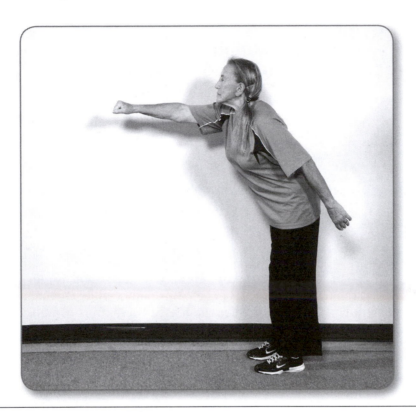

Figure 10.7   The functional reach drill.

Pillow Stands With Changes in Center of Gravity

It's often difficult for older persons to maintain balance on a compliant (spongy) surface. There are numerous commercial devices that provide such a surface, but one of the most economical and least challenging devices you can use is a simple foam pillow available at most discount stores. You can use progressively more difficult stances as your balance improves. As with any of these drills, be sure that your spotter is standing next to you and that a rescue surface such as a wall or chair is available, especially as your positions become more challenging. The following is a balance progression that can be performed on a compliant surface:

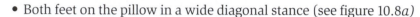

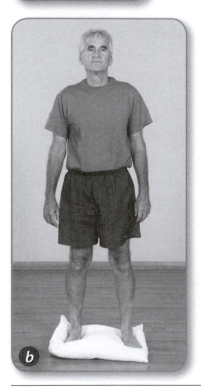

- Both feet on the pillow in a wide diagonal stance (see figure 10.8*a*)
- Both feet on the pillow in a wide stance (see figure 10.8*b*)
- Both feet on the pillow in a narrow stance (see figure 10.8*c*)
- Both feet on the pillow in a tandem stance (see figure 10.8*d*)
- Single-leg stand on the pillow (see figure 10.8*e*)

To this progression you may add the following changes in arm position:

- Arms extended forward or to the side (see figure 10.8*f*)
- Hands at the sides (see figure 10.8*g*)
- Arms crossed over the chest (see figure 10.8*h*)
- Hands held high overhead (see figure 10.8*i*).

In addition to performing each of these stances independently, you can transition from one stance to another while remaining on the pillow to add an even greater challenge. These drills can also be performed on the floor to reduce the challenge or on a foam roller or BOSU ball to increase the challenge.

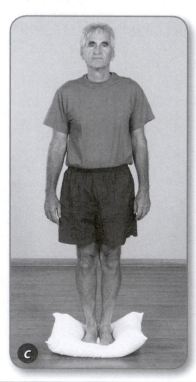

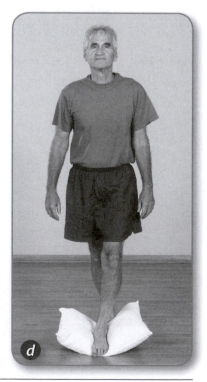

Figure 10.8   Pillow drills showing *(a)* both feet on the pillow in a wide diagonal stance, *(b)* both feet on the pillow in a wide stance, *(c)* both feet on the pillow in a narrow stance, *(d)* both feet on the pillow in a tandem stance,   *(continued)*

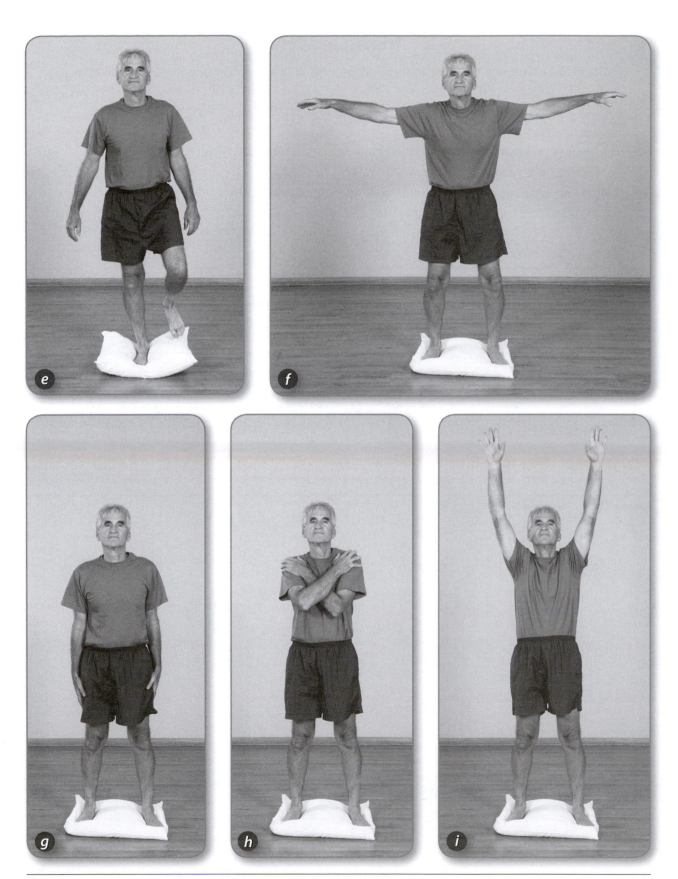

Figure 10.8 *(continued)* *(e)* a single-leg stance, *(f)* arms up, *(g)* hands at the sides, *(h)* arms crossed over the chest, and *(i)* arms overhead.

▰▰▰ Triple-Line Drill ▰▰▰

This drill is set up by placing three 15-foot (4.6 m) lines parallel on the floor about 4 inches (10 cm) apart (see figure 10.9). The idea is to walk down these lines in a specific walking pattern. These walking patterns may include the following:

- Feet outside the three lines
- Feet on either side of the middle line but inside the outer lines
- Feet along the middle line
- Feet crossing the middle line inside the lateral lines
- Feet crossing the middle and lateral lines

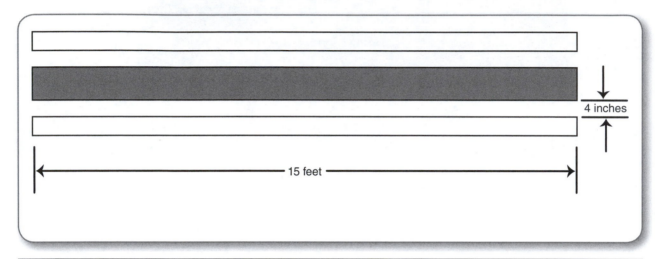

Figure 10.9 The triple-line drill layout.

LINE DRILLS

Line drills increase eye–foot coordination during walking or other forms of locomotion. The drills presented here are modifications of patterns used when training athletes.

Lateral Line Drill

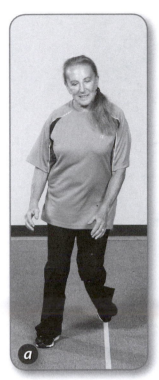

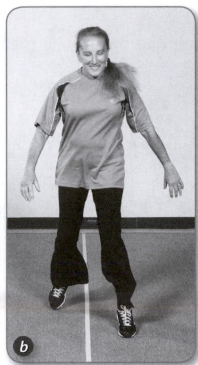

This drill requires a 15-foot (4.6 m) line to be taped on the floor or ground. Start the drill by shuffling from one foot to the other while crossing the line side to side (see figure 10.10a). To increase the difficulty level, try bouncing on the balls of the feet while shuffling (see figure 10.10b). Next, perform the same drill but attempt to minimize the time the foot is in contact with the ground (see figure 10.10c). And finally, move along the line using lateral hops (hop with both feet together; see figure 10.10d).

Figure 10.10   Lateral line drills showing (a) stepping, (b) bouncing, (c) quick bouncing, and (d) hopping.

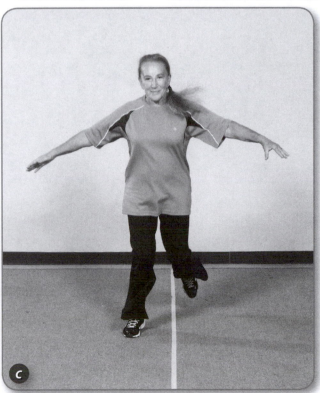

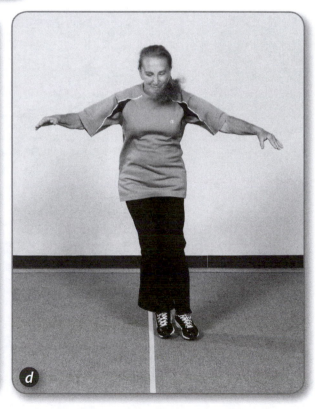

Forward and Backward Passes

This drill can also be performed at different levels of difficulty. Using the 15-foot (4.6 m) line taped on the floor, step forward over the line with one foot and then step back to the original position (see figure 10.11*a*). Next, step over the line with one foot, step over the line with the other foot, and step backward with the first foot, and step backward with the second foot (see figure 10.11*b*). Next, bounce forward across the line with a single foot and then bounce back on the foot behind the line (see figure 10.11*c*). Finally, jump back and forth across the line (see figure 10.11*d*).

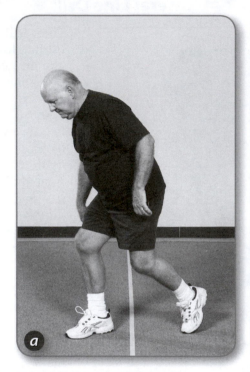
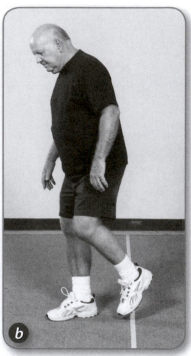

Figure 10.11   Forward and backward passes with *(a)* one foot out and back, *(b)* both feet over and back, *(c)* bouncing forward and back, and *(d)* jumping forward and back.

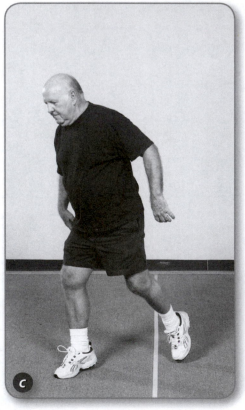
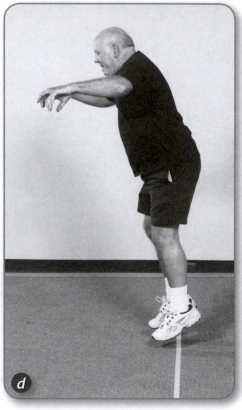

Truckin' Drill

Place a foot on either side of the 15-foot (4.6 m) line and then walk forward, swinging the feet in wide arcs (see figure 10.12). To increase the difficulty level, try the drill while walking backward.

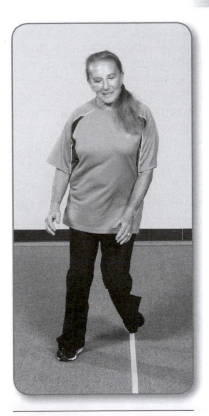

Figure 10.12   The truckin' drill.

Dual Tasking

Each of the line drills can be performed while using some mental exercise as a distraction. For example, you can count backward from 100, recite the alphabet backward, or name all of the states in the United States (and their capitals if you are a geography aficionado). It has clearly been shown that adding a mental task to a physical motor skill creates a significant level of interference and increases the task difficulty for older persons.

AGILITY DRILLS

Agility is the ability to change the body's or any part of the body's direction and position and to do so with coordination and control. While the value of agility is obvious in competitive athletics, its importance is often overlooked in daily life. Avoiding other pedestrians when walking, smoothly turning sideways when walking through a turnstile, and jumping back onto a curb when a car comes around the block all depend on agility. So let's look at some drills to improve this motor skill. Most of these drills use pylons (cones) to map out a course to be run.

Skating Drill

Set up a row of eight cones with 2 to 3 feet (about 1 m) between cones (see figure 10.13). Using wide sliding steps that mimic skating, move in and out of the cones while working your way up the row. Repeat the drill by going back to the starting line.

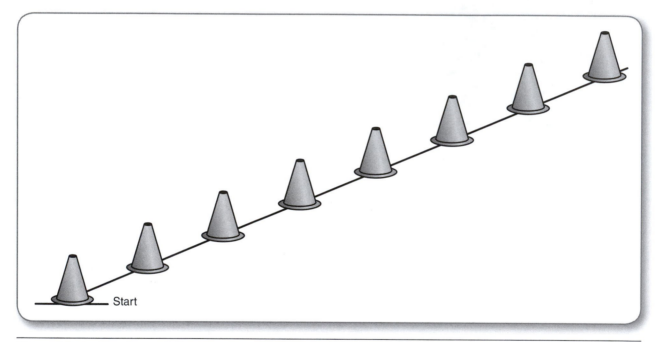

Start

Figure 10.13   The skating drill.

Zigzag Drill

This drill is a spin-off of the zigzag agility test. To set up the course, put four cones on the corners of a 10- × 16-foot (3 × 5 m) rectangle, and then place one more cone in the center of the course (see figure 10.14). Label the cones in the corners of the rectangle as 1, 2, 3, and 4 and label the center cone C. Start the drill at cone 1. Go to cone C, then cone 2, then cone 3, then cone C, then cone 4, and then back to cone 1. You can change the drill by altering the distances between the cones or the movement pattern between the cones.

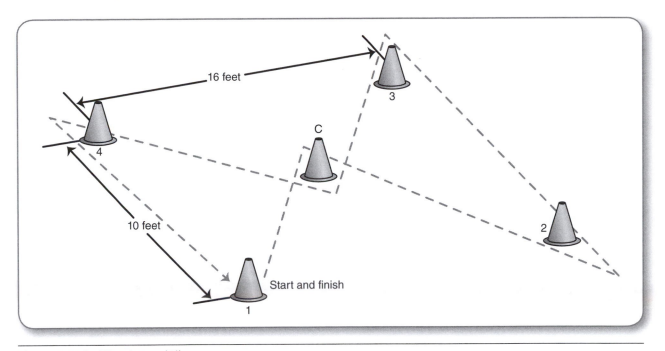

Figure 10.14   The zigzag drill.

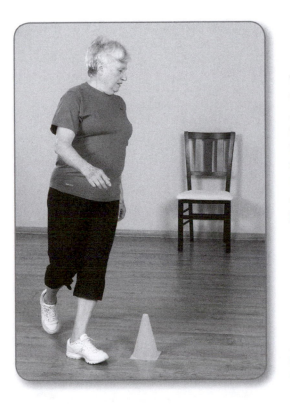

8-Foot (2.4 m) Up-and-Go Drill

This drill is also a reworking of a standard test. Set up the course by placing a chair against a wall and a cone about 8 feet (2.4 m) from the front edge of the chair seat. Sit in the chair with the feet flat on the floor. Then stand up, walk around the cone, and return to sitting as quickly as possible (see figure 10.15). You can modify the drill by changing the distance between the chair and the cone and by performing multiple repetitions.

Figure 10.15   The 8-foot (2.4 m) up-and-go drill.

Cone-Touch Drill

If you have ever played basketball, you may be familiar with drills called *suicides.* Although the name is rather sinister, don't let it prejudice you against this modified version of the drill. To set up the course, place cones along a straight line at distances of 10, 20, and 30 feet (3, 6, and 9 m) away from the starting point (see figure 10.16). To perform the drill, move to the first cone, turn quickly and return to the starting line, go to the second cone and return, and then go to the third cone and return. Be sure to perform the drill as quickly as possible and to touch the cones instead of passing around them.

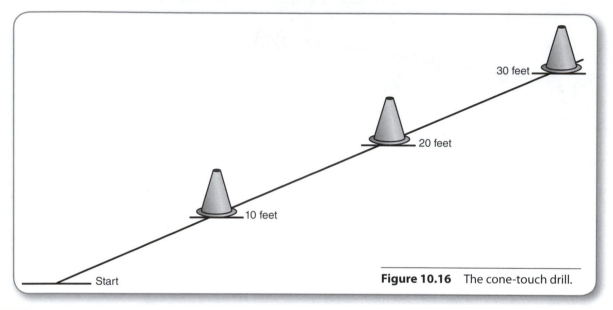

30 feet

20 feet

10 feet

Start

Figure 10.16 The cone-touch drill.

In-and-Out Agility Drill

The course for this drill is a 33-foot (10 m) line with four cones set equidistant along it. Start the drill by passing the right side of the first cone. Pass by the left side of the next cone, the right side of the next cone, and finally the left side of the last cone. Circle the last cone and head back in the other direction, once again alternating sides in an in-and-out pattern (see figure 10.17). For variation you can easily alternate the patterns by skipping cones, reversing directions midway or further along the cones, or performing zigzag patterns between the cones.

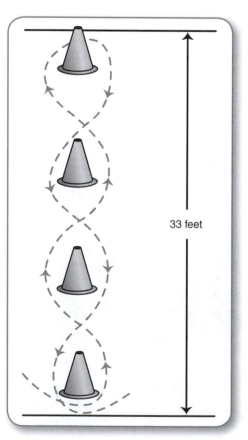

33 feet

Figure 10.17 The in-and-out agility drill.

Lateral Shuffle Drill

Draw a straight line that is approximately 20 feet (6 m) long. Place a mark at the midpoint of the line and a cone at each end. Start at the midpoint and shuffle sideways to one cone and back (see figure 10.18). You can use alternating patterns or you can concentrate on a single side.

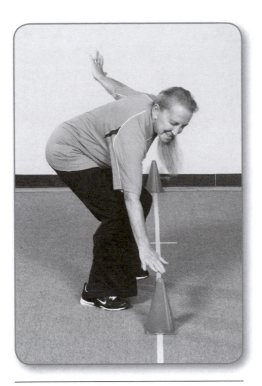

Figure 10.18 The lateral shuffle drill.

Forward and Backward Cone Drill

Using the course described for the lateral shuffle drill, start at one cone and then walk or run to the other cone. Then go around the cone and switch from walking forward to walking backward. Continue to switch walking patterns throughout the drill (see figure 10.19).

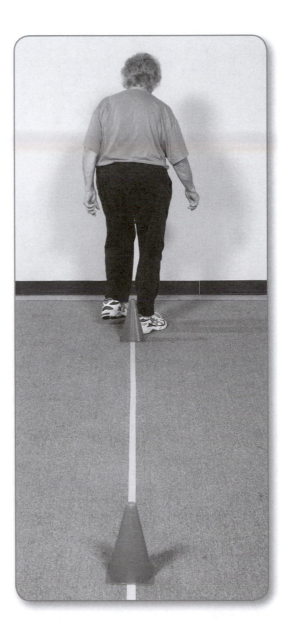

Figure 10.19 The forward and backward cone drill.

LADDER DRILLS

The ladder is one of the most effective exercise tools for improving footwork in competitive athletes. The ladders used for athletes usually have fiber sides and plastic rungs. The ladder drills presented here are a bit more conservative since the ladder is drawn on the floor with paint or tape in order to reduce the potential for injury. Typically the widths between the sides and the rungs are 15 to 18 inches (38-46 cm). The following are drills that I have used in my training sessions. Each of these drills can be performed with different goals in mind. The most common goal is enhanced coordination, which is achieved by using increasingly complex patterns. The second goal might be step amplification, which is accomplished by increasing step height, step length, or step width (see figure 10.20a). The third might be dynamic balance during directional changes, which is accomplished by complex pattern training that requires shifts in body direction (see figure 10.20b). A fourth goal might be foot speed, which is achieved by combining faster movements with less complex patterns.

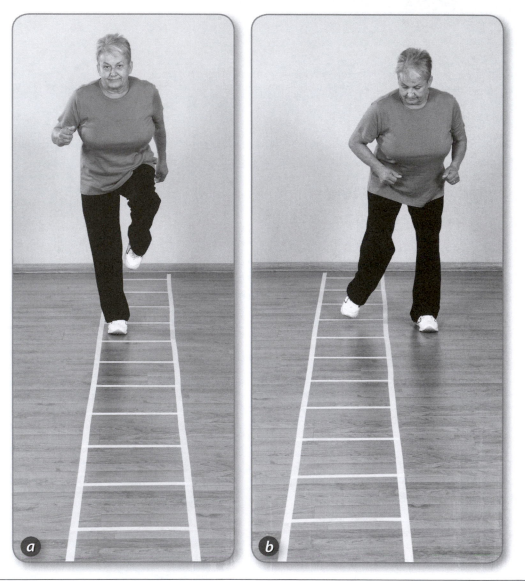

Figure 10.20   A typical ladder drill illustrating (a) high stepping for stride amplification and (b) lateral movements to target balance.

Between-Every-Rung Drill

The between-every-rung drill requires you to step within each space between the rungs on the ladder (see figure 10.21). Since the spaces between the rungs are only 15 inches (38 cm), this means that your step length will be small; however, you should perform the drill at high speed. Therefore, the goal of this drill is to increase movement speed, one of the factors affecting gait speed. You can increase your step height during this drill to increase your ground clearance during normal walking.

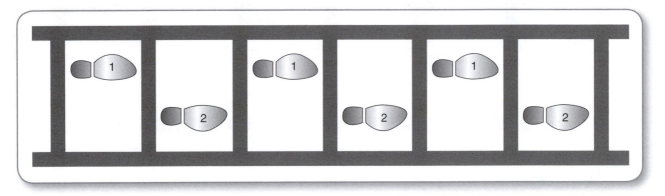

Figure 10.21   The between-every-rung drill.

Two-Between-Every-Rung Drill

The two-between-every-rung drill requires you to take two steps within each space between the rungs of the ladder (see figure 10.22). This requires you to perform the drill at even greater speeds. This drill is also designed to increase movement speed.

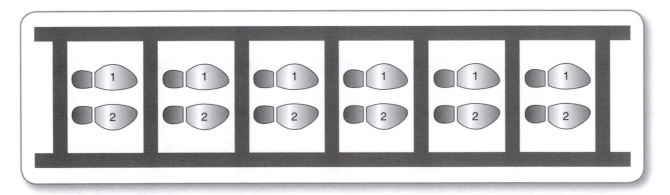

Figure 10.22   The two-between-every-rung drill.

Between-Every-Other-Rung Drill

As the name indicates, this drill requires you to step in the spaces between every other rung on the ladder (see figure 10.23). The step length for this drill is considerably greater than that for the between-every-rung drill. Therefore, this drill focuses on amplifying stride length. Stride length is also important to gait speed.

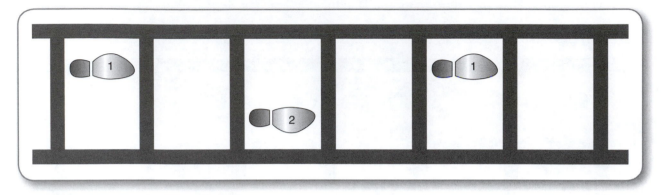

Figure 10.23 The between-every-other-rung drill.

Two-In, Two-Out Drill

The two-in, two-out drill uses two alternating step patterns. The first two steps are into the space between rungs 1 and 2, the second two steps are outside of the space between rungs 2 and 3, and the next two steps are into the space between rungs 3 and 4 (see figure 10.24). This in-and-out movement continues throughout the drill. The purpose of the drill is to train the quick lateral movements that are so important to obstacle negotiation.

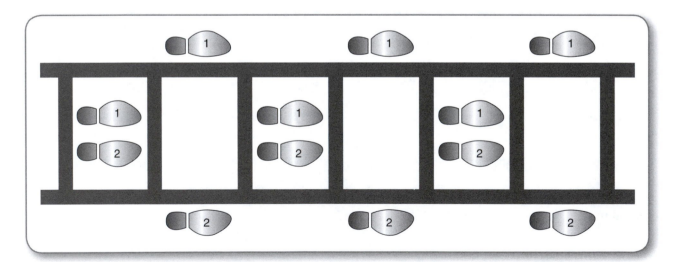

Figure 10.24 The two-in, two-out ladder drill.

In-and-Out-the-Window Drill

Begin the in-and-out-the-window drill by standing along the side of the ladder and facing the space between rungs 1 and 2 (let's call this *space 1*). To begin the drill, step into space 2 with the foot closest to rung 1. Next step with the other foot onto the far side of space 3. Follow with the first foot so that you are again in a parallel stance, this time with your back to the ladder. Now repeat the stepping pattern, this time moving backward through spaces 4 and 5. This will put you at space 5 and return you to the starting parallel stance. Repeat the drill, stepping forward into space 6 (see figure 10.25). This drill mimics the forward and backward movements that are very important in the prevention of falls.

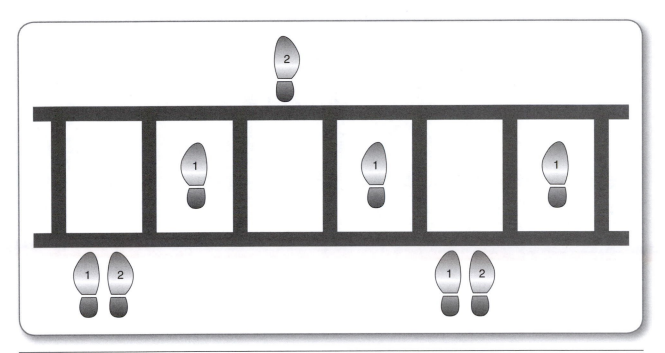

Figure 10.25   The in-and-out-the-window drill.

Lateral Advances

Lateral advances can be practiced in three different patterns (see figure 10.26). Begin all advances by standing in a parallel stance between two rungs of the ladder. The first pattern is to step the right foot into the far right side of each space and then to step the left foot into the left side of the space. The second pattern is to step the right foot into the space and then to shuffle the left foot into the space while quickly moving the right foot to the next space (use a small lateral skip). The third pattern is to use alternating forward and backward crossover steps (cariocas or grapevines). The ability to perform crossover steps without one leg interfering with another is one of the major skills separating younger and older adults.

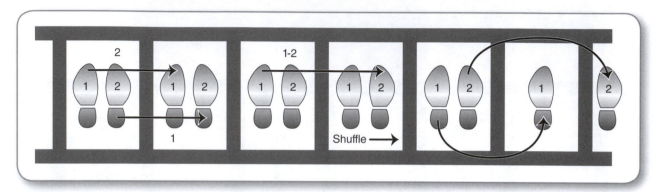

Figure 10.26   Lateral advances.

DRILLS BASED ON ACTIVITIES OF DAILY LIVING

Functional drills work on movement patterns that imitate the activities performed in daily life. Motor learning encodes in the brain in specific patterns, and those patterns need to be trained if they are to be perfected.

▄▄ Chair Stand Drill ▄▄

Rising from and sitting on a chair, bed, or bench are two of the most common ADLs. They require skilled sequential firing of the motor nerves. This drill is merely a spin-off of the chair stand test used to assess leg strength (see figure 10.27). When performing this drill, you can stand as many times as you wish or you can change your speed to provide a sufficient overload or a necessary recovery. The number of stands you use when first beginning the drill will depend on your performance during the 30-second chair stand test. If your test performance puts you in a lower percentile (25th percentile or less), you will most likely have to begin with a low number of stands and do multiple sets with longer recovery periods. Regardless of your conditioning, start conservatively and build across the translational periods. Remember that you can't get your youthful performance back by next Tuesday.

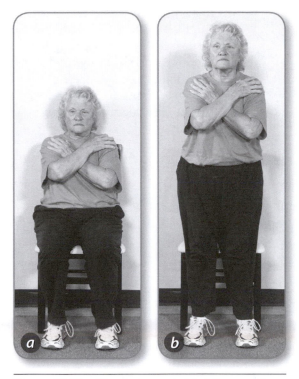

Figure 10.27 The chair stand: *(a)* sitting position and *(b)* standing position.

▄▄ Chair Drills ▄▄

Let's take the chair stand one step forward and look at the chair drills. Think about when you used to play musical chairs. You probably never thought of musical chairs as a great way to increase your physical or motor capacity, but it is. And here's the good news: With these chair drills there will always be a chair available. Several patterns are presented here, but feel free to use your imagination. The inside-circle chair drill (see figure 10.28) and outside-circle chair

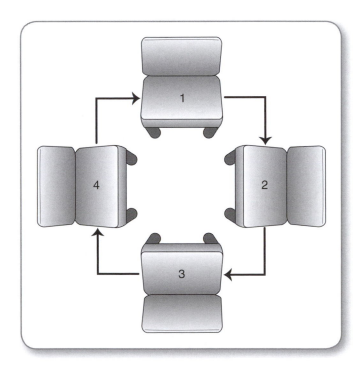

Figure 10.28 The inside-circle chair drill.

drill (see figure 10.29) require you to circle inside or outside of a ring of chairs, sitting and standing as you move from one chair to another. This drill can also be performed with the chairs in a straight line (see figure 10.30). The next drill is the musical chairs drill that you are probably familiar with from your childhood (see figure 10.31). The last drill is the in-and-out chair drill, in which you move between chairs that are facing opposite directions (see figure 10.32). Each of these drills trains leg strength and power while increasing the dynamic balance component of the activity.

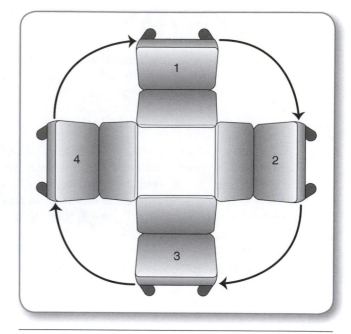

Figure 10.29   The outside-circle chair drill.

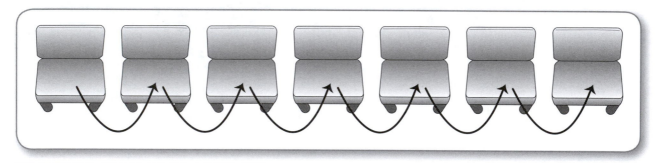

Figure 10.30   The straight-line chair drill.

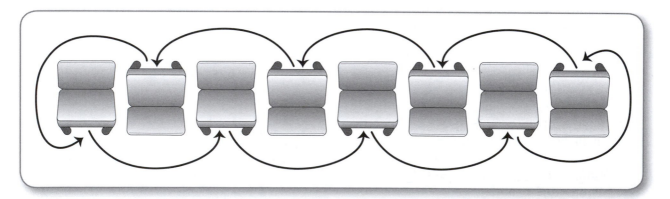

Figure 10.31   The musical chairs drill.

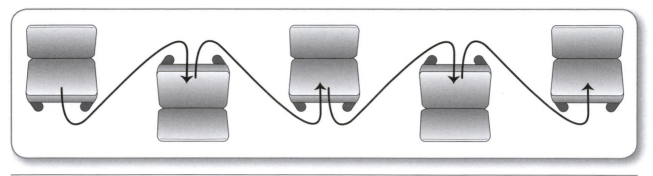

Figure 10.32 The in-and-out chair drill.

Broom Hockey

Sweeping or vacuuming the floor is one of the most common and mundane of the daily housecleaning activities. One option that I developed for training this motor pattern is a drill I call *broom hockey* (see figure 10.33). Using several balls of the same size (e.g., tennis, basketball) and a bucket or other target, use a broom to shoot the balls into the target. You can make this drill more or less difficult by decreasing or increasing the size of the target or increasing or decreasing the distance between you and the target. Another option is to set up a croquet course with cones and use the broom to guide the balls in different patterns through the cones.

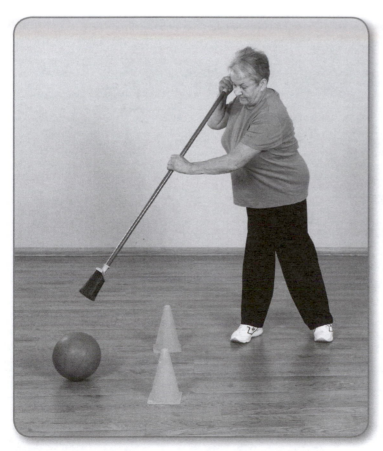

Figure 10.33 Broom hockey.

Step Drill

Stair-climbing is often used to test lower-body power. It is also one of the more challenging ADLs to perform. While running up and down a flight of stairs may bring to mind old memories of stadium drills, the dangers involved in using flights of stairs far outweigh the potential benefits. The step drill presented here uses patterns borrowed from step aerobics to train the climbing pattern and to develop the leg strength, leg power, and dynamic balance components of climbing the stairs. You can use typical aerobic steps and adjust the heights as your client improves. Try this pattern:

1. Step up with one foot, bring the second foot up into a double-leg stance on the step, step down with the first foot, and follow with the second foot into a double-leg stance on the ground (see figure 10.34, *a* and *b*).

2. Step up and down with one foot only, eliminating the double-leg support stance on the step (see figure 10.35, *a* and *b*).

3. Step up with one foot, follow with the double-leg stance on the step, perform a single-knee lift, regain the double-leg stance, and step down (see figure 10.36, *a* and *b*).

4. Perform the pattern just described and add an overhead reach when lifting the knee. Increasing the step height or movement speed can increase the difficulty level. Alternate starting legs. See figure 10.37, *a* and *b*.

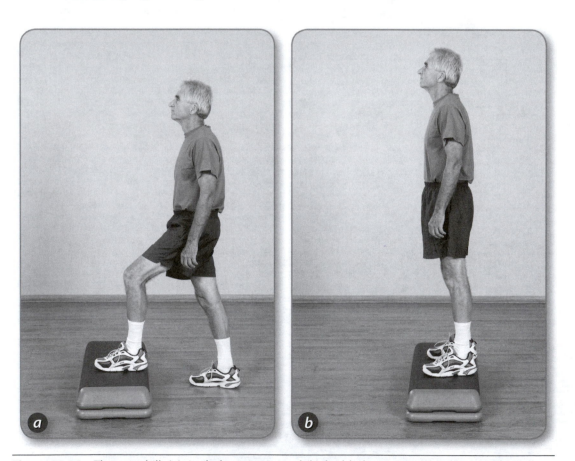

Figure 10.34 The step drill: *(a)* single-leg step-up and *(b)* double-leg stance on the step.

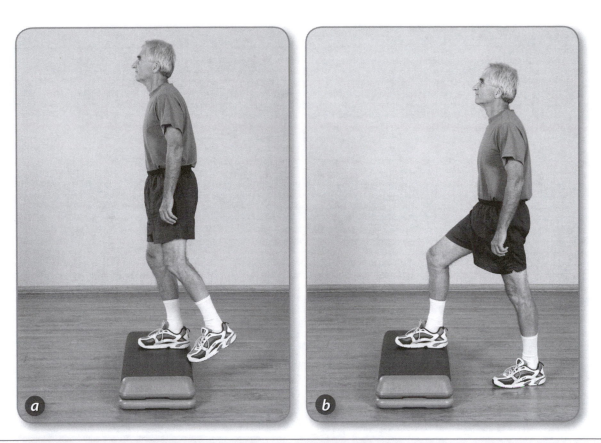

Figure 10.35 The step drill: Using a single leg to *(a)* step up and *(b)* step down.

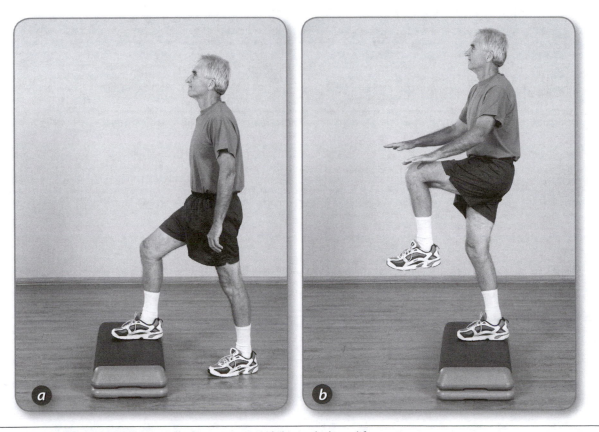

Figure 10.36 The step drill: *(a)* single-leg step-up and *(b)* single-knee lift.

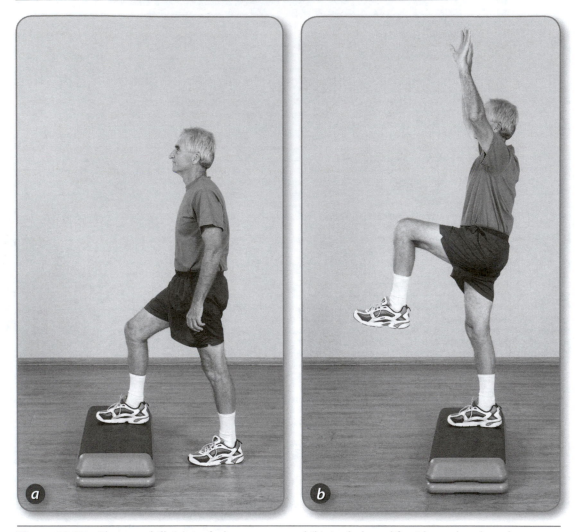

Figure 10.37 The step drill: *(a)* single-leg step-up and *(b)* single-knee lift with overhead reach.

Lateral Step-Up

This is a simple modification of the step drill. In this case, however, the step-up is lateral rather than straight on (figure 10.38). Perform the following patterns:

1. Single-leg step-up, two-leg stance on the step, single-leg step-down, and two-leg stance on the ground

2. Single-leg step-up, single-leg stance on the step, and single-leg step-down

3. Single-leg step-up, double-leg stance on the step, single-leg step-down to the other side of the step, and double-leg stance on the ground

4. Repeat previous pattern with a single-knee lift and overhead reach after the double-leg stance on the step

Follow the precautions presented in the previous step drill. You can use any number of more complex movements to increase the motor challenges offered by these step drills.

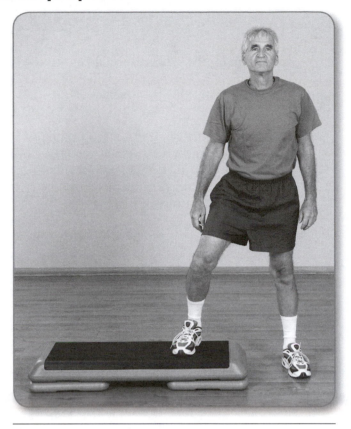

Figure 10.38 Lateral step-up.

Speed and Stride Drill

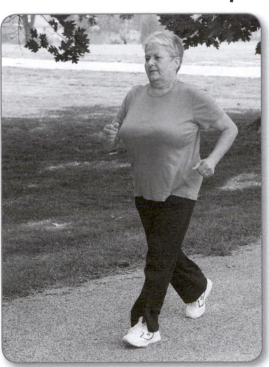

This drill is a modification of the gait training used in the Frailty and Injuries: Cooperative Studies of Intervention Techniques (FICSIT) intervention. It is a way to work on gait patterns while walking a 30-foot (9 m) straight line. When performing this drill, be sure to use proper walking mechanics (see figure 10.39). The concept is to increase stride length (reduce the number of steps necessary to complete the course) and speed (reduce the time necessary to complete the course) while walking the line. Attempt to increase stride length and speed, but do not overreach during the drill.

Figure 10.39 The speed and stride drill.

DRILLS BASED ON INSTRUMENTAL ACTIVITIES OF DAILY LIVING

In addition to ADLs, IADLs should be trained. The drills presented here involve manipulating objects while performing skills common to daily life.

Scarf Drill

This drill is a spin-off of the scarf pickup test used in the Continuous-Scale Physical Functional Performance Tests. Place a number of scarves on the floor in any set or random pattern and then pick them up (see figure 10.40). You can change the difficulty of the movement by increasing the distance between the scarves or picking them up in a specific pattern (one at a time, in pairs, and so on).

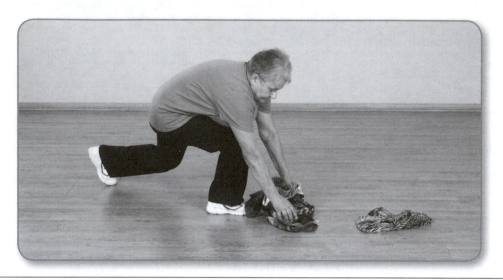

Figure 10.40 The scarf drill.

Book Drills

The book drills presented here use the lunge exercise in a pattern specific to daily activities. The concept behind the drills is to lunge, pick up a book, and move the book to another location. Begin the first drill by standing approximately two stride lengths behind a stack of books. For the rest of the drills, you will need four stacks of books arranged in a square. Each stack should be two stride lengths from the center of the square, which is the starting point for these drills. Here is how to perform the book drills:

1. Lunge forward and pick up the top book on the stack, and then return it to the stack (see figure 10.41*a*).

2. Lunge forward on a diagonal and pick up a book off a stack, and then place it diagonally on the stack at the other forward corner of the square (see figure 10.41*b*).

3. Lunge forward on a diagonal and pick up a book off a stack, and then place it on the stack in the back corner on the same side of the square (see figure 10.41*c*).

4. Lunge forward on a diagonal and pick up a book off a stack, and then place it on the stack in the diagonal back corner of the square (see figure 10.41*d*).

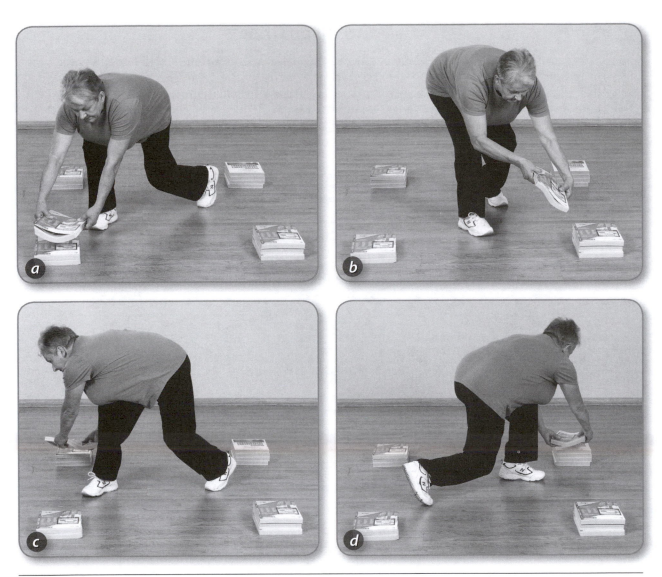

Figure 10.41   The book drills using *(a)* the forward lunge, *(b)* the lateral lunge, *(c)* the backward lunge, and *(d)* the diagonal lunge.

You can control the intensity of the book drills by changing the distance between the books, by piling books higher to make the top book easier to reach or lower to make the top book more difficult to reach, and by changing the size and weight of the books.

Ball-and-Pylon Drills

This set of drills follows the same pattern as the book drills but requires an added degree of motor control (see figure 10.42). The idea is to perform the same progressive patterns described in the book drills but to replace the stacks of books with a tennis ball in the hole on the top of a cone (pylon). The drill can be made easier by using taller cones. In contrast, shorter cones, heavier or larger balls, and greater distances between cones can increase the difficulty.

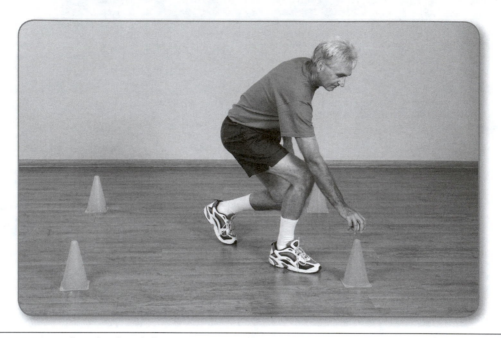

Figure 10.42   Ball-and-pylon drills.

Coin Pickup Drill

This drill is highly dependent on motor skills and not on fitness-based performance. The basic task is to pick up 10 coins as fast as possible (see figure 10.43). The most obvious way to increase the difficulty of the task is to use thinner, smaller coins (dimes) versus larger, thicker coins (half-dollars). The difficulty level can also be increased by using mixed change since the motor pattern must be modified with each coin. The level of difficulty can also be changed by altering the locations of the coins. Coins on the floor are more difficult to deal with than coins on the table. Having coins on the table, a chair, and the floor adds even more difficulty. And finally, the distances between the coins affect difficulty. Coins can not only be moved farther apart but also be placed at unequal distances.

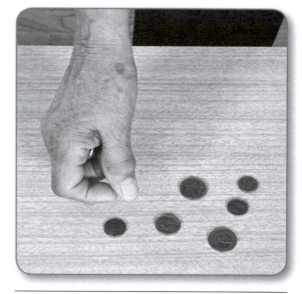

Figure 10.43   The coin pickup drill performed on a table.

Gallon Jug Drill

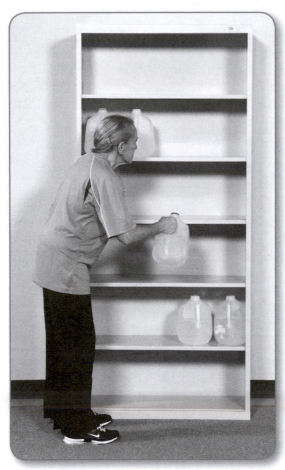

This drill is a modification of the gallon jug shelf test (see figure 10.44). Five 1-gallon (3.8 L) jugs filled with water are placed on a knee-high shelf. A second shelf is placed at shoulder level. The basic drill is to move all of the jugs from the lower shelf to the upper shelf. Now let's think of some modifications. Using smaller jugs decreases the intensity of the drill. Using gallon jugs filled with different amounts of water increases the motor difficulty of the drill. Putting the jugs on the floor adds a greater balance and flexibility challenge. Finally, using multiple shelves with different starting and ending patterns for the jugs defines a more complex movement pattern and significantly increases the motor challenge.

Figure 10.44 The gallon jug drill.

EYE–FOOT COORDINATION DRILLS

We have all heard of eye–hand coordination, but what about eye–foot coordination? Sight is one of the major factors that humans use to adjust movement patterns within an environment. There are direct connections between the cortical and subcortical levels of the brain and the tracks that carry visual information. So let's look at some of the drills that can be used to hardwire these coordination tasks into our neural circuits and make them easier to perform.

Dot or Grid Drills

These drills use visual cues such as numbers or colors and areas such as dots or grids (see figure 10.45). Color or numerical patterns are called out to encourage the client to perform lateral, anterior, and posterior movement shifts in response to the patterns that are called out. In this way the drill does more than simply ask you to follow a visual pattern; it also requires a cognitive component as you link the words you hear with the required color or number.

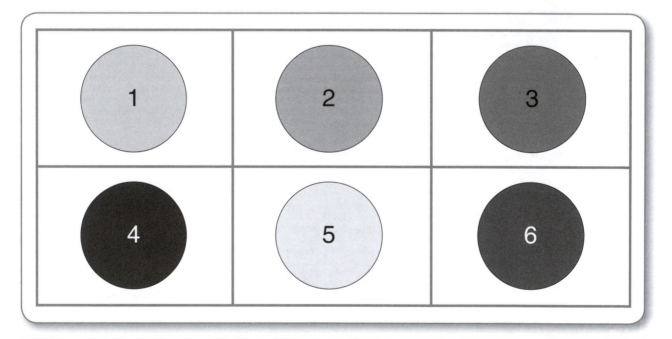

Figure 10.45   An illustration of an eye–foot coordination drill layout showing both color and number based patterns.

Hexagon Drill

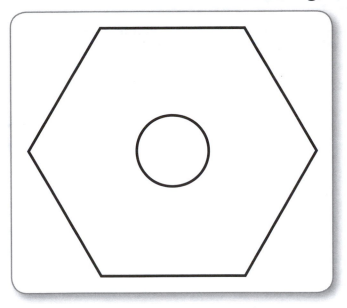

Figure 10.46   The hexagon drill.

Like many of the drills in this chapter, the hexagon drill is a spin-off of an established test, the hexagon test (see figure 10.46). The purpose of the drill is to move at maximum speed across a hexagon marked with tape on the floor. In the classic test, each side is 24 inches (61 cm) long, and each angle is 120°; however, in this drill each side can be lengthened or shortened. Start the drill with both feet together in the middle of the hexagon and face one of the lines marking the sides. Step across the line with both feet, and then step back. While continuing to face the same direction, step over each side of the hexagon and back, thereby completing one repetition of the drill. You may perform single-leg bounces or hops to increase the difficulty level of the drill.

Star Excursion Drill

This is a modification of the test by the same name. The drill is set up by using tape, paint, or a marker to outline a star on the floor. The star is made of four intersecting lines about 2 to 3 inches (5-8 cm) thick and all contained within a 6- × 6-foot (2 × 2 m) square (see figure 10.47). The ends of the lines are labeled as *front, back, left, right, front left, front right, back left,* and *back right.* Begin by standing in the center of the star. To perform the drill, stand on one foot while using the other foot to reach as far as possible along a chosen line. You can use the left or right foot to practice moving around the grid, or you can reach in the direction called out by the trainer.

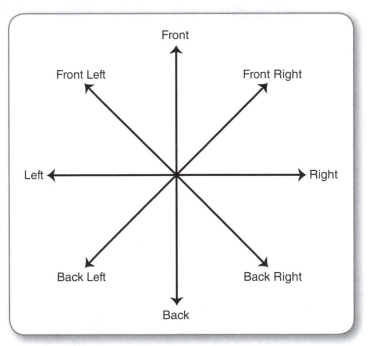

Figure 10.47   The star excursion drill.

BALL DRILLS

Ball drills are excellent ways to practice interacting with objects. These drills are commonly performed using weighted medicine balls; however, playground balls, soccer balls, volleyballs, or basketballs can be used if less resistance is desired. These lighter balls can be used during the early stages of training or at times when the objective of the drill is to improve movement speed rather than strength-related motor training.

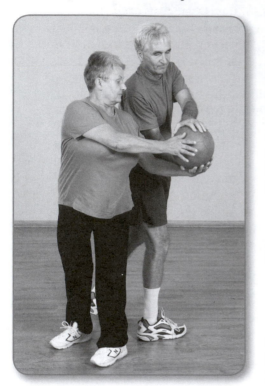

Back-to-Back Handoff

Stand back to back with a partner and hold a ball in both hands (see figure 10.48). Keeping your feet in place, turn to the right, rotating at the waist, and hand the ball to your partner. As your partner brings the ball across the chest, rotate to your other side to receive the ball from your partner as it passed to you. Repeat the handoff a number of times, but be sure to rotate in both directions so that the motor training patterns are practiced bilaterally.

Figure 10.48   The back-to-back handoff.

Chest Pass

Stand, facing a partner, with the knees slightly flexed. Hold the ball close to and high on the chest (see figure 10.49). The first stage of this drill is to extend the ball straight out and then bring it back to the chest without throwing it. The next stage is to throw the ball from the chest to your partner and then receive the return pass. Part of this exercise is slowing the ball down after catching it and bringing it back to the starting position at the chest in preparation for the next throw, so emphasize this eccentric component. Some words of caution. First, begin the drill with a very light (playground) ball. Next, be sure to maintain eye contact with your partner and watch the ball throughout the throw. Third, do not talk until you have stopped the ball and both you and your partner are aware of the stoppage. Too often people are hit because they are not paying attention to the ball or their partner.

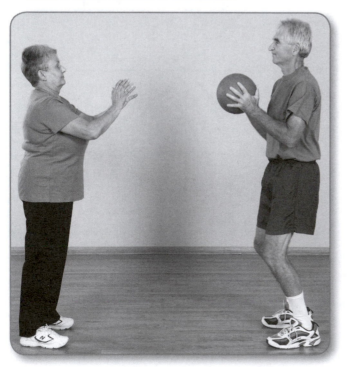
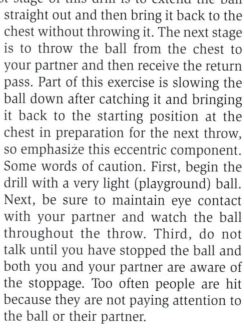

Figure 10.49   The chest pass.

Overhead Throw

Stand with the knees slightly bent and hold a ball overhead. Begin by bending the elbows to bring the ball behind the head and then extend the ball back into the starting position (see figure 10.50). Progress by following this pattern with an overhead throw to a partner.

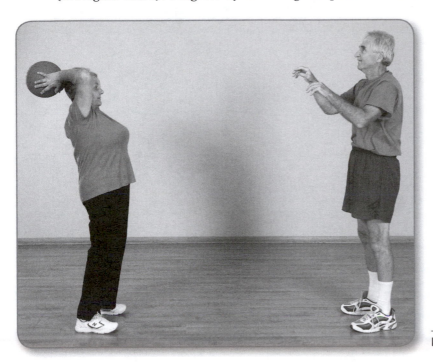

Figure 10.50   The overhead throw.

Lateral Throw

Start by standing with the feet shoulder-width apart and the knees slightly bent (see figure 10.51). Hold the ball next to and slightly below the waist. The arms should be straight. Rotate forward, releasing the ball so that it goes from your right to your partner's right or from your left to your partner's left. Be sure to work both sides equally.

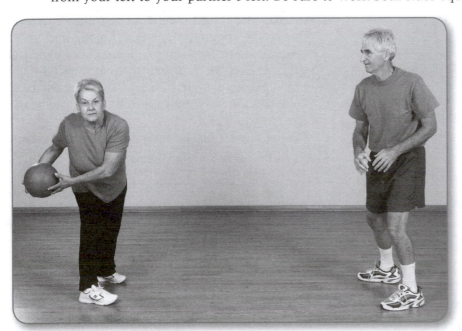

Figure 10.51   The lateral throw.

Soccer Kick

Work with a group of friends and practice kicking a ball in a random pattern to one of your friends (see figure 10.52). Remember to alternate the feet in an attempt to develop motor capacity on both sides. As an alternative to working with friends, the wall can be used for a rebound surface.

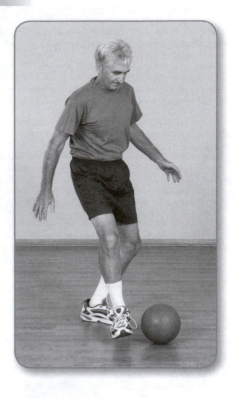

Figure 10.52   The soccer kick.

DANCE MOVEMENTS

It is beyond the scope of this book to examine dances or choreographed routines and their potential to improve balance. However, know that the changes in the direction and speed of movements associated with dance can significantly contribute to balance improvements.

SUMMARY

This chapter has presented the concept of the translational cycle. Remember that translational cycles are intended to

- be complementary to training cycles,
- provide lower-intensity and recovery-oriented training,
- be tapered in as training cycles are tapered out, and
- substitute complexity of movement for intensity of training so that the central nervous system can be trained to facilitate the important movements of daily living.

For exercise interventions to be effective, they must target the specific physiological needs of the individual and change as the client evolves due to the competing effects of aging and exercise. To maximize improvements, the exercise program must incorporate recovery cycles that provide motor pattern training that simulates daily activities. To this end, we have replaced standard recovery periods with translational periods. During these translational periods improvements in fitness parameters such as strength, power, cardiovascular endurance, movement speed, balance, and flexibility can be applied to motor patterns simulating movements associated with independent living, mobility, and fall prevention. These translational periods are as important to our older exercisers as practices on the field or court are to competitive athletes. Thus translational periods should be an integral factor in all exercise interventions for older persons.

Topical Bibliography

Basic Concepts of the Translational Cycle

Ades, P.A., Ballor, D.L., Ashikaga, T., Utton, J.L., & Nair, K.S. (1996). Weight training improves walking endurance in healthy elderly persons: Kinematics. *Ann Intern Med* 124:568-572.

de Vreede, P.L., Samson, M.M., van Meeteren, N.L., Duursma, S.A., & Verhaar, H.J. (2005). Functional-task exercise versus resistance strength exercise to improve daily function in older women: A randomized, controlled trial. *J Am Geriatr Soc* 53:2-10.

de Vreede, P.L., Samson, M.M., van Meeteren, N.L., van der Bom, J.G., Duursma, S.A., & Verhaar, H.J. (2004). Functional tasks exercise versus resistance exercise to improve daily function in older women: A feasibility study. *Arch Phys Med Rehabil* 85:1952-1961.

Dobek, J.C., White, K.N., & Gunter, K.B. (2006). The effect of a novel ADL-based training program on performance of activities of daily living and fitness. *J Aging Phys Act* 15:13-25.

Fiatarone, M.A., O'Neill, E.F., Doyle, N., Clements, K.M., Roberts, S.B., Kehayias, J.J., Lipsitz, L.A., & Evans, W.J. (1993). The Boston FICSIT study: The effects of resistance training and nutritional supplementation on physical frailty in the oldest old. *J Am Geriatr Soc* 41:333-337.

King, M.B., Judge, J.O., Whipple, R.H., & Wolfson, L. (2000). Reliability and responsiveness of two physical performance measures examined in the context of a functional training intervention. *Phys Ther* 80:8-16.

Liu-Ambrose, T., Khan, K.M., Eng, J.J., Janssen, P.A., Lord, S.R., & McKay, H.A. (2004). Resistance and agility training reduce fall risk in women aged 75 to 85 with low bone mass: A 6- month randomized, controlled trial. *JAGS* 52:657-665.

Martin Ginis, K.A., Latimer, A.E., Brawley, L.R., Jung, M.E., & Hicks, A.L. (2006). Weight training to activities of daily living: Helping older adults make a connection. *Med Sci Sports Exerc* 38:116-121.

Nichols, J.F., Hitzelberger, L.M., Sherman, J.G., & Paterson, P. (1995). Effects of resistance training on muscular strength and functional abilities of community-dwelling older adults. *Journal of Aging and Physical Activity* 3:238-250.

Skelton, D.A., Young, A., Greig, C.A., & Malbut, K.E. (1995). Effects of resistance training on strength, power, and selected functional abilities of women aged 75 and older. *Journal of the American Geriatrics Society* 43:1081-1087.

Timonen, L., Rantanen, T., Mäkinen, E., Timonen, T.E., Törmäkangas, T., & Sulkava, R. (2006). Effects of a group-based exercise program on functional abilities in frail older women after hospital discharge. *Aging Clin Exp Res* 18:50-56.

Motor Learning Drills: The Need for Progression

Lundin-Olsson, L., Nyberg, L., & Gustafson, Y. (1997). "Stops walking when talking" as a predictor of falls in elderly people. *Lancet* 349:617.

Melzer, I., Benjuya, N., & Kaplanski, J. (2001). Age-related changes in postural control: Effect of cognitive tasks. *Gerontology* 47:189-194.

Rankin, J.K., Woollacott, M.H., Shumway-Cook, A., & Brown, L.A. (2000). Cognitive influence on postural stability: A neuromuscular analysis in young and older adults. *Journal of Gerontology: Medical Sciences* 55A(3): M112-M119.

Signorile, J.F. (2005). Translational training: Turning fitness gains into functional fitness. *J Active Aging* 4:46-58.

Translational Exercises

Alexander, N.B., & Goldberg, A. (2006). Clinical gait and stepping performance measures in older adults. *Eur Rev Aging Phys Act* 3:20-28.

Aosaki, T., Tsubokawa, H., Ishida, A., Watanabe, K., Graybiel, A.M., & Kimura, M. (1994). Responses of tonically active neurons in the primate's striatum undergo systematic changes during behavioral sensorimotor conditioning. *Journal of Neuroscience* 14:3969-3984.

Cho, B., Scarpace, D., & Alexander, N.B. (2004). Tests of stepping as indicators of mobility, balance, and fall risk in balance-impaired older adults. *J Am Geriatr Soc* 52:1168-1173.

Cress, M.E., Petrella, J.K., Moore, T.L., & Schenkman, M.L. (2005). Continuous-scale physical functional performance test: Validity, reliability, and sensitivity of data for the short version. *Phys Ther* 85:323-335.

Cress, M.E., Buchner, D.M., Questad, K.A., Esselman, P.C., deLateur, B.J., & Schwartz, R.S. (1996). Continuous-scale physical functional performance in healthy older adults: A validation study. *Archives of Physical Medicine and Rehabilitation* 77:1243-1250.

Duncan, P.W., Weiner, D.K., Chandler, J., & Studenski, S. (1990). Functional reach: A new clinical measure of balance. *J Gerontol A Biol Sci Med Sci* 45:M192-M197.

Elble, R.J., Thomas, S., Sienko, H.C., & Colliver, J. (1991). Stride-dependent changes in gait of older people. *J Neurol* 238:1-5.

Guralnik, J.M., Ferrucci, L., Simonsick, E.M., & Salive, M.E. (1995). Lower extremity function in persons over 70 years as a predictor of subsequent disability. *New England Journal of Medicine* 332:556-561.

Jackson, P.L., Lafleur, M.F., Malouin, F., Richards, C.L., & Doyon, J. (2003). Functional cerebral reorganization following motor sequence learning through mental practice with motor imagery. *NeuroImage* 20:1171-1180.

Jones, C.J., Rikli, R.E., & Beam, W.C. (1999). A 30-s chair-stand test as a measure of lower body strength in community-residing older adults. *Research Quarterly for Exercise and Sport* 70:113-117.

Olmsted, L.C., Carcia, C.R., Hertel, J., & Schultz, S.J. (2006). Efficacy of the star excursion balance tests in detecting reach deficits in subjects with chronic ankle instability. *J Ath Train* 37:501-506.

Ory, M., Schechtman, K., Miller, J.P., Hadley, E.C., Fiatarone, M.A., Province, M.A., Arfken, C.L., Morgan, D., Weiss, S., Kaplan, M., & The FICSIT Group (1993). Frailty and injuries in later life: The FICSIT trials. *Journal of the American Geriatrics Society* 41:283-296.

Pacala, J.T., Judge, J.O., & Boult, C. (1996). Factors affecting sample selection in a randomized trial of balance enhancement: The FICSIT Study. *Journal of the American Geriatrics Society* 44:377-382.

Province, M.A., Hadley, E.C., Hornbrook, M.C., Lipsitz, L.A., Miller, J.P., Mulrow, C.D., Ory, M.G., Sattin, R.W., Tinetti, M.E., & Wolf, S.L. (1995). The effects of exercise on falls in elderly patients: A preplanned meta-analysis of the FICSIT trials. *JAMA* 273:1341-1347.

Springer, S., Giladi, N., Peretz, C., Yogev, G., Simon, E.S., & Hausdorff, J.M. (2006). Dual-tasking effects on gait variability: The role of aging, falls, and executive function. *Mov Disord* 21:950-957.

Toulotte, C., Thevenon, A., Watelain, E., & Fabre, C. (2006). Identification of healthy elderly fallers and non-fallers by gait analysis under dual-task conditions. *Clin Rehabil* 20:269-276.

Rikli, R.E., & Jones, C.J. (1999). Development and validation of a functional fitness test for community-residing older adults. *Journal of Aging and Physical Activity* 7:129-161.

Signorile, J.F., Sandler, D.J., Ma, F., Bamel, S.A., Stanziano, D.C., Smith, W., & Roos, B.A. (2007). The gallon jug shelf transfer test: An instrument to evaluate deteriorating function in older adults. *J Aging Phys Act* 15:56-74.

References

Martin Ginis, K.A., Latimer, A.E., Brawley, L.R., Jung, M.E., & Hicks, A.L. (2006). Weight training to activities of daily living: Helping older adults make a connection. *Med Sci Sports Exerc* 38:116-121.

Signorile, J.F. (2005). Translational training: Turning fitness gains into functional fitness. *J Active Aging* 4:46-58.

APPENDIX

Normative Data

Women: Percentile Ranks by Age

	AGE GROUPS (YEARS)						
	60-64	65-69	70-74	75-79	80-84	85-89	90-94
BODY COMPOSITION							
BMI							
10th	33	33.2	31.9	31	30	29	29.5
25th	29.8	30	29.1	28.3	27.4	26.8	27.1
50th	26.3	26.5	26.1	25.4	24.7	24.3	24.1
75th	22.8	23	23.1	22.5	22	21.8	21.1
90th	19.6	19.8	20.3	19.8	19.6	19.5	18.3
Percent body fat							
10th	39.3		41.3		43.3		45.3
25th	35.5		37.5		39.5		41.5
50th	30.9		32.9		34.9		36.9
75th	26.7		28.7		30.7		32.7
90th	21.1		23.1		25.1		27.1
FLEXIBILITY							
Chair sit-and-reach test (in. [cm])							
10th	−3 (−7.6)	−3 (−7.6)	−3.5 (-8.9)	−4 (-10.2)	−4.5 (-11.4)	−4.5 (-11.4)	−7 (-17.8)
25th	−0.5 (−1.3)	−0.5 (−1.3)	−1 (-2.5)	−1.5 (-3.8)	−2 (-5.1)	−2.5 (-6.4)	−4.5 (-11.4)
50th	2 (5.1)	2 (5.1)	1.5 (3.8)	1 (2.54)	0.5 (1.3)	−0.5 (-1.3)	−2 (-5.1)
75th	5 (12.7)	4.5 (11.4)	4 (10.2)	3.5 (8.9)	3 (7.6)	2.5 (6.4)	1 (-2.5)
90th	7 (17.8)	6.5 (16.5)	6 (15.2)	3.5 (8.9)	5 (12.7)	4.5 (11.4)	3.5 (8.9)

(continued)

Women: Percentile Ranks by Age *(continued)*

	AGE GROUPS (YEARS)						
	60-64	**65-69**	**70-74**	**75-79**	**80-84**	**85-89**	**90-94**
FLEXIBILITY							
Back scratch test (in. [cm])							
10th	−5.5 (14.0)	−6 (15.2)	−6.5 (16.5)	−7.5 (17.8)	−8 (-20.3)	−10 (-25.4)	−11.5 (-29.2)
25th	−3 (-7.6)	−3.5 (-8.9)	−4 (-10.2)	−5 (-12.7)	−5.5 (-14.0)	−7 (-17.8)	−8 (-20.3)
50th	−0.5 (-3.8)	−1 (-2.5)	−1.5 (-3.8)	−2 (-5.1)	−2.5 (-6.4)	-3.5 (-8.9)	−4.5 (-11.4)
75th	1.5 (3.8)	1.5 (3.8)	1 (2.5)	0.5 (1.3)	0 (0)	−1 (-2.5)	−1 (-2.5)
90th	4 (10.2)	3.5 (8.9)	3 (7.6)	3 (7.6)	2.5 (6.4)	2 (5.1)	2 (5.1)
Modified trunk rotation test (in. [cm])							
10th	—	22.7 (57.7)		19 (48.3)		17.6 (44.7)	
20th	—	23.6 (59.8)		20.8 (52.8)		19 (48.3)	
50th	—	25.8 (65.5)		26 (66.0)		21 (53.3)	
70th	—	28.5 (72.4)		28.1 (71.4)		23.4 (59.4)	
90th	—	30.7 (78.0)		30 (76.2)		28 (71.1)	
BALANCE							
Single-leg stance balance test (seconds)							
10th	4		0		0		
25th	14		4		0		
50th	25		11		7		
75th	36		19		14		
90th	46		26		21		
Functional reach test (in. [cm])							
10th	11 (27.9)		6 (15.2)				—
25th	12.3 (31.2)		8.1 (20.6)				—

BALANCE						
Functional reach test (in. [cm])						
50th	13.8 (35.1)	10.5 (26.7)				—
75th	15.3 (38.9)	12.9 (32.8)				—
90th	16.6 (42.2)	15 (38.1)				—
8-foot (2.4 m) up-and-go test (seconds)						
10th	6.7	7.1	8	8.3	10	11.1	13.5
25th	6	6.4	7.1	7.4	8.7	9.6	11.5
50th	5.2	5.6	6	6.3	7.2	7.9	9.4
75th	4.4	4.8	4.9	5.2	5.7	6.2	7.3
90th	3.7	4.1	4	4.3	4.4	5.1	5.3
NEUROMUSCULAR PERFORMANCE						
30-second chair stand test (reps)						
10th	9	9	8	7	6	5	2
25th	12	11	10	10	9	8	4
50th	15	14	13	12	11	10	8
75th	17	16	15	15	14	13	11
90th	20	18	18	17	16	15	13
Modified ramp power test (watts)						
5th	96.89	88.16	82.69	66.88	77.02	48.47	48.47
25th	151.28	136.73	116.15	99.82	91.14	65.24	65.24
50th	169.29	163.78	145.15	121.83	107.71	89.05	89.05
75th	213.18	192.88	169.07	149.3	139.57	102.79	102.79
95th	252.22	223.7	203.41	181.53	169.96	137.86	137.86
30-second arm curl test (reps)						
10th	10	10	9	8	8	7	6
25th	13	12	12	11	10	10	8
50th	16	15	15	14	13	12	11
75th	19	18	17	17	16	15	13
90th	22	21	20	20	18	17	16

(continued)

Women: Percentile Ranks by Age (continued)

	AGE GROUPS (YEARS)						
	60-64	**65-69**	**70-74**	**75-79**	**80-84**	**85-89**	**90-94**
	NEUROMUSCULAR PERFORMANCE						
	Gallon jug shelf test (seconds)						
5th	13.2	11.5	13.5	15.2	15.6	18.7	18.7
25th	10.8	9.8	10.8	11.8	12.5	14	14
50th	8.9	9.1	9.6	10.1	11	12.7	12.7
75th	8.1	8.3	8.7	8.9	9.8	11.4	11.4
95th	7.1	7.5	7.7	8	8.7	9.3	9.3
	Usual walking speed test (seconds)						
10th	4.3		4.35		5.22		6.26
25th	3.92		3.99		4.79		5.75
50th	3.53		3.6		4.32		5.18
75th	3.14		3.19		3.83		4.59
90th	2.78		2.79		3.35		4.02
	Maximum walking speed test (seconds)						
10th	3.05		3.15		3.78		4.54
25th	2.83		2.9		3.48		4.18
50th	2.58		2.62		3.14		3.77
75th	2.33		2.33		2.8		3.36
90th	2.11		2.09		2.51		3.01
	CARDIOVASCULAR PERFORMANCE						
	6-minute walk test (yards [meters])						
10th	495 (452.6)	440 (402.3)	420 (384.1)	365 (333.8)	310 (283.5)	260 (237.7)	195 (178.3)
25th	545 (498.4)	500 (457.2)	480 (438.9)	430 (393.2)	385 (352.0)	340 (310.9)	275 (251.5)
50th	605 (553.2)	570 (521.2)	550 (502.9)	510 (466.3)	460 (420.6)	425 (388.6)	350 (320.0)
75th	660 (603.5)	635 (580.6)	615 (562.4)	585 (534.9)	540 (493.8)	510 (466.3)	440 (402.3)
90th	710 (649.2)	695 (635.5)	675 (617.2)	655 (598.9)	610 (557.8)	595 (544.1)	520 (475.5)

Men: Percentile Ranks by Age

	AGE GROUPS (YEARS)						
	60-64	**65-69**	**70-74**	**75-79**	**80-84**	**85-89**	**90-94**
BODY COMPOSITION							
BMI							
10th	32.8	32.9	31.6	31.4	30.5	28	29.6
25th	30.2	30.3	29.2	29	28.4	26.5	27.4
50th	27.4	27.4	26.6	26.4	26.1	24.9	24.9
75th	24.6	24.7	24	23.8	23.8	23.3	22.4
90th	22	22.1	21.6	21.4	21.7	21.8	20.2
Percent body fat							
10th	31.2		33.2		35.2		37.2
25th	27.6		29.6		31.6		33.6
50th	23.5		25.5		27.5		29.5
75th	19.3		21.3		23.3		25.3
90th	15.3		17.3		19.3		21.3
FLEXIBILITY							
Chair sit-and-reach test (in. [cm])							
10th	−6 (-15.2)	−6 (-15.2)	−6.5 (-16.5)	−7 (-17.8)	−8 (-20.3)	−8 (-20.3)	−9 (-22.9)
25th	−2.5 (-6.4)	−3 (-7.6)	−3.5 (-8.9)	−4 (-10.2)	−5.5 (-14.0)	−5.5 (-14.0)	−6.5 (-16.6)
50th	0.5 (1.3)	0 (0.0)	−0.5 (-1.3)	−1 (-2.5)	−2 (-5.1)	−2.5 (-6.4)	−3.5 (-8.9)
75th	4 (10.2)	3 (7.6)	2.5 (6.4)	2 (5.1)	1.5 (3.8)	0.5 (1.3)	0.5 (1.3)
90th	6.5 (16.5)	6 (15.2)	5.5 (14.0)	5 (12.7)	4.5 (11.4)	3 (7.6)	2 (5.1)
Back scratch test (in. [cm])							
10th	−10 (-25.4)	−10.5 (-26.7)	−11 (-27.9)	−12 (-30.5)	−12.5 (-31.8)	−12.5 (-31.8)	−13.5 (-34.3)
25th	−6.5 (-16.5)	−7.5 (19.1)	−8 (-20.3)	−9 (-22.9)	−9.5 (-24.1)	−10 (-25.4)	−10.5 (-26.7)
50th	−3.5 (-8.9)	−4 (-10.2)	−4.5 (-11.4)	−5.5 (-14.0)	−5.5 (-14.0)	−6 (-15.2)	−7 (-17.8)
75th	0 (0.0)	−1 (-2.5)	−1 (-2.5)	−2 (-5.1)	−2 (-5.1)	−3 (-7.6)	−4 (-10.2)
90th	2.5 (6.4)	2 (5.1)	2 (5.1)	1 (2.5)	1 (2.5)	0 (0.0)	−1 (-2.5)

(continued)

Men: Percentile Ranks by Age *(continued)*

	AGE GROUPS (YEARS)						
	60-64	65-69	70-74	75-79	80-84	85-89	90-94

FLEXIBILITY

Modified trunk rotation test (in. [cm])

Percentile	60-64	65-69	70-74	75-79	80-84	85-89	90-94
10th	—	22.7 (57.7)		19.0 (48.3)		17.6 (44.7)	
20th	—	23.6 (59.9)		20.8 (52.8)		19.0 (48.3)	
50th	—	25.8 (65.5)		26.0 (66.0)		21.0 (53.3)	
70th	—	28.5 (72.4)		28.1 (71.4)		23.4 (59,4)	
90th	—	30.7 (78.0)		30.0 (76.2)		28.0 (71.1)	

BALANCE

Single-leg stance balance test (seconds)

Percentile	60-64	65-69	70-74	75-79	80-84	85-89	90-94
10th	7		0		0		
25th	17		8		0		
50th	29		18		6		
75th	40		29		11		
90th	50		38		16		

Functional reach test (in. [cm])

Percentile	60-64	65-69	70-74	75-79	80-84	85-89	90-94
10th	12.1 (30.7)		11.2 (28.5)				—
25th	13.4 (34.0)		12.1 (30.7)				—
50th	14.9 (37.8)		13.2 (33.5)				—
75th	16.4 (41.7)		14.3 (36.3)				—
90th	17.7 (45.0)		15.3 (38.9)				—

8-foot (2.4 m) up-and-go test (seconds)

Percentile	60-64	65-69	70-74	75-79	80-84	85-89	90-94
10th	6.4	6.5	6.8	8.3	8.7	10.5	11.8
25th	5.6	5.7	6.9	7.2	7.6	8.9	10

BALANCE						

8-foot (2.4 m) up-and-go test (seconds)

50th	4.7	5.1	5.3	5.9	6.4	7.2	8.1
75th	3.8	4.3	4.2	4.6	5.2	5.3	6.2
90th	3	3.8	3.6	3.5	4.1	3.9	4.4

NEUROMUSCULAR PERFORMANCE						

30-second chair stand test (reps)

10th	11	9	9	8	7	6	5
25th	14	12	12	11	10	8	7
50th	16	15	15	14	12	11	10
75th	19	18	17	17	15	14	12
90th	22	21	20	19	18	17	15

Modified ramp power test (watts)

5th	117.33	165.35	103.94	86.29	82.57	25.02	25.02
25th	135.73	195.77	169.07	169.02	127.31	73.65	73.65
50th	284.33	259.89	233.88	203.64	206.54	92.51	92.51
75th	339.31	304.9	269.56	252.37	236.49	132.7	132.7
95th	395	343.33	316.76	278.35	303.24	165.16	165.16

30-second arm curl test (reps)

10th	13	12	11	10	10	8	7
25th	16	15	14	13	13	11	10
50th	19	18	17	16	16	14	12
75th	22	21	21	19	19	17	14
90th	25	25	24	22	21	19	17

Gallon jug shelf test (seconds)

5th	12.6	10.9	13.2	14.5	14.8	18.6	18.6
25th	8.3	9	10.2	10.3	11.6	14.8	14.8
50th	7.7	7.9	8.9	9.2	9.8	12.7	12.7
75th	6.8	7.4	8.1	8.7	8.2	10.2	10.2
95th	5.9	5.2	6.7	7.5	7.3	9.4	9.4

(continued)

Men: Percentile Ranks by Age (continued)

	AGE GROUPS (YEARS)						
	60-64	**65-69**	**70-74**	**75-79**	**80-84**	**85-89**	**90-94**
NEUROMUSCULAR PERFORMANCE							
Usual walking speed test (seconds)							
10th	4		4.1		4.92		5.9
25th	3.7		3.78		4.54		5.44
50th	3.36		3.44		4.13		4.95
75th	3		3.09		3.71		4.45
90th	2.7		2.8		3.36		4.03
Maximum walking speed test (seconds)							
10th	2.95		2.7		3.24		3.89
25th	2.67		2.46		2.95		3.54
50th	2.37		2.2		2.64		3.17
75th	2.07		1.94		2.33		2.79
90th	1.8		1.71		2.05		2.46
CARDIOVASCULAR PERFORMANCE							
6-minute walk test (yards [meters])							
10th	555 (507.5)	500 (457.2)	480 (438.9)	395 (361.2)	370 (338.3)	295 (269.7)	215 (196.6)
25th	610 (557.8)	560 (512.1)	545 (498.4)	470 (429.8)	445 (406.9)	380 (347.5)	305 (278.9)
50th	675 (617.2)	630 (576.1)	610 (557.8)	555 (507.5)	525 (480.1)	475 (434.3)	405 (370.3)
75th	735 (672.1)	700 (640.1)	680 (621.8)	640 (585.2)	605 (553.2)	570 (521.2)	500 (457.2)
90th	790 (722.4)	765 (699.5)	745 (681.2)	715 (653.8)	680 (621.8)	660 (603.5)	590 (539.5)

Index

Note: Page numbers followed by an italicized *f* or *t* refer to the figure or table on that page, respectively.

A

abdominal adipose tissue 55
abdominal muscles
  strengthening exercises 191-195
  stretches 97-99
abdominal skinfold measurement 53
acetylcholine 134
active assisted stretching (AAS) 72, 73
  back arm stretch 93
  back scratch stretch 94
  cross-body shoulder 93
  dorsiflexor stretch 94
  leg adductor 85
  overhead trunk twist 97-98
  safety precautions 82
  seated calf stretch 88
  seated cat 96
activities of daily living (ADLs) 15, 16
  conditions affecting 9
  drills based on 281-287
  and flexibility 70, 75, 96
  and muscular endurance 142
  and power 145
  relationship to diagnostic tests 27t,
    28-29
  and resistance training 255-256
  testing performance on 32-33
adaptation 11, 37
adenosine diphosphate (ADP) 39
adenosine triphosphate (ATP) 39
  for anaerobic power 143
  breakdown and resynthesis 40f
adipose tissue 7, 8, 51, 55
ADL-based training 255
ADLs. *See* activities of daily living (ADLs)
aerobic enzymes 137
aerobic glycolysis 39
aerobic power 143
Aerobics (Cooper) 209
aerobic training. *See* cardiovascular
    training
Agaston, Arthur 226
age concepts 4
agility
  and balance 119
  drills 272
agility training
  effects on neuromuscular junction 137
  and fall probability 125
  programs 124-125
aging
  facets of 5f, 28
  and hormone levels 135
  and physical capacity 3
  successfully 5
aging curves 3, 5
  bending with exercise 12, 13f
  cardiovascular 11
  connective tissue 7-9, 11
  neuromuscular 5-7, 13f
alcohol consumption 118
Altena, T.S. 216
American College of Sports Medicine
    (ACSM) 23
anabolic hormones 135
anaerobic energy systems 137
anaerobic enzymes 137
anaerobic exercises 220
anaerobic glycolysis 39, 143
anaerobic power 42, 143
andropause 135

B

ankle flexibility test 78-79
ankle ROM 71, 73, 78
anterior cruciate ligament 8f
"A Perspective on Exercise Prescription"
    (Weber) 23
aquatic training 221, 223
  drag forces 223, 230
  effects on cardiovascular fitness 230
  effects on flexibility 74
  equipment 230
  high-speed work 146
  water depth 230
arm curl test 151-152
arteriovenous oxygen difference 210
arthritis 9. *See also* osteoarthritis
  aquatic training for patients with 74
  and range of motion 70
a-v(O$_2$)difference 210

back exercises 173
back scratch stretch 94, 95
back scratch test 77-78
balance
  and agility 119
  and base of support 118-119
  and center of gravity 118-119
  conditions affecting 9
  equilibrium 119
  and falls 117
  functional balance class content 126t
  maintenance strategies 119, 120f, 121
  in seated position 125
  testing 121-124
  training 124-126
balance drills 264-268
balance platforms 126
balance recovery
  change-in-support reactions 120f
  fixed-support reactions 120f
  rapid limb movement 124
ball-and-pylon drills 290
ball drills 294-296
ballistic stretching 71
Bannister, Edward 240
base of support
  and balance 118-119
  dynamic 126t
bench press
  flat 170
  inclined 172
Benton, Melissa 115
Bernard, Claude 37
beta-oxidation 39
biceps curl 184
bioenergetic specificity 39, 41
biomechanical specificity 39t, 41-43
The Biomechanics of Sports Techniques
    (Hay) 119
block periodization 244-245, 246
blood cells 11
blood composition 11
blood glucose utilization 137
blood lipid profiles 213, 216
blood pressure. *See also* hypertension
  and cardiovascular exercise 213-214
  and falls 118
body composition
  and interval training 61-62
  measurement methods 51
  and mixed training 62-63

resistance training effects 58-61
body density (BD)
  calculation for men 54
  calculation for women 55
body fat 8. *See also* adipose tissue; body
    composition
  changes with age 9f
  consequences of 47
  percentage by age and gender 47f
body mass index (BMI) 48, 55
body weight. *See also* obesity
  changes with age 8, 9f
  loss of lean mass 8, 14
  as marker of frailty 14
  and mortality 49
bone. *See also* fractures
  aging curves 10f
  cells 105
  cortex 105
  cortical 105
  density 8, 10f, 106-107, 110f
  density testing 111-112
  diameter 107, 108f
  geometry 107-108, 110
  growth and loss by age 107f
  lacuna 105
  lamellae 105, 106f
  marrow 106
  minerals in 107
  quality 107
  reengineering 107-108
  response to training 112-115
  strength factors 8, 106
  structure 105-106, 109f
  trabecular 105-106
  wall thickness and diameter 108f
bone–ligament junctions 9
bone loss. *See* osteoporosis
book drills 288-289
Borer, Katarina 112
Borg RPE scale 226
BOSU balls 266
brain restructuring 255
breathing rate 38
bridge exercise 193
broom hockey 283
Bulat, Tatjana 125
bursitis 9

C

calcium
  flow inside muscles 134-135, 137
  low intake 115
  and vitamin D 115
calf muscles 166
calf stretches 88, 89f
caloric burn 57, 58, 59-60
Canadian Centre for Activity and Aging 133
Cao, Zhen-Bo 125
cardiac output 211
cardiovascular disease 47, 55, 213
cardiovascular endurance 142
cardiovascular system 11
  aging curves 11f, 12f
cardiovascular training. *See also* interval
    training
  benefits of 209-214
  EPOC after 62
  equipment 221-223
  periodization in 227
  program design 219

cardiovascular training. *See also* interval
  training *(continued)*
    protocols 224
    steady state 62, 224-225
    types of exercise 219-221
    for weight loss 57
cartilage 9, 10*f*
Case Western Reserve University 215
cat stretch 97
center of gravity 264, 266
    in balance recovery reactions 120*f*
    and base of support 119*f*
    and falls 120
central nervous system 255. *See also*
    nervous system
central obesity 212
chair drills 281-282, 283*f*
chair sit-and-reach test 69, 76-77
chair stand drill 281
chair stand tests 148-149
chest fly 172
chest press, seated 170
chest skinfold measurement 52
cholesterol levels 212, 213, 216
chronological age 4
circuit training 59, 229. *See also* interval
    training
cognition 118
coin pickup drill 290
collagen 7, 70, 107
concentric strength 139
congestive heart disease (CHD) 49*f*
connective tissues. *See also* adipose tissue;
    bone
    adaptation 11
    aging curves 8*f*, 9*f*, 10*f*
    blood as 11
    cartilage 9, 10*f*
    elasticity 7, 8*f*
    properties and gender 8
    strength 7, 8*f*
    types of 7, 8
contractile specificity 43
Cooper, Kenneth 209, 218
coordination
    and balance training 126*t*
    eye-foot drills 269, 292-293
    eye-hand 125
    ladder drills 276
core musculature 191
core stretches 96-99
    cat stretch 96, 97
    cross-legged forward stretch 96
    knee crossover 99
    lateral reach 99
    lying tuck 97
    seated overhead trunk twist 97-98
creatine phosphate system 39, 143
crunches 191

D
dance movements 296
delayed-onset muscle soreness (DOMS) 74
deltoids 172, 180
dense connective tissue 7
diabetes mellitus 48, 59, 212, 231
diagnostic testing. *See* tests
diamond analogy 4-5
diet 57, 115
dog walking 217
dorsiflexors
    exercises 168-169
    stretches 89-90
    testing 78-79
drag forces 223, 230
Duysens, J. 121
DXA 11
dynamic axial resistance device (DARD) 168
dynamic constant resistance 43, 138
dynamic flexibility 69
dynamic stretching 71
dynamometers 139

E
elastic cartilage 9
elastin 7
elliptical trainers 223
endurance. *See* cardiovascular endurance;
    muscular endurance
energy demands 39
energy expenditure 39, 59, 61*f*
energy systems 39, 40*f*
environment
    of failure 24
    and falls 118
    and homeostasis 15, 37
    internal and external 14-15, 17*f*
    for training 146
enzymes 39
EPOC. *See* excess postexercise oxygen
    consumption (EPOC)
equipment. *See* exercise equipment
Eriksen, L. 215
erythrocytes 11
excess postexercise oxygen consumption
    (EPOC) 57
    after aerobic exercise 62
    and exercise intensity 57, 58*f*
    with resistance training 59, 60
exercise. *See also* intensity
    acute response to 37-38
    duration 57
    effectiveness of 57-58
    versus training 38
    training response to 38
exercise diagnosis 17-18, 23. *See also* tests
    analysis of needs 24-25
    general *versus* specific 24
    sample diagnostic sheet 26*t*
exercise equipment 146, 221-223
exercise prescription 5, 23
    based on diagnosis 17, 23-24, 29
    evolving client needs 16, 30
    individualized 14, 16, 17
    mix of anaerobic and aerobic work 41
    model for 18*f*
    and specificity 38
    targeting fitness variables 17*f*
exercise specificity 17, 38-39
    bioenergetic specificity 39, 41
    biomechanical specificity 39*t*, 41-43
    contractile specificity 43
    joint specificity 41
    load 42-43
    movement pattern 43
    muscle specificity 41
    practical example of 63
    speed 41-42
external environment 14
eye-foot coordination drills 292-293

F
falls
    consequences of 116-117
    factors associated with 117
    financial costs of 117
    and flexibility 70-71
    frequency 115-116
    and muscular endurance 142
    and power 145
    prevention strategies 42, 71
    and sarcopenic obesity 50-51
fast twitch muscle fibers 7*f*
    changes with age 6
    cross-sectional area 133
fat burning zone 57-58
fat free mass (FFM) 55
    changes with age 9*f*
    increase with resistance training 57, 59
fatigue
    of central nervous system 243
    during daily cycles 244
    and injury 240, 243
    lower-body 142
    and neuroendocrine disruption 243

and overtraining 243
    sources by training cycle 242*t*
    and supercompensation curve 240
    during time-based training cycles 242-
    243
fat mass (FM) 55
fat utilization 59
feedback mechanisms 37
fibrocartilage 9
fibromyalgia 221
Finkelstein, Eric 50
fitness–fatigue model 240, 241*f*
fitness levels 229
fitness variables 17*f*
flat bench press 170-171
Fleg, Jerome 11
flexibility. *See also* stretching
    causes of decline with aging 70
    effects of aquatic training on 74
    and fall probability 70-71
    implications of decline with aging 8
    and performance of ADLs 70
    testing 69, 76-79
    and translational cycles 81
    types 69
flexibility training
    benefits of 70
    effect on performance 74-75
    effect on ROM when performed alone
    73-74
    exercises 81
    and injury prevention 74
    with other modalities 74, 80
    periodizing 80
    program design 80-81
    versus stretching 70
fly exercise 172
foam rollers 266
footwear 118
force–velocity curve 144*f*, 146, 147*f*
fractures
    and bone health 8, 108, 110, 111
    from falling 117
    results of 111
    risk factors for 112
    risk of 111
frailty
    complexity of 13
    definitions of 12-13
    degrees of 14
    dimensionality 14
    factors associated with 13
    fitness variables 17*f*
    and leg strength 139
    physical performance as marker of
    13-14
    and physical reserve 14, 16*f*
    as a syndrome 13
    and vulnerability 14
Frailty and Injuries: Cooperative Studies of
    Intervention Techniques (FICSIT) 287
"Frailty and Its Definition" (Rockwood) 13
Frank-Starling law of the heart 211
functional age 4
functional drills 281-287
functional reach drill 265
functional reach test 122-123
functional reserve capacity 14, 37*f*
Functional Status Questionnaire 32

G
gait speed 139
gait speed test 153-154
gait training 287
gallon jug drill 291
gallon jug shelf test 24, 25*f*, 152-153, 291
gastrocnemius muscles 88, 89*f*, 166
gender
    and body fat 47*f*
    and connective tissue properties 8
    and obesity 48*f*
get-up-and-go test 122

gluteal muscle stretching 87, 88
Golgi tendon organs (GTOs) 72
goniometers 79*f*
grip strength 139
growth hormone 135, 137

H

Habbu, Shrinivas 49
Haltom, Ronald 60
hamstrings
  exercises 160-161
  stretches 84-85, 96
Hansen, Jennie Chin 116
Harvard step test 255
Haversian canal 105
Hay, James 119
HDL. *See* high-density lipoprotein (HDL)
health costs 55, 117
heart attacks 213
heart rate
  to assess intensity 226
  decline with age 12*f*, 211
  response to running 38*t*
  and VO₂peak 11
heart rate variability 214, 217
heel raise 166-167
hemoglobin 11
hexagon drill 293
hexagon test 293
high blood pressure. *See* hypertension
high-density lipoprotein (HDL) 63, 212, 213, 216
high-speed training 145-146
  building strength base 146-147
  environment 146
  equipment for 146
  optimal loading 146
hip abductors 165-166
hip adductors 164-165
hip circumference 56
hip extensors 163
hip extensor stretches 87-88
hip flexors 162
hip fractures 117, 145
hip replacements 82, 87
hip ROM 71
hip rotator exercise 193
Hoeger, W. 78
homeostasis 15, 37
hormone replacement therapy (HRT) 115
hormones
  resistance training effects 137
  and sarcopenia 135
hyaline cartilage 9
hypertension 48, 212, 213-214
hypertrophy 60, 61, 135, 137, 139

I

IADLs. *See* instrumental activities of daily living (IADLs)
IGF. *See* insulin-like growth factor (IGF)
iliac crest 53
independence 48
  and frailty 14, 16
  and muscular strength 139
  and obesity 49-50
injuries
  and fatigue 240, 243
  incidence and obesity 51
  prevention with stretching 74
  risk factors 8
  from stretching 71, 92, 95
inner ear sensation 117
instrumental activities of daily living (IADLs) 16
  drills based on 288-291
  examples 15
  and sarcopenic obesity 49-50
insulin-like growth factor (IGF) 135, 137
insulin resistance 212
  dose-response relationship to exercise 216*f*

effect of cardiovascular exercise 212
  versus proper response to insulin 213*f*
  training method for 215
Insulin Resistance Atherosclerosis Study 215
intensity
  assessing 226
  and EPOC 58*f*
  improving VO₂max 214-215
  during interval training 226, 229*f*
  manipulating 228, 258, 260
  with periodization 247*f*
  in steady-state training 224
internal environment 14
intertester reliability 28
interval training
  and body composition 61-62
  cycle length 225-226
  designing workouts 228, 229*f*
  EPOC with 62
  intensity 226, 229*f*
  nested intervals 227
  number of intervals 226-227
  oxygen consumption patterns 228*f*
  variations in 227, 228
  work-recovery cycles 227
intervertebral discs 9
invulnerability 15
isoinertial contractions 43
isoinertial strength 138
isokinetic dynamometers 139
isokinetic strength 139
isometrics 43, 71
isometric strength 139
isotonic contractions 43
Iyengar yoga 74

J

Jean Mayer USDA Human Nutrition Research Center 47
Johnson, E. 73
joint angle specificity 41
joints. *See also* range of motion (ROM)
  degeneration 8
  lubrication 7
  surfaces 9
Jones, C.J. 148, 151, 218
Journal on Active Aging (Signorile) 257

K

kinetic movement chains 141, 255
knee crossover stretch 99
knee joint 10*f*
Kokkinos, P.F. 216

L

ladder drills 276-280
lateral raise 178
lateral reach 99
latissimus dorsi 175
lat pull-down 175
Lawton IADL Scale 32
LDL. *See* low-density lipoprotein (LDL)
leg curl 160-161
leg extension 157
leg extension power 14, 15*f*
leg press 156
leg strength 139
leg stretches
  abductors 86-87
  adductors 85-86
  back lotus 86
  butterfly 85
  calf 88, 89*f*
  dorsiflexors 89-90
  full plantar flexion 90
  hamstrings 84-85
  hurdler's stretch 84
  lying leg extension 84
  quadriceps 83
  seated lotus 86
  side lunges 85
leukocytes 11

Lexell, John 5
ligaments 7
line drills 269-271
lipid profile 213, 216
lipoproteins 213
Liu-Ambrose, Teresa 125
load specificity 42-43
long-distance runners 39
loose connective tissue 7
low-density lipoprotein (LDL) 213
lower back pain 96
lower leg 166-167
lunges 85, 159-160
lung ventilation 209-210

M

magnesium 115
Maki, B.E. 124
McIlroy, W.E. 124
mechanical power 143
medications 118
medicine balls 294
menopause 135
metabolic power 40*f*, 143
metabolic rate 59
metabolic syndrome 47, 212, 231
metabolism 40*f*
midaxillary skinfold measurement 52
Miyashita, M. 216
mobility
  conditions affecting 9
  with decreased flexibility 8
  and falls 117
Modified Katz ADL Scale 32
modified ramp power test 149-151
modified trunk rotation test 78
mortality
  and body weight 49
  and leg strength 139
motor learning 32
motor nerves 6
motor patterns
  and resistance training 141
  specificity 43
  training to sweep floors 42*f*
  during translational process 19
motor units 6
  decrease in numbers 134
  healthy *versus* degenerating 135*f*
  resistance training effects 137
  size changes with age 134
movement complexity 260
movement pattern specificity 43
movement speed. *See* speed
multitasking 126*t*
muscle contractions 43, 134-135
muscle fatigue. *See* fatigue
muscle fibers
  age-related changes 5-7, 135
  change in type with training 138*f*
  cross-sectional areas 6*f*, 7*f*, 133, 137
  number of 6*f*
  resistance training effects 137, 138*f*
  types 6
muscle mass 7, 8, 14. *See also* sarcopenia
muscle proteins 135
muscles. *See also* motor units; sarcopenia
  aging curves for 5-7
  atrophy 6
  hypertrophy 61, 135, 137
  repair 135, 137
muscle specificity 41
muscle spindles 72
muscular endurance 41
  and activities of daily living 142
  decline with age 142
  and falls 142
  resistance training for 142
  targeting 59, 138
muscular strength
  and falls 117, 139

muscular strength *(continued)*
  and independence 139
  loss 7
  maximal lifting tests (1RM) 152
  measuring 138-139
  resistance training for 139-141
myelin sheath 134
myosin 135
myosin ATPase 135, 137

N

Nagi Scale 32
National Institute of Diabetes and Digestive and Kidney Diseases 55
National Institutes of Health (NIH) 55, 110
National Osteoporosis Foundation 110, 111
National Safety Council 116
neck stretches 91-92
nervous system restructuring 255
neuromuscular junction
  resistance training effects 137
  structural changes 134, 136f
neuromuscular system
  aging curve with exercise 13f
  causes of sarcopenia 133-135
  normal aging curves 5-7
  resistance training effects 137
Nienhuis, B. 121
Norcross, Jason 51
nutritional status 13, 14

O

obesity. *See also* sarcopenic obesity
  by age and gender 48f
  apple-shaped 212
  consequences of 48
  and injuries 51
  male-pattern 212
  and mortality 49
  prevalence 48
obesity epidemic 48
obesity paradox 48-49
oblique stretches 87, 97-99
occupational therapy 255
optimal load 42, 146
orthostatic hypotension 118
osteoarthritis 10f, 48, 70, 221
osteocytes 105
osteons 105
osteopenia 110
  consequences of 111
  prevalence 111
  and stretching precautions 82
osteoporosis 8
  consequences of 111
  definitions 110-111
  and fractures 8, 110
  prevalence 111
  prevention 112-115
  rate of bone loss 106, 107f
  and stretching precautions 82
overhead press 177
overload
  effect on nervous system 255
  principle of 37
  and training effect 241f
overload stress 37
overtraining 148, 239, 243
overuse injuries 240, 243
oxygen consumption 221. *See also* VO₂max; VO₂peak
  postexercise 57
  testing 11
oxygen pulse
  aging curve 12f
  and VO₂peak 11

P

periodization 18, 148
  applied to clients 248-253
  block strategy 244-245, 246

building phase 247f
  in cardiovascular training 227
  classic linear 244, 245f, 246
  daily cycle 244
  event cycle 243-244
  in flexibility training 80
  models of 247f
  nonlinear 244, 245f, 246
  peaking phase 247f
  taper phase 246, 247-248
  and translational cycles 256
periosteal apposition 107
peripheral nervous system 255. *See also* nervous system
peripheral sensation 117
Phillips, Wayne 59
phosphate 115
physical activity 9
physical conditioning 19
physical disability 221
Physical Performance Tests (PPT) 32
physical reserve 14, 15f, 16
physical vulnerability 15, 16
physiological age 4
plantar flexion 78-79, 90
plasma 11
plyometrics 115
PNF. *See* proprioceptive neuromuscular facilitation (PNF)
pool workouts. *See* aquatic training
postmenopausal women
  bone density 106, 115
  bone diameter 107
  calcium intake 115
power
  and activities of daily living 145
  definition 143
  and falls 145
  and levers 147f
  lever systems 147f
  loss in 7
  mechanism of loss 145
  resistance training for 145-146, 148
prescription 23
prevention 16, 23
proprioception 124, 142
proprioceptive neuromuscular facilitation (PNF) 71-72
  duration of stretch 76
  effectiveness of 75
  for stretching neck 92

Q

quadriceps
  exercises for 156-160
  stretches 83, 90
quadruped exercise 194
quality of life 9, 24, 50

R

ramp test 149-151
range of motion (ROM)
  and connective tissue properties 8, 70
  and flexibility 69, 70
  increasing with external resistance 73
  and likelihood of falling 71
  and strength 41
rate of perceived exertion (RPE) 226
reaction time
  and agility training 125
  and falls 117
reciprocal inhibition 72, 73f, 75
recovery 32. *See also* interval training
  after injury 145
  from fatigue 241
  during resistance training 60
  and testing 32
  as a training tool 18, 19
  and translational process 19
rehabilitation 16, 145, 255
reliability 28

resistance training
  and ADL performance 255-256
  aerobic *versus* anaerobic 42-43
  biochemical effects 137
  and body composition 58-59
  bone response to 114
  breathing method 155
  building a base 146-147
  cardiovascular effects 229
  circuit training 59-60
  effect on nervous system 255
  equipment 146, 155
  exercises 155
  load amount 61, 139, 146
  load application direction 114
  and metabolic rate change 58-59
  motor patterns 141
  movement speed 60, 145-146
  muscle groups targeted 140-141
  for muscular endurance 142
  for muscular strength 139-141
  neuromuscular effects 137
  for power 145-148
  protocols 59-61
  recovery time 60
  repetitions 59, 139
  and sarcopenia 135, 137, 138
  sessions per week 59, 140
  sets 59, 60, 139-140
  standard recommendations 138t
resting metabolic rate (RMR) 59
reticular connective tissue 7
rhabdomyolysis 244
RIkli, R.E. 151, 218
Robling, A.G. 114
Rockwood, Kenneth 13
Romberg's test 122
Rosow-Breslau Functional Health Scale 32
rotator cuff
  external rotation 182
  and injury to 95
  internal rotation 180
  stretches 92, 93
Roubenoff, Ronenn 47, 133
Roybal-Allard, Lucille 116
RPE. *See* rate of perceived exertion (RPE)
running 220
  acute and long-term response to 38t
  energy demands 39, 224
  on treadmills 222

S

safety precautions
  active assisted stretching (AAS) 82
  neck stretches 92
  performing squats 159
  rails 264
  shoulder stretches 95
  use of spotters 264
Saliba, Debra 16
sarcopenia 6
  biochemical causes 135
  clinical definition 133
  contributing factors to 134f
  neuromuscular causes 133-135
  prevalence 133
  and resistance training 135, 137, 138
sarcopenic obesity 8, 47
  effect on IADL performance 49-50
  and fall probability 50-51
  training interventions for 57
sarcoplasmic reticule 134-135
satellite cells 135, 137
Sayers, S.P. 145
scarf drill 288
scarf pickup test 288
seated balance 125
seated chest press 170
seated twist 87, 98
shoulder exercises 177-180
shoulder flexibility 77

shoulder stretches
  anterior rotators 93-94
  behind-the-back 94
  doorway stretch 94
  downward rotators 94-95
  external rotators 93
  internal rotators 92
  kneeling chest and shoulder 94
  overhead back 94
  rotator cuff 92, 95
  safety considerations 95
Shrier, Ian 75
shrug 179
side plank 192
Signorile, J.F. 226, 257
single-leg stance balance test 121-122
Siri formula 55
sit-and-reach test 69, 76-77, 96, 97t
skeletal muscle 5-7. *See also* muscles
Skelton, D.A. 145
skill-based training 248
skinfold measurements 51-54
slow twitch fibers 6
slow twitch muscle fibers 7f
soccer kick 296
soleus muscles 88
somatopause 135
The South Beach Diet Supercharged (Agaston &Signorile) 226
specificity. *See* exercise specificity
speed
  definition 143
  during resistance training 60
  specificity 41-42
  strength 143
spongy bone 105
Sprigle, S. 125
squats 61f, 158-159
stability balls 85, 172, 191, 195
stable equilibrium 119
stair climbers 223
stair climbing 15f, 149, 284
staleness 239
stance stability 126t
star excursion drill 293
static flexibility 69
static stretching 71, 75
stationary cycles 222-223
step aerobics 255
step drills 284-287
step taper 248
strain-stress curve 69, 70f
strength. *See* muscular strength
stretches. *See also* active assisted stretching (AAS); leg stretches
  for chest 94
  for core 96-99
  hip extensors 87-88
  for low back 96-97
  for neck 91-92
  for shoulders 92-95
stretching. *See also* flexibility training
  agonist contract–relax (ACR) technique 72
  ballistic movements 75, 82
  breathing during 82
  comparison of types 75
  contract–relax technique 71
  contract–relax with agonist contract (CRAC) technique 72
  delayed response to 69-70
  effect on performance 74-75
  for hip replacement clients 82
  holding time 75-76
  immediate response to 69, 72-73
  injury during 71
  and injury prevention 74
  partner-assisted 71
  passive *versus* active 71
  soreness after 82
  and stress-strain curve 69-70

types of 71-72
  and viscoelastic stress relaxation 72
  warming up body 82
stretch reflex 72
stroke 213
subcutaneous fat 51, 57, 59
subscapular skinfold measurement 54
supercompensation curve 239, 240f
superman exercise 195
suprailiac skinfold measurement 53
sweat production 38
swimming. *See* aquatic training
synaptic cleft 134
syndrome X 212

T
tai chi 74, 124
Talanian, J.L. 215
taper 80, 248-249
tendons 7-8, 8, 81
Terjung, R.L. 211
testing triangle 28, 29f
testosterone 135, 137
tests
  diagnostic battery 25, 26t
  effectiveness measures 28-29
  feedback to clients 30
  norm comparisons 31
  of performance of ADLs 32-33
  preliminary 29-30
  purpose of 30-31
  relationship to ADLs 27t, 28
  reliability 28
  sensitivity 28
  validity 28
  when to administer 29-32, 31f
thigh skinfold measurement 53
Thorpe, Roland 217
thrombocytes 11
Tinetti balance test 122
toe point 90
toe raise 168-169
training. *See also* resistance training
  carryover effects from 246t
  versus exercise 37, 38
  intensity 258, 260
  load 42-43
  matching translational cycles 262-263
  mixed 62-63
  movement complexity 260
  skill-based 248
  specificity 38-39
  targeted 18, 31, 245, 246
  and testing 31
  volume 260
training age 4
training cycles 32, 242t. *See also* periodization
training methods
  to address heart rate variability 217
  for central obesity 215
  for clients with high blood pressure 216-217
  to improve lipid profile 216
  and insulin resistance 215, 216f
training response 38
translational cycles 19, 32, 256
  components to manipulate 258, 259f
  design factors 258f
  and flexibility 81
  matching training 262-263
  and motor pattern training 255
  and periodization 256
  timing of 257
translational exercises 263
trapezius muscle 179, 180
Trapp, E.G. 61
treadmills 221-222
triceps
  extension 187
  kickback 189

push-down 186
triceps skinfold measurement 54
triglycerides 212
trunk rotation test 78
trunk twist 97-98
Tsuzuku, S. 59
type I,II muscle fibers 6, 7f

U
up-and-go test 24, 25f, 122
upper back 173
upper-body strength 151

V
validity
  in testing 28-29
  types of 28t
vastus lateralis muscle 7
velocity 143
vestibular sensation 117
vestibular stimulation 126t
video games 126
visceral fat 57, 212
vision, impaired 112, 117
vitamin D
  and calcium 115
  deficiency 112
  for osteoporosis prevention 115, 126
Volkmann's canals 105
volume
  manipulating 228, 260
  with periodization 247f
  in steady-state training 224
$\dot{V}O_2$max
  definition of 11
  and delivery of blood 211-212
  and diffusion capacity 210
  and extraction of oxygen from blood 210-211
  and intensity 215
  and lung ventilation 209-210
  measuring 11
  patterns during interval training 228f
  reasons for drop with age 209
  training methods to improve 214-215
$\dot{V}O_2$peak 11

W
waist circumference 55-57
waist-to-hip ratio 55-57
walking
  as activity of daily living 15
  the dog 217
  effect on nervous system 255
  pace and heart rate 227
  patterns and falls 8-9, 71
  as physical activity 4, 57, 217
  power 27t, 145
  speed 50, 145, 166
  and stretching 74
  tests 27t, 32, 153-154, 218-219
  on treadmills 221, 222
walking speed test 153-154
Weber, Herb 23
Weerdesteyn, V. 121
weight. *See* body weight
weight shifting 126t
weight training. *See* resistance training
Whipple, R. 145
White, Andrea 115
whole-body vibration (WBV) 113, 126
Wilder, Gene 255
Woods, K. 74
work-recovery ratios 225
wrist curl 184

Y
yoga 74, 75

Z
Ziuraitis, Joana 59

About the Author

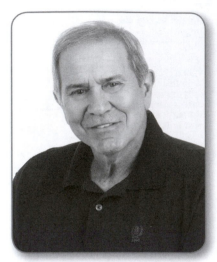

Joseph F. Signorile, PhD, is a professor in the department of kinesiology and sport sciences at the University of Miami in Coral Gables, Florida. He is a research health science specialist for the Miami Veterans Affairs Medical Center and has served as senior researcher at the Stein Gerontological Institute of the Miami Jewish Home and Hospital for the Aged.

Dr. Signorile's research interests include prescriptive periodization training for older individuals, diagnostic test development for exercise prescription, electromyographic analysis of sport- and activity-specific training, and evaluation of training techniques concentrating on power development. He has written over 50 refereed articles and book chapters and presented at countless national and international scientific and industry meetings.

Dr. Signorile is a member of the University of Miami graduate faculty and serves on its research council and the graduate school committee for doctoral curriculum evaluation. He serves on the board of the International Council on Active Aging. He is also a member of the American College of Sports Medicine, the American Geriatrics Society, and the National Strength and Conditioning Association.

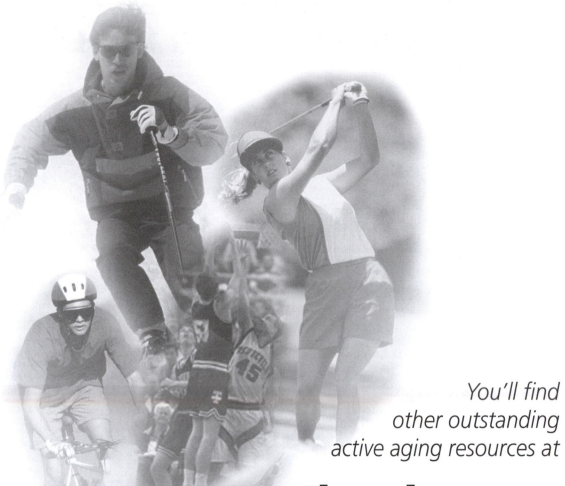

Accessing the Diagnostic Testing Battery on the DVD

The diagnostic testing battery can only be viewed on a computer with a DVD-ROM drive. To access the spreadsheet, use a program that can open Excel 2003 spreadsheets and follow these instructions:

To access from Windows®,

1. Insert the DVD into your DVD-ROM drive.
2. Open "My Computer," right click on the DVD-ROM drive, and select "Explore" or "Open in New Window."
3. Select "Diagnostic Testing Battery."
4. Select the spreadsheet and copy it to your hard drive.

To access from a Macintosh® computer,

1. Insert the DVD into your DVD-ROM drive.
2. Double-click on the DVD icon on your desktop.
3. Select "Diagnostic Testing Battery."
4. Select the spreadsheet and copy it to your hard drive.